T0361866

The International Library of Psychology

CONDITIONS OF NERVOUS ANXIETY AND THEIR TREATMENT

Founded by C. K. Ogden

The International Library of Psychology

ABNORMAL AND CLINICAL PSYCHOLOGY
In 19 Volumes

CONDITIONS OF NERVOUS ANXIETY AND THEIR TREATMENT

W STEKEL

Introduction by Samuel Lowy

First published in 1923 by
Routledge

Reprinted 1999, 2000, 2001, 2002 by
Routledge
2 Park Square, Milton Park, Abingdon, Oxon, OX14 4RN

Transferred to Digital Printing 2007

Routledge is an imprint of the Taylor & Francis Group

© 1923 W Stekel
Translated by Rosalie Gabler

The publishers have made every effort to contact authors/copyright holders
of the works reprinted in the *International Library of Psychology*.
This has not been possible in every case, however, and we would
welcome correspondence from those individuals/companies
we have been unable to trace.

These reprints are taken from original copies of each book. In many cases
the condition of these originals is not perfect. The publisher has gone to
great lengths to ensure the quality of these reprints, but wishes to point
out that certain characteristics of the original copies will, of necessity, be
apparent in reprints thereof.

British Library Cataloguing in Publication Data
A CIP catalogue record for this book
is available from the British Library

Conditions of Nervous Anxiety and their Treatment
ISBN 0415-20934-X
Abnormal and Clinical Psychology: 19 Volumes
ISBN 0415-21123-9
The International Library of Psychology: 204 Volumes
ISBN 0415-19132-7

AUTHOR'S PREFACE TO THE ENGLISH EDITION

THE present edition of this book is an abridgment of the third German edition. *Habent sua fata libelli!* The first German edition was honoured with a Preface by my former teacher, Professor Freud, introducing me to the scientific public as one of his first pupils and assistants. I shared the destinies of his genius while all the world was ridiculing the message of the new prophet. With him I drank the bitter cup—convinced, enchanted, and enraptured, recognizing the tremendous importance of the new science. I fought and struggled in the front rank unreservedly and inexhaustibly with the fanaticism of a devotee.

At that time I was a medical practitioner, with a practice that kept me busy night and day. Among the many patients coming under my treatment I observed a large proportion whose maladies were not organic, as usually diagnosed, but neurotic, especially disguises of morbid fears. This material is the foundation of the present volume. It is written, not only for neurologists but also for practitioners by a practitioner.

This book, which has won so many friends for psychanalysis, was the origin of my differences with Freud. An explanation of this schism requires a brief review of the history of psychanalysis. In the early days of the science, Freud asserted publicly that anxiety states are not curable by psychanalysis. He differentiated phobias as a constitutional disease from anxiety neuroses (*Angstneurosen*), the latter being the consequence, according to his law, of sexual abuses. He differentiated " actual neurosis " from psycho-neurosis. The former he asserted to be caused by sexual abuses, the latter by psychic disturbances.

I could not agree with this conclusion for the following reasons : Firstly, I found that *every* state of morbid fear was psychically determined. Secondly, I was not able to find the so-called neurasthenia of Freud at all. In every case of actual neurosis I found the psychic cause, and came to the conclusion that every neurosis is caused by a psychic conflict. Freud defended his law with the blind obstinacy so common to genius, finally proposing to me to call the phobias " anxiety hysteria."

In my first edition I yielded to his suggestions, and in the second edition, I tried to make a compromise between the facts and the wish of my teacher. This edition conforms to established law : *all neuroses are psychic diseases.*

I was astonished to find that many cases diagnosed by other physicians as heart-trouble, asthma, stomach trouble, appendicitis, irritations of the skin, tics, cramps, etc., were caused by mental conflicts. These facts had been overlooked because physicians have not understood the " organic language of the soul." This phrase means that neurotics have a wonderful ability to express their mental states in a symbolic language of the bodily organs. Such heart troubles as palpitations, aches, irregularity of rhythm, and the like, may be the consequences of disturbances of the affections. Such stomach troubles as vomiting, loss of appetite, pains, and so on, may result from some disgusting psychic experience repressed and hidden in the unconscious. Vaginism in women is due to resistance against a forced marriage ; the reader will find plenty of cases in this book. I could with perfect propriety, change the title of this book to " The Organic Language of the Soul." Indeed, this is a true language with all the variations of idiom, dialect, slang, argot, stuttering, stammering, lisping, and the rest.

This book was the first, and remains the only, systematic collection of facts of morbid states on which a true science of psychanalysis can be founded. Such a collection could have been made only on the basis of a private practice in general medicine. It could never have been done in a clinic. Now that I am a specialist I seldom see the kind of material on which this book rests. It is quite evident that every successful psychanalyst must—besides a thorough neurological foundation—have had a previous experience of several years as a general practitioner. Otherwise he will have no understanding of his patients' troubles as dependant upon family life, their social relations, their struggles for bread and butter, and other factors of environment.

Besides the influence of sexual life as a cause of the neuroses— sufficiently emphasized by Freudians—this book shows the importance of ambition, religious feelings, and the instinct of self-preservation in this sense. Without a thorough knowledge of *all* the factors at the basis of a neurosis no one can understand it.

This book is the first volume of a work entitled " Disturbances of the Impulses and the Emotions " (*Störungen des Trieb-und Affektlebens*), of which seven volumes have already appeared in German. Translations of the other volumes by Dr. S. van Teslaar are ready and will be at the service of English physicians in a short time. The complete work will comprise ten volumes. Although each volume can be read and understood independently, a grasp of the whole subject requires a knowledge of all of them.

In conclusion, I wish to say that I am profoundly grateful to my teacher Freud who made the first, most difficult, and most important explorations in the unexplored regions of the neuroses. But I remember the golden words of Nietzsche : " You are ungrateful to your teacher, if you are not able to go beyond him."

WILHELM STEKEL.

BAD GASTEIN.

TRANSLATOR'S NOTE

My grateful thanks are due to Dr. Arnold Eiloart, Mr. Jennings White, M.A., and Miss Muriel Passingham for their kindness and valuable help with the translation.

ROSALIE GABLER

CONTENTS

B

SECOND PART—THE PHOBIAS

THIRD PART—GENERAL

INTRODUCTION

By Samuel Lowy, M.D. (Prague)

Associate Ch. Assistant in the
Department for Psychological Medicine, St. Bartholomew's Hospital

The mental conflict. The fundamental thesis of this work is that the central factor in the causation of psychoneuroses is the mental conflict. This may sound a truism to many readers. In the earlier phases of Freud's psychoanalysis, however, and to a considerable extent even later, this concept was not so popular as it is to-day. Likewise, the interplay between personality traits and the social atmosphere has not always received the attention it does now by psychotherapists of all colouring. Among the pioneer psychoanalysts it was the author of this book who advocated the supplementing of what used to be then the analysis of the libido with the examination of the patient's socio-cultural background and ideology. Admittedly in this volume this angle is not yet elaborated as well as in later works of the author. His insight into the complexities of the psyche developed with growing experience.

Frustration. It is, however, not only the interest in the historical development of analytical theory and therapy which may be satisfied by the perusal of this volume. Fundamental discoveries and formulations are not made invalid by the riches of subsequent research. Following the author's lively discussion as well as his arguments against certain concepts held by others, the reader may feel impelled to examine the problems for himself. Furthermore, in the perspective of present-day knowledge some theories discarded by the author may appear still of value though in a modified sense.

Thus it is an indisputable observation that libidinal frustration predisposes some individuals to anxiety reactions. Stekel proved right in explaining that such "physical" tension may stimulate a variety of phantasies which in turn result in serious mental conflicts. Subconscious death wishes against relatives occur more readily under the pressure of instinctual frustration, or dissatisfaction in general. Unbiased observation could not fail to reveal that frustration of the personality in spheres other than libidinal may likewise upset the psychoaffective balance and lead to anxiety and its various symptomatic manifestations.

The competition of tendencies and polar tension. In a later work (*Doubt and Compulsion*) the author has shown that the mental conflict is not always, or solely, that between instinctual urge and social morality. The personality possesses a number of guiding principles, dynamic motives, aims and trends. Most of these are remote from concrete reality, and are also "crossing" each other's line. The difficulty in achieving a working harmony among them results in psychoneurotic potentials.

Thus, a person may be dominated excessively by the desire to please his father; or, by the idea of surpassing him or any other member of his family; or, by the tendency to annul, in imagination, an embarrassing fact. Moreover, the desire for freedom from moral and social obligations may be parallelled by an equally strong tendency for asceticism. Besides such wish-elements there is a number of trends enforced by concrete realities and the implied tasks of life. Those belonging to the sphere of imagination are, to varying extents, in contrast to those rooted in external realities; and if the former category occupies the mental functioning to an excess, a tendency to intense day-dreaming results. The author speaks about "polar tension" within the psyche in view of the gap between integrating and disintegrating processes. This tension is the breeding ground of psychoneuroses as well as vegetative disturbances with subsequent structural damage. Compulsion neuroses and psychogenic epilepsy are explained by Stekel by the utmost intensity of the polar tension.

Organic predisposition. We must not ignore that functional deficiency of the nervous centres may be responsible for the failure in limiting sufficiently the spheres of phantasy. Likewise, the tolerance of frustration in various personality spheres may be intrinsically smaller than average. Yet, even in such cases, it is possible to an extent to relieve the psyche by training the patient in recognizing and rejecting some of his fictitious goals and combating reverie.

Ignored or unconscious elements. Indubitably it is possible in frequent cases to carry out psychoanalytical treatment on a comparatively superficial level; that is, by dealing with such processes as love and hatred, sex, ambition and failure, latent homosexuality, and other wish elements consciously recognizable though elaborated subconsciously. Practice has confirmed Stekel's contention that the aetiological factors are elements of the conscious mind ignored to varying degrees, but not early infantile complexes deeply unconscious from the outset and recoverable only by interpretation. Nevertheless, the analytical approach is necessary because of repression, symbolic disguises, and the unconscious resistance to treatment.

Admittedly all sorts of emotional trouble are bound to spread into the deeper layers and affect the "microscopical" elements in so far as they really exist. Some obsessional and delusional formations as well as dream elements do suggest, e.g., the dynamic existence of so-called oral and anal tendencies. The question is only whether in the course of average treatment we need to deal explicitly with such and comparable "complexes"; and if so, to what extent.

Stekel's analytical therapy. The analytical psychotherapy developed by this author differs greatly from psychoanalysis in the current sense. His approach is characterized by the analysis of disturbing elements that are contents of conscious thought but are carried over into subconscious spheres and elaborated there by associative symbolisms; further, by a thorough investigation of the patient's attitude to the problems of *good* and *evil,* and the polar tension ensuing from this source; and lastly, by the unmasking of day-dreams produced excessively and rich in symbolic disguises. The initiative is always that of the physician, his greatest helper being his capacity for understanding the infinite variety of substitute formations.

Limited analysis and educative psychosynthesis. Re-educative training of the mind is one of the main tasks of active psychoanalysis—as the author called his method. In his opinion, the psychoneurotic does not suffer so much from past impressions as from irrational modes of facing the present and contemplating the future. The divining of neurotic guiding motives is the only way of achieving results in a comparatively limited period of analysis. The majority of cases reported by the author in the ten volumes of *The Disorders of the Instincts and Emotions* were helped in 40-120 sessions. He emphasized, for almost three decades, that long analyses stimulate infantilism and dependence; and that the unconscious resistance is bound to increase if early return to full activity is not to be the therapeutic aim from the outset. This has recently been recognized by other authors (cf. F. Alexander and T. M. French, *Studies in Psychosomatic Medicine;* and *Psychoanalytic Therapy*).

It is, nevertheless, true that the best knowledge of symbolism, and the most complete grasp of the case at an early phase of the analysis, cannot dispense with a certain length of treatment. In some pctients this may require even a year with three weekly sessions. (Dr. Stekel preferred daily treatments for a lesser period, believing that resistance is thus more effectively combated.) In terms of current knowledge, we may assume that the alternating course of "transferences" requires sufficient opportunity for unfolding themselves. Moreover, a certain measure of gratification implied in the analytical process seems to be needed by many patients to be able to utilize the interpretations as well as the logical re-education. In the somewhat simplified formula of Stekel, the patient expects to receive the love and attention that was denied to him by certain persons significant for his life. We must also recognize that a change-over in psycho-affective dynamics requires time, irrespective of any interpretable motive.

Site of the organ-neurosis. The first half of this volume consists of a rich assembly of organ-neuroses. The author conceives them in the main as anxiety neuroses due to moral conflicts. He explains the particular localization of the complaint by a variety of determinants. (1) Organic predisposition, as a rule reinforced by a pertinent idea. Thus, a person with proneness to muscular spasms may suffer from psychoneurotic pains in the leg and be hereby prevented from going somewhere he ought not to according to his conscience. (2) Popular associations of various emotions with certain organs. Thus, conflicts of love, in particular of sexuality, affect frequently the heart region; those due to criminal wishes lead to headaches, the brain being the site of such disapproved thoughts. (3) Somatization of current meta-phorical phrases such as "to turn a blind eye", or "a sickening behaviour", etc. (4) The role of the organ in the case history. Thus the hand may be affected through the sense of guilt related to masturbation, or owing to the idea to attack somebody. Resistance to a certain occupation may betray itself by the organ chosen by the neurosis. (5) The principle of *jus talionis* (an eye for an eye) may determine the kind of self-punishment. Thus, a mother after parting with her illegitimate child took ill with difficult swallowing because tormented by the idea that the infant might not receive sufficient food [see also (4)]. (6) Symbolic substitution in accordance with psychoanalytical formulas. For instance, displacement from the genital region to the abdomen, legs, or throat may lead to sensations there following a sexual conflict. Neuroses of the eye may combine this mechanism with the significance of the eye to perceive scenes of shocking character. (7) Subconscious asceticism is responsible for many cases of habitual indigestion, as well as other discomforts preventing average enjoyments. [This ascetic tendency is due not simply to a sense of guilt, but substantially to the need for intense religious-ethical experience in persons who are not capable of achieving it by conscious spiritual activity.] (8) The ordinary somatic accompaniments of fear or libidinal excitement may be mobilized by unconscious elements; such are increase of cardiac and vasomotor activity, forced respiration, tremor, enteric hyper- or hypoactivity, etc.

Psychotherapy in clinical medicine. W. Stekel knew already three decades ago that mental factors may be decisive in arterial hypertension; that even in organic damage of the heart the attacks and general incapacity may decrease after psychotherapy; that the enlarged thyroid may become smaller in the course of psychoanalysis; that habitual bronchitis is based, very frequently, on emotional disturbance, or dislike of work; in 1926 he was already treating patients with pulmonary tuberculosis with a view to aiding their recovery by alleviating psychoneurotic potentials. All these observations have been amply confirmed later and systematic research extended to the whole field of medicine. Thus E. Wittkower relieved the pain of angina pectoris patients even though organic damage was present (cf. A. T. M. Wilson, in Individual Psychology Pamphlets, No. 20, 1938). The same author (together with Petow and Polonow) investigated the problem of bronchial asthma from the angle of psychotherapy and psychogenesis (cf. *Z. Klin. Med.*, 1929 and 1932).

Organdialect. The author of this notion seems to be Alfred Adler (1914). He applied to organ manifestations his conception of neurotic symptoms which he interpreted as protests and defences against the specific roles and tasks of man and woman as well as social life in general. In Part II, Ch. 1 of his *The Neurotic Constitution* there is an instructive scheme showing how a number of complaints in a woman manifested her dislike to be a sexual partner to her husband, a female bearing children, and a mother looking after her family. Her constipation, for example, is conceived as a parallel to her past vaginism, a kind of symbolically "blocking up" her body. It is assumed that constitutional inferiority of the bowels was intensified by spasms due to the emotional motive mentioned.

The pathogenic "id". One of the earliest pioneers of psychosomatic medicine in the narrower sense was G. Groddek (1918). In his belief the depth personality (*id*) can cause organic illnesses in support of certain intelligible tendencies. His own sciatica and gout improved after his recognizing their role in isolating him. Endocrine and genital disorders in women may be the outcome of aversion to pregnancy thus made impossible. He also claimed the reduction of his enlarged thyroid after coming to terms in self-analysis with his infantile wish for becoming pregnant (big with child).

Cannon's theory of psychosomatic phenomena. The involvement of somatic functions by mental processes has been more accurately explained by W. B. Cannon's *emergency theory* (1915). He refers to the danger situations of animals whose organism responds in rage and fear with preparation to fight and flight. This is done by intensified blood circulation and pressure, vasoconstriction, shortening of the clotting time, and mobilization of sugar, the energy supply for muscle and brain. This basic psychosomatic response is considered the disposition from which the manifoldness of affectogenic organ-responses has developed.

Clearly, there is no such a utilitarian sense in the infinite variety of psychosomatic involvements in the human being. Apart from the desirability of sufficient energy supply in effort, the impact of emotionality on the soma is more disturbing than vitalizing. We may only say that the organism appears to react to its mental processes and conflicts as though these were internalized objects of task and danger. In fact, however, no internalized anxiety can develop without fear of the external world. Competitiveness for bread, comfort, appreciation and love, as well as the fear of being denied these objects, is a rich source of effort, concern and struggle. Thus anxiety with its circulatory and other somatic accompaniments refers to both the external and internal obstacles to a satisfactory life.

Gastrointestinal syndromes and the struggle for existence. From here we may proceed to the understanding of psychosomatic ailments of the digestive system. Food is part of the external world; and nutrition, with all its component aspects, is a function more prominent in conscious awareness than respiration or circulation. Moreover, this function is closely tied up with the concern for the elementary needs of life and, in extension of this feeling, with that for security and appreciation. Stressful situations, intensifying the continual undercurrent of fear about one's future and obligations, are frequently accompanied by disturbances of the alimentary system. It has been the impression of the present writer that repetitive attacks of indigestion, that is the beginning of the habitual nature of the somatic complaint, coincide with the realization by the patient that his personal limitations and struggles might become permanent. Mental life as a whole is thus but continual aiming, effort, defence and struggle, and therefore a true parallel to the emergency situations of animals.

The oral-receptive wishes. The explanation put forward here by the writer is not that held currently by most psychoanalysts dealing with psychosomatic medicine. F. Alexander and his fellow workers contend that the aetiological force at the root of psychosomatic ailments of the digestive system is the pressure by oral-receptive wishes, the craving for their gratification in persons who outwardly suppress them and who suffer from the unconscious sense of guilt for harbouring such wishes. The over-motility and hypersecretion of the stomach—as if receiving food, the equivalent of love in infancy—is the work of this suppressed, though dynamic current. A similar affective background has been claimed for the increased mobilization of sugar in diabetics. This line of interpretation has been applied to constipation and colitis, suitably modifying the mental formula (cf. *Studies in Psychosomatic Medicine*).

Psychotherapy in bronchial asthma. French and Johnson (in *Studies* etc.) state that in patients with psychogenic asthma "there seems to run as a continuous undercurrent, more or less deeply repressed, a fear of estrangement from the mother. The cause of this fear is usually the patient's own forbidden impulses which he thinks will offend the mother." Here we may be reminded of Stekel's claiming the cure of some patients with asthmatic attacks, after their "intrauterine phantasies" have been brought to consciousness and the associated elements analysed.

Dunbar's personality profiles in various clinical syndromes. Another approach—based on investigations on a large scale—is that of F. Dunbar (*Psychosomatic Diagnosis*). Groups of patients suffering from certain syndromes were examined in respect of a number of personality aspects. Such were the family history, education, previous illnesses, mode of carrying out one's occupation, social relationships, sexual adjustment, attitude towards family, pattern of general behaviour, neurotic traits and addictions, and the life situation before

B*

as well as the reaction to the current illness. Surprisingly, fracture patients, originally included as controls, turned out to have their own characteristics as a group. Clinical syndromes investigated were: coronary disease, hypertensive cardiovascular disease, anginal attacks, arrhythmias, rheumatic fever and arthritis, rheumatic heart disease, and diabetes; further, groups with overlapping syndromes. The "areas of focal conflicts and characteristic reactions" have been found more or less different and specific.

Thus, the coronary patient "attempts to be and subdue authority" and identifies himself with authority and pertinent concepts. The sick person with angina is characterized by "rivalry with authority", but "he tends to be as good and as superior rather than surpassing the person in authority"; further, by a tendency "to be his own boss rather than to boss others", etc.

An important role is attributed to having been "exposed" to a certain illness of relatives or close friends. Thus the significance of heredity may be much less than thought, and the personal closeness to a sick relative with frequent "exposure" to his illness the main aetiological factor. [Conscious rejection of such an identification and of the implied fear probably counters this morbid influence.—S.L.]

Dunbar's observations have proved that relapses or deterioration are much less frequent if psychotherapy is given besides the organic treatment, as compared with the respective control group treated solely on current medical lines. The knowledge of the various "personality profiles" may facilitate the therapeutic approach of the particular patient. The period required for such a psychotherapy is, as a rule, much less than in psychoneuroses.

This implies a certain difference in technique and planning of the therapeutic procedure, a fact not sufficiently realized by the average expert in psychotherapy. We are driven to the conclusion that appropriate psychotherapy in organic ailments in essence relieves the psychosoma and enables the autonomous forces of healing to operate. This in turn leads us to recognize in the psychological aetiology of somatic syndromes above all the *stress factor*, irrespective of the particular mental contents involved. The selection of the organ affected is not determined by its physical inferiority but, as we may assume, by its increased proneness to psychosomatic responses. Many patients suffer from a succession of various syndromes, each being the trouble at a certain period of life. This phenomenon is unexplainable by a fixed organic inferiority of a particular anatomical structure. If the mental stress involves an organ anatomically inferior, it does so through the additional psychosomatic proneness.

Remarkable is also the observation that if a psychosomatic illness is improved by medical or surgical treatment, the ignored psychoaffective contributor may lead, sooner or later, to a severe neurotic or depressive picture. In a case observed by the writer, stammer was the complaint in childhood, severe allergic asthma the trouble in youth, and anxiety states with some depression the incapacitating condition in early manhood. All this appeared to be due to the rather difficult relationship between son and father as well as to additional complications.

Stekel's case histories. Dunbar's work inspires confidence in particular through her presentations being free from simplifications. She does not ignore the multisidedness of character aspects in the patients examined by her and her fellow workers. In this respect her approach bears a resemblance to that of Stekel in his analysis of compulsive formations and hypochondriac sensations; he regards them as multiply determined, and the psychoaffective polar tension in such cases as resulting from the personality structure in the face of a number of problems, events and complexes.

The organ neuroses dealt with in this volume, however, were approached by him more simply, in that a particular trauma or difficulty was considered the main object of analysis. The therapeutic success seems to justify this mode of treatment in suitable cases. Even in our period, with the more frequent occurrence of compulsion and character neuroses, one comes across cases closely resembling those of Stekel. The perusal of this volume is, therefore, bound to benefit the student of psychiatry of the present. The significance of the moral conflict as well as that of psychoneurotic symbolism is abundantly illustrated by the case histories included.

The author's presentation is characterized by a sequence of formulas on the same problem, each carrying the discussion further, at times apparently without reference to what has been said earlier. This may not compare with the neat systems of other authors. The reader, however, is compensated by the liveliness of the discussion, by the absence of vague hypotheses, and by a wealth of ideas as well as a considerable number of interesting cases.

This introduction was written at the suggestion of Mrs. Hilda Stekel (London), who had been a close fellow worker of the author for many years. She thinks it is necessary to supplement this volume by important particulars contained in the improved 4th edition (1924) of the German original, as well as by a review of progress in psychosomatic medicine, a field to which Dr. W. Stekel had devoted so much practical interest.

LONDON,
November, 1949.

FIRST PART

ANXIETY NEUROSIS

CHAPTER I

GENERAL POINTS OF VIEW

THIS book is written by a medical practitioner for the Profession. Its purpose is to describe the origin and treatment of nervous anxiety conditions as clearly, briefly and thoroughly as possible, and to instruct us in the understanding of the enormous power of psychological forces. It is intended as an introduction to psycho-therapy, that great art which forms the basis of all medical practice.

We have so long enjoyed the fruits of biological discoveries that we have entirely forgotten that man has also a soul. In the progress made in chemistry, physics, bacteriology and pathology we have left the psychic component of disease out of account, and have seriously neglected the investigation of the human psyche; but the amazing experiences of life lead us back into the domain of psychology, proving to us that a thorough knowledge of the human psyche is of supreme importance. *A good doctor must be a good psychologist*, he must have a thorough knowledge of men.

And now to our theme! What has been hitherto known about Anxiety? It passed for a feeling of displeasure, of expectation, a higher degree of fear. Fear and anxiety were regarded by doctors in the same sense. This was Löwenfeld's view, to whom we are indebted for the most profound treatise on anxiety conditions.[1] " According to the ordinary use of language, fear indicates a lesser degree, and anxiety a higher degree of the emotional condition of painful anticipation characterised by a feeling of dread." He speaks indiscriminately too of fear and anxiety conditions without giving any criterion of their intensity.

If, however, we wished to make accurate linguistic distinctions, we should differentiate between *fear* and *anxiety*. We should regard fear as an unpleasant emotion with a logical basis serving the instinct of self-preservation. Fear has always reference to some particular object. One is afraid of burglars, another of violence. The feeling of displeasure can always be traced to some

---

[1] Die psychischen Zwangerscheinungen. Wiesbaden, 1899.

particular cause. We dread the "Unknown." *Anxiety is the neurotic sister of fear.* We awake in the night with a vague feeling of oppression and palpitation and we call this unpleasant feeling "anxiety." Anxiety is by no means a higher degree of fear. A higher degree of fear is *fright.* Fear is the chronic, fright the acute, condition. Fright increases again to terror when it takes away the individual's capacity for conscious action. Fear, fright and terror are all manifestations of *one* instinct—the instinct of self-preservation. In fact Möbius[1] describes Fear as the most important manifestation of the instinct of self-preservation. "If, in pathological conditions, the instinct is weakened, the longing for death supervenes and the pale mists of twilight seem to cover all that was once bright and lovely."

Anxiety also is an expression of the instinct of self-preservation with this one difference : it manifests the presence of a "*repressed*" instinct. It is the product of so-called "*repression.*"

This brings us for the first time to the expressions "suppression" and "repression," which are not familiar to every doctor. They are, however, easily comprehensible, especially when the impulsive is under consideration. All progress, all development, all civilisation, *e.g.*, education, morality, good manners, etc., is based on repression. The impulsive life has been very little investigated, and one must agree with Möbius when he says, "The misapprehension of the human impulsive life is a veritable *testimonium paupertatis* for psychologists, and nothing is more pitiable than the theory about 'ideas that act and fight like little mannikins in the soul.' "

The instinctive life explains a remarkable fact. We have previously spoken of the feeling of Anxiety as an unpleasant feeling. This is really not correct. Anxiety-feeling can be, under certain circumstances, a pleasurable feeling, *e.g.*, the delicious trepidation with which children listen to a fairy-tale—the tale of Hans who went out into the world to learn to "shiver and shake" is a proof of this. And we gain a still deeper insight into this subject from the fact that "feelings of anxiety" can sometimes serve to inspire works of art. The remarkable discovery that feelings of anxiety are so often linked up with feelings of sexual pleasure provides food for reflection. *Janet* regards this type of sexual excitement as a deviation from fear. But this explanation is not satisfactory to us. We can already perceive the dawn of a realisation that between fear and the sexual impulse there must exist certain intimate connections.[2]

Freud, in his epoch-making investigations upon the "Quellen der infantilen Sexualität" (Drei Abhandlungen zur Sexualtheorie,

---

[1] "Die Hoffnungslosigkeit aller Psychologie." Halle. a.d. S. 1906.

[2] In the wonderful tale of Hans, who went forth to learn to shiver and shake, he is taught this art for the first time by his wife. The fairy-tale therefore confirms the fact, discovered by Freud, of the connection between sexual excitement and anxiety.

Wien, 1905) points out that all intensive affects, even the excitement caused by fright, encroach on sexuality, a fact which may contribute to the understanding of the pathogenic functioning of such emotions. "In the school child," he says, "the anxiety due to examinations, the tension produced by some difficult problem, may have very serious consequences both as regards his relations to the school and to the outbreak of sexual manifestations, in so far as such conditions very often engender a feeling of excitement which leads to the manipulation of the sex organs or to something in the nature of an emission with all their disturbing consequences. The sexually exciting functioning of affects which are displeasurable in themselves: anxiety, trepidations, horror, very often persist in after life and this is possibly the explanation of the fact that so many people seek the opportunity for such sensations if only certain accompanying conditions, belonging to the phantasy life (reading, attending theatres) lessen the intensity of the unpleasant emotions."

This brings us into the realm of the psychopathology of Masochism and Sadism which would lead us too far away from our present theme. We shall have sufficient opportunity when quoting cases to trace the connection with this subject.

We only wish to indicate that the connection between Anxiety and Sexuality is very often apparent without any disguise. This is illustrated by the case of a patient suffering from examination anxiety who always had one, or even several, emissions during each examination. *Löwenfeld* (Sexualleben und Nervenleiden—Wiesbaden, J. F., Bergmann) records similar instances. They must be familiar to every experienced nerve-specialist. In some cases patients seek anxiety as a means to effect an orgasm. They arrange for artificial shocks, dangerous situations which stimulate their emotions. (Compare my essay "*Der Neurotiker als Schauspieler.*" Zentralbl. I. Bd. I. Heft). Feré describes a very interesting case of a very similar character. A patient seeks dangerous situations in which he may be surprised, or discovered, for the purpose of obtaining a violent orgasm. (La peur et l'explosion sexuelle. Revue de médecine 1907, I. Heft).

It is, of course, obvious to the experienced that such cases are the repetition of infantile pleasurable experiences.

Anxiety and sex-impulse are intimately connected. The sex impulse, like various other impulses, makes its appearance in association with counter impulses. The sex-impulse is always accompanied by the instinct of self-preservation and its counterimpulse, the Death-impulse. In fact the sex-impulse may be directly identified with the instinct of self-preservation. "Sich ausleben" means in the language of the common folk, "to live oneself out," to satisfy one's sexual instinct. Furthermore, coitus, as the Viennese philosopher, *Swoboda*[1] aptly expresses it, is a partial death.

[1] Die Perioden im menschlichen Organismus in ihrer psychologischen und biologischen Bedeutung. Wien 1904, *Deuticke.*

The begetting of another being involves the surrender of *our* right to existence. Love and death are closely connected. The greater the development of the instinct of self-preservation, the more likely is the individual to become a prey to the feelings of fear. It is the suppression of this instinct of self-preservation, linked with the sex-impulse, which leads to anxiety. Anxiety is always the result of repression.

Anxiety then is the reaction against the pressing forward of the death impulse engendered by the suppression of the sex or self-preservation instinct.

In short, all anxiety is ultimately the fear of annihilation of the ego—is, in fact, the fear of death.

Although I previously agreed with Freud that all anxiety was of sexual origin, the experiences of the World War have taught me that the instinct of self-preservation can produce anxiety without its sexual component. All those who tremble, tremble for their lives. The trembling of those frightened by the War is a motor fixation of anxiety—is fear of annihilation, is reaction of the instinct of self-preservation against the dangers which threaten the ego.[1]

On the other hand the analysis of the various anxiety states reveals that every neurotic is afraid of himself.

Anxiety, therefore, can also be fear of oneself, i.e., fear of one's own criminal impulses. The desire for death (the longing to commit suicide), is a manifestation of anxiety.[2]

I may claim the credit of having built up the real psychology of neurotic anxiety by the amplification and persistent application of *Freud's* teaching and also by some modification to avoid certain of his errors, as I have demonstrated by my numerous clinical illustrations. I am certainly indebted to Freud for having paved the way. He drew a definite distinction between " *Angstneurose* " (Anxiety-neurosis) and other neuroses. Sexual etiology is clearly demonstrated in Anxiety-neurosis. But we will deal more fully with this subject later, and will now turn our attention to a few practical illustrations of the nature of repression. We shall thereby gain an insight into the foundations of modern psychotherapeutics.

[1] The fixation of the trembling neurosis in favour of certain pretensions as a consequence of covetousness and for the purpose of personal aggrandisement is a secondary symptom.

[2] A lady who felt an imperative desire to throw herself from the top story on to the pavement below, was frightened to look down into the street even from the ground-floor window.

CHAPTER II

THE NATURE OF REPRESSION[1]

OUR culture is built upon territory conquered inch by inch after laborious struggles. Fœtid water had to be diverted ; marshes drained ; primeval forests cleared and mighty dykes constructed. Culture is repression—a well-functioning inhibition.

What applies to humanity in general applies equally to men. Repression enables us to live the life of a civilized man who is willing to comply with all the ethical and social demands of his age. It is also the key to that inner culture, the life on a higher plane, which distinguishes us from the common herd.

Repression is not always a desirable acquisition to our existence. On the contrary. He who is not able to trace his thoughts back to their most obscure origins, and their most minute associations will never be able to free himself from them. Repression without the aid of consciousness is the cause of countless diseases ; it is not a relief but a burden. The matter that lies hidden beneath the threshold of consciousness may, when stirred up, shake us to the depths. *We can only forget that which we have consciously known.*

In the histories of innumerable patients we shall see what an important rôle repression plays in the etiology of neuroses. One must take care not to confuse the mere forgetting of indifferent impressions, with repression. Repression presupposes an affect, some painful, unpleasant emotion. Forgetfulness, which is the result of repression is a dynamic psychic activity—as distinct from ordinary forgetting.

In repression the affect remains undiminished. It has been merely diverted from the sphere of consciousness into the unconscious, or into the pre-conscious, or it has found a surrogate (Affect-displacement). This substitution by its concealment of the affect in the unconscious renders the affect unassailable. Forgetfulness on the contrary implies a diminution of the affect. Remembrance, like attention, is essentially an affective process (*Bleuler*). In repression the attention appears to be diverted from the object which is charged with affect to some other object. This Repression is an active process, an act of will, in contradistinction from " forgetting." *By repression we understand an apparent forgetting*

[1] Partly from my booklet, " Die Ursachen der Nervosität." (Paul Knepler, Wien).

when from motives of displeasure we do not *wish* to think of a particular idea.

Repression is seldom entirely successful. Indeed, successful repression, the complete forgetting of an event, of an impulse, or of a phantasy can seldom be traced. Affect-toned events are the more difficult to repress in proportion to the strength of the affect. If, however, the attempt is successful, we speak of it as successful repression, as *suppression*. Neuroses are the result of *unsuccessful repression*, as we shall see. The affect is not insulated,[1] it is only diverted. The symptoms are then a compromise between affect and repression.

Suppression has, however, rendered the psychic material concerned entirely worthless. The suppression, the successful repression, can never give rise to a neurosis. Ineffective repression may be compared with hysterical amnesia. In hypnosis or in dreams apparently forgotten impressions reappear. We will not at present go into the question of whether or not that form of hysteria common to us all plays the leading part in repression.

Recent investigations have convinced me that Freud's assumption that in repression there is a *real* amnesia is mistaken. It is a question of "*Not wanting to see*," while Freud interprets it as "*Incapacity to see*." The idea concerned is not *unconscious*, but *pre-conscious*. It is relegated from the visual field of our attention, to the periphery, so that the result is a limitation of the mental field of vision. The neurotic is like a man suffering from torticollis, who must always look in one direction because he is unable to turn his head the other way. The neurotic also looks in a wrong direction which accounts for his "incapacity to see," which is always shown by analysis to be a desire not to see. In the same way many a man does not want to see the infidelity of his wife. He represses all thoughts suggestive of her unfaithfulness. He is eventually able to convince himself that he believes her to be faithful.

An excellent example of repression is given by *Janet* : "A young girl of nineteen is subject to attacks of somnambulism, in which she talks of money, thieves and fire, and calls a certain ' Lucien ' to her assistance. When awake she has absolutely no idea of the meaning of it all, and maintains that she has had no experience in which fire, theft and ' Lucien ' played a part. As she came to the hospital alone we have no means of verifying her statement and are forced to assume that it is a case of " délire imaginaire." Six months later her parents came up from the country, called on us and related the dramatic incident which was the origin of the nervous attacks. She was in service at a castle which was one night burgled and set on fire ; she was rescued by a gardener of the name of Lucien. Now how could this young person have forgotten such an important occurrence ? Why did she never speak of it in

[1] Auschalten = insulate, electrical term.

giving an account of her life ? How can such a remarkable lapse of memory be reconciled with the development of a secret remembrance which revived the experience during the attacks of somnambulism ? That is the important question. (Les Nevroses, *p.* 4.)

Modern psychotherapy has undertaken to trace the origin of these repressions, to release them and thereby cure the patient.

It is hidden thoughts that produce the various neurotic symptoms. The strong sense of guilt expresses itself in ill-humours which are only puzzling as long as the inner cause remains unknown. The most remarkable part about this condition is that *the neurotic does not know himself where the shoe pinches.* But that no longer surprises us when we realise that the unpleasant thoughts have been banished from his consciousness and repressed, and that he does not *want* to know the truth. The art of the physician consists in removing these repressions and in getting the patient to acknowledge the truth fearlessly. This is a difficult task and generally requires a long technical process which we call " psychanalysis."[1]

It seldom happens that we can take a patient unawares and thereby immediately relieve him of his repression. In fact, the modern doctor of the soul prefers not to practise this treatment, although some cases could undoubtedly be cured in one sitting. We shall meet with some examples of this. The following example of a case of this nature coming within my own experience, may serve as an introduction to psycho therapeutic methods. It deals with a patient suffering from Agoraphobia. (Platzangst).

No. 1.—A tall, well-built man, twenty years of age, came to my consulting-room to see me about his fear of open spaces. Various hydrotherapeutic and electrotherapeutic treatments had been tried without success. I asked him to describe his anxiety symptoms ; they were typical. The patient stopped at every open place, began to shake, and no power on earth could induce him to cross alone. But he could manage it accompanied by another person. I questioned him in regard to all the circumstances that might have been conducive to the neurosis, and we came to his sex-life. I will take this opportunity of drawing the reader's attention to an excellent remark of Freud's. Freud had learned by experience that many doctors although ignorant of psycho-therapeutic methods, nevertheless seek the root of neuroses in the sex-life, and simply advise the patient to give free rein to his sex-impulses in the hope that this may effect a cure. " But this is not the point," says Freud. " The sexual need and privation is only one factor in the mechanism of neurosis. If it were the only one, debauchery and not disease would be the result. The other indispensible factor, which is only too readily overlooked, is the sexual aversion of neurotics, their incapacity to love, that psychic condition which I have called ' repression.' *The disease arises out of the conflict between the two tendencies* and in consequence, any counsel to indulge in sexual activity in cases of psychoneurosis, can seldom be regarded as wise."

Let us, therefore, bear this fact in mind.[2] Our patient showed very little

---

[1] At the suggestion of *Pfister* the expression Psycho-analysis is altered to Psychanalysis in my works.

[2] How much harm is done by doctors because they are so prone to regard every neurotic symptom as the result of sexual needs ! I have met women who were advised, in consequence of " compulsion-neurosis " to form a

interest in women. He had never been in love in his life, and had never felt any need for it. On one or two occasions he had tried sexual intercourse, without experiencing any particular sensation. This admission involuntarily gave rise to the suspicion that this was a case of homosexuality. The patient emphatically denied this, although he was otherwise quite open in his confessions. He would not even admit partial homosexual tendencies, which so often find expression in erotic homosexual dreams. In such cases one is not far wrong in deducing some fixation of sexual life. And who could be more appropriate as the object of this fixation than some person in the immediate environment on whom the child has already fixed his love ? I asked him innocently if he were fond of his parents.

" Tremendously," he replied. His eyes lighted up and his whole face became animated. " My mother rather more so than my father."

" Are your parents poor ? "

" Very poor. I support them."

" What is your profession ? "

" I am a cashier in a large Banking House."

" Does much money pass through your hands ? "

" Yes, millions of kronen every day."

The understanding of his anxiety neurosis flashed upon me. *The man must have been playing with the idea of seizing a few millions and going off with them.* I put the unexpected question : " Have you never thought to yourself, here am I up to the arms in gold while my poor parents are in want ? "

" Oh, yes, I've often thought that."

" And have you never felt tempted to go off with the money so that your parents' remaining years may be free from care ? "

The patient suddenly turned pale, considered a while, and then said frankly : " Yes, the idea has occurred to me, but I always suppressed it immediately."

" Naturally," I replied, " as any honourable man would do." We chat a while longer and eventually he asks my advice. I tell him quite frankly that his malady has arisen from the repression of the desire to run away with a large sum of money. " I can only see one means of curing you : you must exchange your position of cashier for another which may perhaps entail more work but less temptation." He declared that it was out of the question, that it would arouse suspicion, which I denied, in view of his neurotic condition that prohibited any occupation dealing with accounts and money.

Here we have the repressed desire as the cause of anxiety. The open place symbolises the great unknown future, the ocean across which he would flee to America. Every neurotic is an actor, playing a particular scene. Our neurotic *acted* at the open space the flight to America.[1]

We see from this first example that anxiety is not directly connected with the sex-life. It is obvious in this instance that the patient is afraid of his own criminal impulses. The fact that he contemplates the theft for the benefit of the mother cannot be considered the primary factor in his anxiety. He acts the flight to America and trembles because in his imagination he is caught by the police. If he were confident of success he would probably not be afraid. By this example my definition " The neurotic is a criminal without

" liaison." The result was the aggravation of the disease. For neurotics are excessively moral people, inwardly religious and reproach themselves for the bare thought of sin.

[1] Cp. my opinion : Der Neurotiker als Schauspieler. Zentralblatt für Psychoanalyse I. Jahrg. H.1, and the essay " Schauspieler des Lebens " in Nervöse Leute (Verlag Paul Knepler, Wien).

the courage to commit a crime " may be more readily understood. After six months I heard from his family that he had given up his position and was entirely cured of his trouble. I do not know whether I shall ever see him again. And that is the strange thing about psychic cures : whereas in other successful cures the patients praise the Doctor and are only too glad to recommend him to others, they preserve the strictest secrecy as regards their psychic cures, which they owe to the psychotherapist.

In the first place, he has penetrated into the secret places of their minds, and revealed the criminal within, that dwells in every one ; secondly, they fear he may betray the unflattering picture thus exposed. So they make their revelations as in a confessional, look upon the Doctor as a Father-Confessor whom they will never see again, and after the cure is complete avoid him. I must, however, hasten to acknowledge that there are exceptional patients who visit the doctor from time to time to free themselves from some minor ailment.

Let us turn to another case :—

No. 2 concerns a lady who came to consult me about a remarkable peculiarity. She could not remain in a room without a second person being present, who also must not be a stranger but some near relative of her husband. The suggestion of employing psycho-analytical treatment met with opposition because the treatment must only be carried out in the presence of her husband. Now confession in the presence of a third party is an utter impossibility. I attempted, nevertheless, to gain a closer insight into the nature of the affliction.

The patient had been quite healthy until her marriage eight years before. Then it transpired that her husband was impotent for several years after the marriage and could not perform the sexual function. His condition had now improved so that he was able to fulfil his marital duties, although only moderately, and she became the mother of a child. She was of a lively imaginative disposition, and had been fond, ever since her youth, of dreaming, reading novels, etc., and her ideal of manliness certainly did not coincide with her real husband. She was obviously sexually unsatisfied and was subject to frequent neurotic phantasies. The mechanism of the anxiety was now quite apparent. Her devotion and passionate love for her husband were struggling against her desire to be unfaithful to him. She may have felt an inward leaning to be unfaithful to him on the first occasion that she was left alone with some other man and the lack of strength to resist his wooing and as a reaction against this impulse—manifested in this case as anxiety—arose the dread of being left alone in a room. Her husband, or some relative had to be there to protect her honour. Anxiety as the guardian of honour.

This case proves that anxiety serves as a " self-protective " measure to save the moral ego from destruction. This self-protection increases with the insistence of the impulses. In this case first the servant girl was sufficient protection for her, then any female relative, then a female relative of the husband must be present ; and lastly the poor woman seized her husband's hand and implored him not to leave her and not to go to the office. She only felt safe when she held his hand. Imagine the struggles which must take place in this woman's mind. On one side she is beset by impulses, by passionate desires and longings for love and complete satisfaction, which are vetoed on the other hand by moral inhibitions. The neurosis was the salvation of her moral ego.

This example clearly demonstrates how the conflict between sexual inclination and sexual aversion is capable of producing the neurotic symptoms.

These two cases may suffice to justify the great importance of psychotherapy for the practice of medicine. *Psychic diseases can only be cured by psychic methods.* The detailed analyses in these pages will demonstrate to the doctor what means must be employed in dealing with these complicated phenomena. I will mention another case which I cured with the assistance of a Father-Confessor and in which I myself did not play the part of father-confessor but left that rôle to the church :—

No. 3.—A lady consulted me in regard to attacks of trembling and fainting fits, from which she had suffered since her childhood. The attacks were preceded by excessive anxiety. The first attack took place on Christmas eve while she was at prayer.

I at once offered to tell her the place where the attacks started.

" I wonder whether you can guess that ? "

" *Forgive us our trespasses !*—that might have been the place,"—and so it was.

The girl of fourteen was disgracefully treated by a music master. She had allowed him to do what he liked with her, except coitus, because she believed she was abnormally formed (a common form of anxiety among girls) ! She was very devout and pious, and the conflict between piety and sin had given rise to the attack. The repetition of this attack during recent years pointed to a similar conflict. This proved to be so. She confessed that she had had a liaison with the husband of her greatest friend. Psychanalytic treatment was not possible as the lady could only remain in Vienna a few days.

I asked her if she was still religious. She replied, " Yes," but said it was quite a year since she had been to Confession. I advised her to go, and expressed the hope that if she could find a wise, judicious father-confessor, the attacks would certainly disappear. But so much depends upon the priest. If he is also a doctor of the soul (unfortunately he is not always that) he can read the heart of the sufferer, and a reassuring word from him may remove the whole psychical burden and relieve the conflict. He strengthens the inhibitions either one way or the other. If he pictures terrifying prospects to her, if he threatens with hell and punishment, he will make the illness worse, and increase the conflict, so that at length it becomes almost incurable. But in this case all went as I hoped. The patient went to Confession, and the mysterious attacks, although they had resisted a three months' stay at a well known Hydropathic Institution, disappeared after a single Confession. What *my* part was in this success, is not for me to say.

Perhaps a remark may not be out of place here, concerning the relationship of religion and neurosis. All neurotics are at heart religious. Their ideal is " *Pleasure without guilt.*" Belief has been overcome by the intellect, but is deeply rooted in the emotions. Or more precisely : Faith is rooted in the infantile ; and only through psychanalysis can the conflict be resolved. The patients can neither believe nor disbelieve. They must be brought to do one or the other.

A really religious man can become well merely through confession, that is, if he has faith, knows what is amiss, and what he desires. Unfortunately, this is not often the case; the neurotic is seldom conscious of his criminal desires.

What the Confessional of the Church is to the religious, so the confessional of the doctor must be to all those whose souls are suffering. Karl Marhold (1907), rightly says, without passing sentence on the worth of confession, that in the Protestant countries of German nationality, suicide is more frequent than in the Roman Catholic countries. Yet how few men, modern men, can make use of the benefit of confession! For such the physician must become the sympathetic priest—the priest whom Nietzsche in the " Fröhlichen Wissenschaft," so strikingly describes : " The people venerate an entirely different type of man. . . . namely, the serious, simple, chaste, priestly nature. . . . Before whom they can pour forth their hearts with impunity, by whom they can obtain release from their secrets, their cares, and from things that are even worse. Here there is a *great need ; also for spiritual sewers with thoroughly cleansing water ; a need for powerful streams of love,* pure, strong hearts prepared to sacrifice themselves in such service which is outside the department of public health."

The psychotherapist who investigates repressions, must be of a like chaste and earnest nature. With such a mind we can speak of all things, even of things that other people would condemn as "beastliness." We cannot choose the cause of a neurosis. We must accept it as bountiful Mother Nature gives it to us. But let us not wrong nature! Nature has nothing to do with neurosis. Civilisation is alone to blame, because it assumes that it can violate nature with impunity. All illnesses are at base nothing else than sins against nature.

I consider that the three former examples illustrate the relationship between repression and anxiety.

It is interesting that even great men, whose deeds fill us with admiration, could not prevent feelings of anxiety. Augustus Cæsar's whole body trembled when it began to thunder. He fled to the deepest cellar in his palace, and covered his head with thick furs, so that he might not hear the thunder-claps. Erasmus was horrified if he saw a fish, and Pascal was afraid of a thousand and one things. Frederick the Great had an aversion for all new clothing, or new uniforms. He frequently nearly fainted when he had to put on a new coat. Bernardin de Saint-Pierre, the author of " Paul and Virginia," Newton, and Paganini were frightened and sick on encountering water. Mozart ran away at the sound of a trumpet or hunting horn. Schopenhauer trembled at the sight of a razor. Carlyle never dared to set foot in a shop ; although a keen critic of heroes and heroic deeds, he was afraid of an ordinary shop-keeper. Edgar Allan Poe, Musset, Schumann and Chopin were all afraid of the dark. Dostojewski all through his life trembled before a something incomprehensible, inconceivable, that would one day stand before him, as "something real, loathsome, and full of horror." Finally, Maupassant had a fear and horror of open doors. Those who know the relationship between genius and neurosis, will not be surprised at this. Compare my writing, " Dichtung und Neurose." " Grenzfragen des Nerven und Seelenlebens." J. F. Bergmann, 1909.

CHAPTER III

BASIC CONCEPTS OF ANXIETY NEUROSIS

"UEBER die Berechtigung, von der Neurasthenie einen bestimmten Symptomenkomplex als Angstneurose abzutrennen " is the work by Freud[1] which set out to prove that a great number of so-called neurasthenics indicate an illness different to the typical neurasthenic. This clinical picture *Freud* calls " anxiety neurosis," after the chief symptom, anxiety, around which all the other symptoms are grouped, and holds that the clinical picture cannot always be clearly recognised nor easily diagnosed. There are, for instance, a great number of symptoms which appear as anxiety equivalents, without being accompanied by the affect of anxiety, a circumstance to which E. Hecker[2] has already called attention. Once we know the typical symptoms or anxiety equivalents of the anxiety neurosis, then it should not be difficult, with some experience, also to discover the less distinct cases of anxiety neurosis.

Freud names " anxiety neurosis" and " neurasthenia," "Actual Neuroses," because, in his view, they arise from some harmful form of sexual life. He takes neurasthenia to be the result of excessive masturbation ; anxiety neurosis the result of frustrated excitation.

The separation of anxiety neurosis and neurasthenia contradicts actual psychotherapeutic experience. *Freud's* anxiety neurosis cannot be separated from neurasthenia. More exact analysis points to the fact that every neurasthenia is interpenetrated by anxiety neurotic symptoms. Anxiety neurosis really embraces the complete picture of neurasthenia. There remains compulsion neurosis, psychopathic inferiority, and light psychosis (dementia præcox). I call all neuroses : *Parapathias.*

In this terminology one looks in vain for hysteria. This is the great truth : there is only one neurosis with different forms of expression. One can think of anxiety neurosis as hysteria, and of hysteria as anxiety neurosis. But we will return to this subject later on. It would perhaps be more reasonable to call these maladies after the French custom, psychasthenia, for this does justice to the fact, that without the co-operation of the psyche the neurosis would not occur. *There is no actual neurosis,* in the sense of Freud's

---

[1] Neurologisches Zentralblatt, 1895, und in den " Beiträgen zur Neurosenlehre," Bd. I, Franz Deuticke. Wien und Leipzig, 1910.

[2] "Uber larvierte und abortive Angstzustände bei Neurasthenie." Zentralblatt für Nervenheilkunde, 1893.

conception; there are only *psycho-neuroses*, and really only *one psycho-neurosis* with different forms of expression and degrees of intensity.

Nevertheless, on didactic grounds, it is advisable to retain Freud's classification for the present.

I will here, first of all, sketch in outline the clinical picture, as Freud has determined it.

A *never failing cardinal symptom is a general irritability*, manifested by abnormal reaction to all stimuli without and within. This irritability is extended to all the sense-organs, especially, as Freud emphasizes, to the sense of hearing, so that such an auditory hyperæsthesia may arise, causing insomnia.

A further symptom is the *great absence of mind* and *forgetfulness* of these patients. Most of them complain that they can neither concentrate nor remember names; they easily forget orders and resolutions, so that they become frightened at the decrease of their mental powers. They show the well-known symptom, "fear of insanity."

In addition, these patients suffer from a state of "*Anxious expectation*." This condition is aptly described by Löwenfeld[1] as follows :—

"The most harmless undertaking, such as going for a walk or drive in unfavourable weather, leads to exaggerated fear for body and life; a passing pain in any part of the body brings thoughts of severe illness. The belated return of any relation calls up the worst forebodings. A noise in the house will immediately suggest thieves and murderers, a business transaction of small importance leads to extreme fear of complications and disaster. It is easy to understand, that with all these extreme anxieties, their lives can seldom be cheerful. They see, for the most part, how groundless and ridiculous their fears are, and often try, with all the energy of their rational ego, to defend themselves against the compulsive nature of their fears, generally, however, without much success.

The abnormal disposition to anxiety does not always show itself in the same way on those different occasions which generally produce fear and hesitation. Besides those cases in which, there being a very slight possibility of harm, fears of a lesser or more serious degree appear on many different occasions, e.g., general anxiety. we also meet other cases in which the anxiety disposition is principally or exclusively manifested in a single sphere of personal interest.

Löwenfeld distinguishes the following forms of anxiety conditions :—"(a) *Anxiety which specially concerns one's own health*, hypochondriacal anxiety. This appears in peculiarities conditioned either by heredity or by educational influences of the environment. It can also develop as the result of psychic upheavals, and other experiences harmful to the nervous system. (b) *Moral Anxiety*, in which the most harmless action or omission forms the starting

[1] Die Psychischen Zwangserscheinungen. J. F. Bergmann, Wiesbaden.

point for moral or religious scruples, which very frequently become an exceedingly fruitful source of compulsion ideas. A sub-species of this special anxiety is concerned with the standard of the social conventions, and leads to an immoderate fear of offence against politeness or morality, also to extreme pedantry in manners and in the whole conduct of life. (c) *An abnormal anxiety in reference to the health of near relatives* (children, parents, husband or wife). One notices this form especially after severe mental stress caused by illness or death in the family. Such are roused to a painful state of agitation over the most trifling illness in the family, while they pay insufficient attention to their own physical sufferings. (d) *Abnormal anxiety concerning one's affairs or profession.* To these belong the pessimists and those who take a black view of things. They see loss or disadvantage everywhere, and out of insignificant difficulties; make for themselves endless troubles."

Dr. Wilhelm Strohmayer (" Die Beziehungen Der Sexualität zu Angstzuständen," Journal für Psychologie und Neurologie, Band XII, Heft 2.3, 1908) emphasizes the disturbances of the *ego-feelings.* He says : " Of special interest to me, in these patients, were conditions which stand in the closest relation to anxiety ; *and which are characterized by a diminished ego-feeling in the association of ideas, or by a momentary inability to bring certain feelings or conceptions into normal associative relations with the ego-consciousness.* The peculiar conditions like anxiety appear in the form of attacks. It is often difficult to decide which was prior, whether anxiety or disorder of the ego-feeling. The patients say they cannot feel their ego, or that on account of the attacks it no longer resembles their normal ego. Their orientation in time and place is quite correct ; but for their own person they have a feeling of " strangeness," as if someone else thinks, feels, or acts for them. Their own body, face, voice, appear strange to them. The same patients distinguish from these symptoms, a second : they become partially conscious of their own personality, or a disturbing inability to associate organic feeling with the ego-consciousness. They feel the head, the arms, the hands, but as something outside the accustomed feelings of the body, or as an isolated part in strange dimensions. Finally, there is yet another variety to be considered : a strange emptiness in the head ; the ego-feeling remains unaltered, but the outer world has a changed aspect. Suddenly, all the surroundings become ' so completely altered,' ' so strange,' ' so comical.' In spite of complete orientation, the surroundings lack the quality of recognition. Sometimes there is connected with it a feeling of remoteness and diminution. These conditions were always accompanied in my patients by extreme anxiety, because they believed, that ' madness stared them in the face.' "[1]

[1] " A. Pick (Neurol. Zentralbl, 1903, Nr. 1) has explained similar conditions through an attack of agnosia. He has also had experience with patients who are epileptics and hysterical, who often without positive psychosensory

" *The most striking symptom of anxiety neurosis is the anxiety attack.* The attacks can come on suddenly and unexpectedly with great psychical disturbance, or by the gradual increase of rudimentary attacks. The patients feel that their end is approaching, they fear a stroke, feel that something is entangled in their brain, ' the head feels as if it would burst,' they are going mad, the heart seems to stop, somebody is throttling them and interferes with their breathing ; just as a dying man must feel. All the symptoms that usually accompany the affect of fear or horror may also accompany an anxiety attack. The patients pale, lose their balance, and must lie down. They fight in vain for words and breath (vox faucibus haesit !). The arms and legs shake as in fever. Many patients shake violently, sweat breaks out from the whole body, the hair bristles, and the back creeps with coldness (cutis anserina). An abnormal secretion of urine causes an involuntary emptying of the bladder, or a violent disturbance of the bowels expresses itself in tenesmus, passing of wind, spasms and diarrhœa ; this also produces involuntary evacuation. The pupils of the eyes dilate (according to Fliess, usually the left). The secretion of saliva ceases to flow,[1] and the mouth becomes dry. Often there follows attacks of faintness, migraine, giddiness or tachicardia of great intensity, various pains occur in the heart, chest, head ; neuralgia, stomach-ache, and so on. All these phenomena can appear in the simplest to the gravest form, isolated, or in manifold combinations and variations."[2]

Quite as important as the understanding of the acute anxiety attack in its pronounced form is a thorough knowledge of the rudimentary anxiety attack, the so-called " *anxiety equivalents.*" There is quite a scale of such rudimentary attacks, from simple discomfort and sudden depression, from an attack of sudden tiredness right up to extreme faintness and sudden collapse, thereby

anæsthesia or paræsthesia, complain of a feeling of strangeness in their surroundings." Löwenfeld (Die psychischen Zwangerscheinugen. Wiesbaden, 1904) classifies these symptoms under " Zwangsgefül des Fremdartigen " and " Zwangspfindungen." In a new work, (" Über traumartige und verwandte Zustände," Zentrabl, F. Nervenhlk. Psych., 1909. Bd. XX.) the same author draws attention to the importance of the affect underlying the phenomena. Cf. the Chapter " The Feeling of Strangeness in Life and in the Dream " in my book, " Die Sprache des Traumes " (The Language of Dreams) J. F. Bergmann, 1911.

[1] " In India there is said to be a custom of discovering a thief. All the domestics are called together and some grains of rice are put into the mouth of each. The one whose rice remains dry is judged to be the thief, since anxiety stops the secretion of saliva." Alois Pick, " Zur Kenntnis der Neurosen des Verdauungstraktes." (Med. Klinik, 1909, Nr. 40.)

[2] One of my patients, when shouted at, or at a sudden noise, or during an anxiety attack, feels fear in the region of the nates. He also has there a sensation of heat and cold, numbness, and the feeling, " Now, I'm done for." Obviously this anxiety expresses the most important anxiety-complex ; homosexuality. The anxiety attacks the erogenous zones, which are forbidden.

alarming the whole household.   The physician and those surrounding the patient have to work hard to relieve the disorder.   The knowledge of the rudimentary anxiety attack is of great significance to the practitioner.

Freud mentions the following equivalents of the anxiety attacks : (*a*) Disorders of the heart, palpitation with short arhythmia, with longer lasting tachycardia, up to a condition of such severe weakness, that the distinction from organic affections of the heart is not always easy ; pseudo angina pectoris (no light task for diagnosis !). (*b*) Disorders of the breathing, several forms of nervous dyspnœa, attacks like asthma, and so on.   Freud mentions that even these attacks are not always accompanied by recognisable anxiety. (*c*) Attacks of excessive sweating, often at night.   (*d*) Attacks of trembling and shaking, which may easily be mistaken for hysteria. (*e*) Attacks of bulimia, often combined with giddiness.   (*f*) Sudden attacks of diarrhœa.   (*g*) Attacks of locomotor giddiness. (*h*) Attacks of so-called congestion, practically all that was formerly called vasomotor neurasthenia.   (*i*) Attacks of paræsthesia (these seldom without anxiety).   (*j*) Sudden fright on awakening from sleep (as if falling from a mountain).   (*k*) Sudden urge for micturition.   (*l*) Muscular cramp.

I should like to add to this list some important further additions :—(*m*) Sudden deep sighs, the result of breathlessness, often amounting to air-hunger.   (*n*) The sudden on-coming of a feeling of weariness, that can amount to faintness.   (*o*) Vomiting and stomach-ache (very important symptoms !), also painful flatulency with the noisy passing of large quantities of wind.   (*p*) The fingers suddenly becoming dead, or the whole hand, or arm. (*q*) Migrâine.   (*r*) Great restlessness, aimless running about.

How do such anxiety equivalents originate ?   We can only say now that some symptoms manifestly obtrude and represent the whole picture of the anxiety neurosis.   Certainly by a more careful examination, many other symptoms can be found (irritability, anxious expectation, and so on), thereby rapidly proving the typical picture of an anxiety neurosis.

For the cause of the anxiety neurosis there are several injurious developments of the sexual life to be considered.   *Freud* (*l.c.*) treats the conditions of men and women separately.   According to his experience the anxiety neurosis with women occurs in the following circumstances :—

" (*a*) As virginal anxiety or the anxiety of adolescence.   A number of observations of undoubted significance have shown him, that a first meeting[1] with the sexual problem, or similarly, the sudden disclosure of that which was formerly concealed,

---

[1] Certainly it is not the first meeting.   In childhood there were important sexual experiences and phantasies, which fell under a complete amnesia by repression.   After puberty, psychanalysis revives the memories and removes the repressions.

the seeing a sexual act, sexually exciting information or a lecture, can produce an anxiety neurosis in a girl approaching maturity.

" (b) As anxiety of the newly married.   Young women, who with the first cohabitation remain anæsthetic, often develop anxiety neurosis, which disappears when it gives place to the normal feeling.

" (c) As anxiety of women whose husbands suffer from ejaculatio præcox, or very reduced potency ; and

" (d) Of women whose husbands practice coitus interruptus or reservatus.   These cases go together, for we can be assured by the analysis of a great number of examples that it all depends upon whether the woman obtains satisfaction in coitus or not : in the latter case the conditions for an anxiety neurosis are present ; on the other hand, the woman escapes the neurosis if the man who is troubled with ejaculatio præcox can repeat the congress imme-diately afterwards with better results.   The congressus reservatus with the condom does not harm the woman if she is easily aroused and the man very potent ; otherwise, this sort of preventive inter-course is no less harmful.   Coitus interruptus is almost always harmful ; but for the woman it is only harmful if the man is thought-less, that is, if he interrupts as soon as the ejaculation approaches, without troubling about the state of the woman.   If on the con-trary, the man waits for the satisfaction of the woman, then such a coitus has for her the same significance as a normal one : but in that case, the man is the victim of an anxiety neurosis.

" (e) As anxiety of widows and those who abstain intentionally. Not seldom in typical combination with compulsory ideas.

" (f) As anxiety in climacterium during the last great increase of the sexual need."

Freud places men in the following groups which likewise have their analogies among women :—

" (a) Anxiety of the intentional abstainer, frequently combined with symptoms of defence (compulsory ideas, hysteria).   The motives which could account for intentional abstinence would also account for a number of peculiarities, hereditary traits and so on of this category.

" (b) Anxiety of men with frustrated desires (during courtship). The men who (out of fear of the consequence of sexual intercourse) satisfy themselves with touching and looking at women.   This group of conditions, which can likewise be transferred to the other sex unaltered, (courtship with sexual abstinence) supply the clearest cases of neurosis.

" (c) Anxiety neuroses of men who practice coitus interruptus. As already remarked, coitus interruptus is harmful to the woman if consideration is not shown for her satisfaction.   It is also harmful for the man, if he, in order to satisfy the woman, manages by force of will, to delay the ejaculation.   In this way we can understand why among married people given to this practice, usually only one of them suffer. Coitus interruptus seldom creates in men a pure anxiety neurosis, but usually a mixture with neurasthenia.

"(d) Anxiety of men in senium. There are men, who like women, show a climacterium, and at the time of their descending potency, and increasing libido, manifest anxiety neurosis."

"Finally"—*Freud* remarks—"I must include two cases that serve for both sexes :—

"(e) The neurasthenics, who practise masturbation, develop an anxiety neurosis as soon as they give up their mode of sexual satisfaction. These people have made themselves particularly incapable of bearing abstinence."

Freud emphasizes here as an important point in the anxiety neuroses, that any remarkable development of it can only arise with men who have remained still potent and with women who are not anæsthetic. "With neurasthenics who have already seriously depreciated their potency, the anxiety neurosis in cases of abstinence, is very mild and is limited mainly to hypochondria and slight chronic giddiness. The majority of women must be considered as potent ; a really impotent, that means, anæsthetic woman, is likewise not easily accessible to anxiety neurosis and bears the afore-mentioned disadvantages extremely well."[1]

"(f) The last ætiological conditions to be mentioned do not appear to be of an especially sexual nature. The anxiety neurosis originates in both sexes through over-work, exhaustion and strain ; for example, night-duty, tending the sick, and even after severe illness."

It will be seen from our material that the latter is only the releasing cause. An already exhausted body cannot withstand the attack of a neurosis that has already been preparing for a long time. For a single example will show us that the individual on such an occasion is brought into severe psychical conflict, sufficient to disturb the psychic equilibrium.

The deeper I penetrate into the nature of the so-called "*neuroses*" so much the stronger becomes my conviction that it only concerns disorders of the feelings, thus, "*parapathia.*" Above all, one must never be satisfied with a superficial anamnesia, but must always employ profound analytic investigation to find the basic truth.

---

[1] This passage contains a number of errors, that must be corrected. It is not true that neurasthenics have harmed (by masturbation) their potency severely. In the fourth volume of this work (" Die Impotenz des Mannes ") I have corrected this error of *Freud*. It does not correspond to experience that the anxiety neurosis of impotent neurasthenics is limited to slight giddiness and hypochondria. *Freud* has drawn a premature conclusion from few experiences. To maintain that impotent (anæsthetic) women are not easily accessible to anxiety neurosis, and bear the injury well, is absolutely wrong. They bear this injury well, only for so long as they do not desire satisfaction. In most cases these anæsthetic women are consumed by the desire for satisfaction and disclose the gravest symptoms of anxiety. There are numberless examples in Volume III : especially instructive is, " Die Analyse einer Messalina."

In earlier editions I have supplemented *Freud's* statements :—

(*g*) There are a large number of variations in the practice of *coitus prolongatus* or of prolonging the orgasm. I am reminded of a case in which a man read a newspaper or a novel, thereby prolonging the act up to half-an-hour. Another counted up to a thousand. The third repeated the Roman Emperors. All these men suffered from an anxiety neurosis. In the same way women try to suppress the Libido, in order to prevent pregnancy and thereby become liable to a severe anxiety neurosis.

(*h*) Many men have the remarkable idea that the loss of the sperm is very harmful and robs the body of its best energy. Such men practise *coitus sine ejaculatione*, a particularly harmful form of cohabitation. *Coitus interruptus sine ejaculatione* is, more frequently than one would suppose, the cause of an anxiety neurosis.

(*i*) Also, " *masturbatio interrupta* " and " *pollutio interrupta* " play their part in originating an anxiety neurosis. *Rohleder* has been the first to call attention to this very important and frequent form of masturbatio interrupta (Zeitschrift für Sexualwissenschaft, 1908, Nr. 8, und, " Vorlesungen über den Geschlechtstrieb und das gesamte Geschlechtsleben des Menschen "). The pollutio interrupta was first described by *P. Näcka* (Einiges über Pollutionen. Neurol. Centralbl, 1909. Nr. 20, und Ueber die pollutio interrupta, Münch, med. Wochenschr, 1909, Nr. 34.)

(*j*) Masturbatio prolongata is another cause of anxiety neurosis. For instance, one of my patients could practise masturbation ten times in a night, without allowing an ejaculation. He showed symptoms of a severe anxiety neurosis. While on the other hand, I knew a young man of medium strength who could practise masturbation with ejaculation, five to ten times in an hour, without showing any neurotic symptoms. As soon as he ceased the practice of onanism, he developed severe neurotic symptoms. That is an experience that any physician can easily note.

(*k*) Further, an anxiety neurosis can originate, if a man or a woman imagines another person, during cohabitation, or uses phantasy in order to obtain the orgasm.

(*l*) One often meets men, who carry on a normal coitus, but nevertheless suffer from anxiety neurosis. If one investigates for any length of time—for these intimate things do not come up in the first hours of talk—one realises that one is treating persons whose sexual desires strive after some different kind of satisfaction. For instance, a married homosexual will, despite the so-called normal satisfaction, suffer from an anxiety neurosis : so to a pervert woman the normal coitus is an act of onanism. (*Relative abstinence !*)

How does. Freud describe the etiology of anxiety neurosis ? He believes that the libido is converted into anxiety in some mysterious (chemical or organic) manner. I have again and again

been able to prove the relationship which Freud has described, and tempted by these facts, I accepted this libido theory.
After a more precise investigation of all the facts, I have completely abandoned it.
I do not believe that physical harm comes to the nervous system by means of frustrated excitation.
I have found in every anxiety neurosis a psychical cause.
I conveyed these facts to Freud and he proposed to distinguish two sorts of anxiety neuroses : one with a pure somatic basis, *Freud's* genuine anxiety neurosis, and one with a psychical basis, which he terms " anxiety hysteria." But in the second edition of this work (*page* 22) I wrote : " I may here, however, emphasize that the distinction between anxiety neurosis and anxiety hysteria is more clearly worked out in this book from a theoretical point of view than from practical experience. The sexual disorder contains within itself the germ of the psychic conflict. The unsatisfied man will long for other objects from which he expects full satisfaction ; the same with the unsatisfied woman. This produces in marriage a series of traumatic wish-phantasies, which create a torturing sense of guilt.
" That is really the germ of the whole truth. *There is no anxiety neurosis*, only an *anxiety hysteria.* Or we will call anxiety neurosis every psychical suffering in which the effect of the anxiety is in any way somatically expressed. I retain the expression anxiety neurosis, not in Freud's meaning of " actual neurosis," but as psycho-neurosis. Illness in which the anxiety is expressed somatically (mostly mono-symptomatic) we will treat of as anxiety neurosis, while according to an old custom, we will treat the complicated psychical anxiety conditions as *phobias.*
All symptoms of an anxiety neurosis can be explained by a " psychical conflict."
I return to the formula which I first used in my pamphlet of 1908, " Die Ursachen der Nervosität " : " Every Neurosis originates through a psychical conflict ! "
This psychical conflict explains the great irritability of the anxiety neurotics. They are—as are all unsatisfied and unhappy people—in a continual ferment. They show an increased affectivity and *sensitiveness*, which are indicated by touchiness and irritability. Their absence of mind and forgetfulness can also be explained by psychic factors. People who are continually occupied with themselves, think inwardly, and those whose affectivity is focussed on their complexes, cannot turn their attention to anything except their complexes. Anxious expectation is the result of their inward distraction.
We must learn to understand truly the nature of anxiety. Anxiety is a wish of the inner man that is always censored and rejected by the moral self. When two wishes fight in a man's breast, wishes that show a tendency to bipolarity—the one as a

sign of social obedience in the service of culture, the other as a rebel in the power of the life of impulse—*the stronger wish asserts itself, and the weaker appears in consciousness as anxiety.* Anxiety is repressed desire. That distinguishes anxiety from fear. The anxiety is only *apparently* not attached to an obiect. The object is merely concealed from consciousness.

Anxious expectation corresponds to the unfulfilled wish. I have already in the second edition drawn attention to the psychical roots of anxiety after exhaustion (Point (*f*) of Freud's thesis). I said there (*page* 12) : " This form of anxiety neurosis can according to the latest experience be traced back to psychical causes only.—Of course one must take into account that many of the people who act as nurse must live in a state of abstinence, for example, the wife who attends her sick husband, and so on. Very often in these cases there exists a repressed death-wish. The evil wish : ' Oh, if only the patient would die, then I should be free and all possibilities open to me ' flashes for a second through the mind, and becomes the source of an extreme feeling of guilt. They atone for this by showing excessive anxiety and care for the patient, and in the case of death express it by a prolonged (unnaturally severe) grief."

The more precise and profound investigation of my material has convinced me that the anxiety neurosis is always caused by psychical factors, and that the so-called frustrated excitation, lacking such a conflict, has no harmful tendencies. I have observed men who have practised coitus interruptus for many years, and found satisfaction in it. They were exempt from all signs of anxiety neurosis. This also confirms the observations of Havelock Ellis which he expresses in his " Geschlecht und Gesellschaft " (II. Teil, Würzburg, Kurt Kabitsch, 1911). It treats of the so-called sect, " Male continence," founded by Noyes. Every man was the husband of every woman, but he was only allowed to beget children by one. There were certainly two kinds of cohabitation, a propogative and non-propogative. It was the duty of the man to prolong the coitus for an hour, which was obtained by delaying the orgasm. Most of the members of the sect were perfectly healthy, only two, who had carried it to excess, showed slight signs of nervous disorder. This interesting observation shows, that excluding wish-phantasies and the psychic conflict, coitus interruptus is, in and for itself, somatically an indifferent procedure.

I have known men who were able to extend coitus for an hour, and, finally, to accomplish coitus in anum, irrumatio or coitus inter mammas with ejaculation. I have not been able to find in these men more nervous symptoms, if they are free from psychic conflicts, than in other men who practise normal intercourse.

The basic condition is, that the man should find his sexual satisfaction from the woman he loves and desires. If this is not the case, then dissatisfaction and weariness result, and after coitus a variety of symptoms and pains will appear ; these are, however, all psychically determined, as are the various troubles after masturbation.

Every unsatisfied man who is filled with wish-phantasies that his sexual partner cannot satisfy, becomes liable to an anxiety neurosis ; also the successful repression of criminality leads to an anxiety neurosis, as shown by the example of the cashier, on page 8.

We come then to a single formula for the sexual etiology of anxiety neuroses : it runs as follows :—

Every individual who cannot find a form of sexual satisfaction adequate to himself, or is in severe psychical conflict between criminality and morality *suffers from an anxiety neurosis.*

An anxiety neurosis is the disease of a bad conscience. It might be a bad conscience arising from tabooed sexual impulses, or from a bad social conscience. It can always be proved that the ideal-self of the individual has come into conflict with his impulsive self.

Where the instinct of self-preservation and the conscience, *i.e.,* the sum of all inhibitive ideas which interpose themselves between impulse and action, clash, the conditions for an anxiety neurosis have been established.

CHAPTER IV

CLINICAL PICTURE OF ANXIETY NEUROSIS: THE ANXIETY ATTACK

WE are still in the dark as to the part played by the ductless glands in anxiety neuroses. But we may assume that the organism is under the influence of toxins which eliminate certain inhibitions and release suppressed tendencies, a process which results in reaction formations of a psychical nature that are eventally manifested in fear of the strength of one's own impulses. Unsatisfied sex instincts stimulate the imaginative faculties of the individual and by the resultant sensual phantasies tend to produce fresh conflicts between moral duty and erotic need. *Two factors are therefore working in conjunction for the creation of the clinical picture of anxiety neuroses, the somatic and the psychic.* I do not agree with Freud's theory that anxiety represents a complete metamorphosis of the libido, as, in the common form of anxiety neuroses the psychic factor (the suppression of the sexual and criminal instincts) plays a necessary part.

My conception of the constitutional factor of neuroses, which I have called " Psychic disorders," is by no means limited to the disturbances of the internal secretions above mentioned.

I regard the neurotic as a "reaction phenomenon." He is distinguished by exceptionally strongly-marked appetites. All his impulses, and of course the sex-impulse, are more strongly developed and are not in accordance with the demands of culture.[1] His criminality is also more strongly defined than it is with most people. What are we to understand by this criminality? Merely the a-social (egoistic) dispositions which are perpetually endeavouring to procure enhanced pleasure for the ego. The neurotic lacks " esprit de corps," the subordination to the requirements of culture. He remains the psychic anarchist, whose impulse-life cannot be reconciled with the dictates of culture. His "will to power" has been hypertrophically developed, his egotism is without bounds, his affectivity is always increased. The atavistic sexual emotions in particular are instrumental in bringing the individual into severe conflict with morality. The neurotic has to contend against sadistic, necrophilic, cannibalistic, mysophilic tendencies, and must expend so much energy in the suppression of these impulses that he is socially quite worthless. He is also a

[1] Discussed in detail for the first time in my book, " Die Träume der Dichter." Eine vergleichende Untersuchung der Treibkräfte bei Dichtern, Neurotikern und Verbrechern. I. F. Bergmann, 1912.

prey to morbid ambition, exaggerated sensitiveness, and a feeling of inferiority which originates in the imminent sense of guilt. The fear of himself, and the a-social impulses drive the patient to take defensive measures (self protection) among which anxiety plays a dominant part.

An anxiety neurosis results in an individual when he is physically and psychically disposed by his own impulses to come into severe conflict with the conventions of life and society.

The anxiety neurosis is the social reaction against the a-social imperatives of the impulses.

The anxiety attack forms the centre of the anxiety neurosis. It is scarcely less important than the great hysterical attack. It also has the same psychic etiology.

Freud is justified in pointing out that the symptoms of the anxiety attack exhibit to some extent surrogates of the specific action of the sexual excitement omitted. He says: "In confirmation of my theory I would remind the reader that in normal coitus the excitement finds expression in accelerated breathing, palpitation of the heart, sweating, congestion, etc. In the corresponding anxiety attack of the neurosis we observe dyspnœa, palpitation, etc., isolated and intensified."

The serious anxiety attack, as in cases of anxiety neuroses, actually does show a remarkable resemblance to the phenomena of coitus. The latter, however, is capable of a thousand different variations.

Equally variable are the phenomena of the anxiety attack. Only one symptom is common to all. A vague, torturing inexpressible fear of death. In some cases the anxiety alone predominates in the conscious mind. The patients complain of feelings of anxiety and localise these in various places. One feels it in the heart, another in the breast, a third in the stomach, a fourth even in the bladder, a fifth in the head,[1] and some only experience a dull sense of depression. (Note the expressions used to convey a feeling of anxiety, all of which imply a certain constriction. Angst equals enge. Beklemmung equals Klamm.)

The anxiety attack may occur quite suddenly or after certain psychic premonitions. It is sometimes preceded by irritability, or slight ill humour. The patients are depressed, or in a bad temper on that day. But that is not the rule. For the anxiety attack can appear suddenly like a thunderbolt out of a cloudless sky. At all events a detailed psychanalysis always reveals an affect emerging from the unconscious. It is then that we find the secret associations leading from some apparently harmless impression, or from the dream-picture to the *repressed painful* thought.

[1] Cramer (" Zur Symptomatologie und Therapie der Angst," Deutsch. med. Wochenschr., 1910, Nr. 32) asserts that, with a very few exceptions, he has never met a patient who has localised the anxiety in the head, the legs or any other part of the body but the region of the heart. This is contrary to my experience.

The attack imitates the phenomena of coitus. The patients complain of an oppressive feeling in the chest, the breathing appears to be laboured, the heart beats painfully, they begin to pant and make all kinds of uneasy movements. They turn pale, the pulse is feeble and rapid—often arhythmical—these symptoms are followed by ague (shivering fits), cramp, paræsthesia and an urge to urinate and defæcate.

Every attack is, however, not so easily recognisable as such. The anxiety may be latent and some correlative symptom exhibited—for example, palpitation. We call this an " anxiety equivalent." Here also the sex life is the determining factor in the attack.

Of the concomitant phenomena of anxiety equivalents one is especially characteristic. A woman predisposed to Dyspnœa is more liable to nervous asthma as an equivalent than one whose chief symptom is palpitation. The latter will be more likely to suffer from violent palpitation of the heart as anxiety equivalent, which in its turn will produce, by excitement, the hypochondriacal illusion that she has heart disease—thus fostering the anxiety. We shall have an opportunity of dealing with the rudiments of anxiety in the following chapters.

In anxiety attacks the " locus minoris resistentiæ " is chosen as the point of fixation and the organic manifestation of the anxiety. A man inclined to disorders of the bowels will react with a diarrhœa or colic—a man with a nervous heart will evince a marked tendency to cardiac affections ; in fact, anxiety can manifest as pseudo-strokes or fainting fits. The "inferior organ" (Adler) is generally the seat of the transformation of anxiety into physical symptoms.

The anxiety attack not only simulates coitus but also death. " Birth and death," " coitus and dying " are nevertheless the polar counterparts of one and the same complex. Some anxiety attacks are not, however, comprehensible unless we realise that the patient is actually going through his own death. There are people who die a thousand times before their death. All these neurotics are tortured by a perpetual dread of death. During the anxiety attack they call for a doctor, take leave of their relatives, and make their final arrangements. The tragic scene is very often of a pronouncedly hysterical character.

We may mention that this fear of death is in many instances the outcome of a guilty conscience. It is noticeable in those unconsciously pious, who, while professing to be free-thinkers, are haunted by the fear of retribution as the hour approaches when they must stand before the " Divine Judge." This fear of retribution is naïvely expressed by Hölty, in his well-known song :

" Ub' immer Treu' und Redlichkeit   " Dann wirst du wie auf grünen Au'n
    Bis an dein kühles Grab—   Durchs Pilgerleben geh'n ;
    Und weiche keinen Finger breit   Dann kannst du sonder Furcht und
    Von Gottes Wegen ab.   Grau'n
                                      Dem Tod ins Auge seh'n."

But as no man is capable of leading such a life that he never swerves a finger's breadth from God's appointed paths, the thought of his last hour must needs be fraught with " Angst und Grau'n."

Also the " criminal complex " and the guilty conscience may be expressed in violent anxiety attacks.

But enough of theory. I consider it to be more satisfactory to illustrate the various questions as they arise through the medium of examples, taken from the daily life of the practitioner. As a preliminary step in the exploration of the vast region of nervous disorders I will give a few cases of simple transparent anxiety neurosis.

No. 7.—Mrs. I. I., a thirty year old widow, organically quite sound, sitting with her family one evening, was feeling perfectly well and happy. The chapter of a book in which she was engrossed suddenly inspired her to read portions of it aloud to her brother. She had hardly begun when she was seized with a sudden sense of uneasiness. To reassure herself, and to allay her fears, she continued to read although her eyes were streaming and her voice was breaking. When her brother asked what ailed her she burst into tears, and was very downcast and miserable. Her mind was filled with the blackest thoughts. She dared not go to bed because she was afraid to sleep ; she was terrified lest she should never get up again ; everything began to flicker before her eyes, hot waves ran over her body ; she was convinced that she must be sickening for some fever. But the thermometer revealed a perfectly normal temperature. She was suddenly seized with the alarming premonition that she would never see her beloved little daughter again, and she began to torture herself with doubts as to what will become of the child when she is gone. She was in a pitiful state as if she were " really seriously ill." The next day she came to me with the request to examine her thoroughly so that by timely intervention her premature death might be averted.

On examination I found the organs to be perfectly sound. There were also no traces of hereditary trouble. (Only in a diminishing proportion of anxiety neuroses do hereditary influences come into question). I was naturally interested in the book which she had been reading because it was here that I hoped to find associations with the repressed phantasy-complex which obsessed her. The word " complex " was coined by Bleuler and has been adopted as legal currency by the language of psycho-therapy to express the fact established by Freud, of the repression of a particular group of ideas. It was, in point of fact, a love scene which she had been reading with such enthusiasm, and which made her realise the lovelessness of her own life. This scene must have had a violent effect on the sexual emotions, by way of contrast. She was, as we have seen, a widow, and had lived a life of complete abstinence for two years. During the last year she had made the acquaintance of a man who had made a very favourable impression on her and with whom she had fallen in love. Erotic dreams in which this man played a part became more and more frequent, and these were followed by indescribable depression and irritability. She ceased to find pleasure in being beautifully dressed (very characteristic !), art no longer interested her, until she finally reached a pitch of nervous anticipation in which she felt she was about to experience something that would throw her completely off her mental balance. About three or four weeks previously she had had an interview with the man in question, which, however, only resulted in frustrated excitement. During the last few months she had suffered now and again from a slight feeling of uneasiness and palpitation. Since then her condition had grown worse from day to day until the twenty-eighth day—(we shall learn presently the significance of this date for the advent of the attack)—when she was seized with the first acute attack after the reading. I saw the patient again after a further three months. She was perfectly well. Anxiety attacks and nervous fears had entirely vanished. We need hardly mention that she had plucked up courage to overcome various prejudices and had given herself to the man of her choice.[1]

The mechanism of the origin of this anxiety neuro: is is clearly apparent in this example. In great libidos the anxiety neurosis develops gradually as a consequence of enforced abstinence, until at some critical juncture, over-excitement brings it to a head. But let us turn to a second example. In the course of our investigations we shall have ample opportunity to consider this question in detail.

No. 8.—Mr. S. N. was one day taken very ill in the street. It happened to be a Sunday and he was walking through the Ring with his fiancée in the direction of the Art Museum. He was obliged to enter a doorway and lean against the wall to save himself from falling. He felt as if he were going to vomit—as if he would die. After a few moments the attack passed over and he felt perfectly well again. Curiously enough his fiancée experienced the same sensations scarcely half an hour later in the Museum. Everything seemed to grow dark, she was obliged to sit down quickly and begged to be taken to the air. They both came to consult me on the same day. In such a case as this, one is naturally inclined to attribute the indisposition to some poisonous matter in the food, especially as Mr. S. N. had had symptoms of nausea and later on had a violent attack of diarrhœa. Nothing, however, could be traced in the food to which the circumstances could be attributed. Both parties, moreover, felt perfectly well after the attack. Mr. S. N. admitted that he suffered considerably from the exigencies of the engagement. He is of an exceptionally highly sexed and passionate temperament and was formerly accustomed to sexual union several times a week. He has now been completely abstinent for fourteen months for fear of infection and also because he found it impossible to copulate with another woman. An attempt at a puella publica was unsuccessful and he could not effect an erection, whereas when his fiancée was merely present in the same room with him he was positively tormented with violent erections. This attack was twice repeated but in a lesser degree after he had had resort to bromide, hydropathic cures and had remained apart from his fiancée for some considerable time on the advice of his Doctor. On the other hand the diarrhœa increased and yielded to no remedies. Especially on leaving his fiancée when on his way home to his flat which was some distance off was he troubled in this way, and was always sure of having to pay a couple of visits to cafés. He often awoke in the night with attacks of fright, and began to suffer from periodic insomnia. The fiancée was not in particularly good health either. She suffered from nervous anxiety, palpitation, giddiness, paræsthesia. *A week after the marriage both he and his bride had no further trouble from these symptoms.* It was a case of anxiety neurosis resulting from the conjunction of abstinence with an increased libido.

[1] Eventually I learnt the most important *constituent* of this anxiety. She had at that time a second suitor who had said to her : " If it were not for your child I would marry you on the spot." The phrase, " What will become of the child when I am gone ? " is a hypocritical inversion of her own criminal designs on the child's life (thoughts against the child) and should read : " If the child were not alive you would now be the happy possessor of a husband. *Kill it !* " Anxiety is the reaction against this criminal desire. Similar motives are to be found in Janet's case (No. 12). Every escape is the endeavour to escape from the ego, from one's own innermost evil thoughts ; every useless excitement which manifests itself in such acts as throwing the furniture about, breaking vases, is a substitute for some criminal act. There are actually patients who make lunging movements with the hand as if they were stabbing someone, clench their fist as if to strike, or simulate strangling.

The psychic conflict was also very apparent. Both suffered under the abstinence. They felt an urgent desire to consummate their love before the ceremony. Counter-impulses fought for ascendancy in the minds of both bride and bridegroom. The diarrhœa is explained from his peculiarity of being overcome by an urge for defæcation immediately before coitus. This unpleasant tendency did not cease until he had had intercourse several times with his partner. It disappeared entirely after marriage. The conflict between the " Ideal Ego " and the " Impulse Ego " is to be seen in this case also.

No. 9.—Mr. L. W. is subject, after the death of his wife, to slight fits of depression and frequent attacks of distressing nervous anxiety which he cannot account for. He feels that it will not be long before he joins his wife. He is also alarmed by the frequent presence of blood in the urine. He sleeps very badly and is haunted by the thought of death. He is afraid of " he knows not what," and can hardly await the morning. This is a typical anxiety neurosis. Anxiety neuroses may often be met with in men who have reached the senium. The psychic factor conducing to this condition is the sense of shame which these people feel at still being subject to the importunities of the libido ! Anxiety neuroses occur in old men who are still under the influence of a powerful libido. The patient one day surprised me by asking whether it would be harmful if he were to indulge in sexual intercourse once a week. Since his wife's death he has lived the life of an ascetic and is troubled by the most violent erections. I allow him moderate sexual intercourse with certain precautions. He feels distinctly better thereafter and forms an attachment whereby intercourse takes place several times a week in a perfectly normal manner. All symptoms of anxiety vanish and the hæmorrhage of the bladder decreased considerably and took place at longer intervals in comparison with the former condition. His appearance is brisker, he is as if endowed with a second youth. Even to-day, though seventy-four years of age, he still feels the necessity for weekly sexual intercourse, without which he is unable to sleep.[1]

Psychic conflict : He desired the death of the wife he loved. He longed for change and for young girls. He felt constrained to suppress the inclination to rejoice at his freedom gained by his wife's death. The sense of guilt (law of Talion) made him fear the retribution of God. " You are rejoicing at your wife's death and God will punish you."

Here the anxiety is not of a purely libidinous character—otherwise it would have occurred during the three years abstinence while his wife was ill and he was unable to sleep with her—it was the result of a guilty conscience.

Let us consider a case of distinctly hysterical structure.

No. 10.—Mr. A. W., aged fifty-two, complains of epileptic fits. He tells me that he sprang out of bed one night with a terrible cry. He felt that by crying out he would save himself from being stunned and suffocated. This occurred at the Hotel. His brother, who was sleeping with him at the time, thought something awful must have happened and " nearly died of fright." This attack took place on November 5th, 1907. The first attack occurred on June 25th, 1905, the second on June 12th, 1906, as in this instance, without apparent cause. There is also a general disposition to scream in his sleep. He describes this as " minor attacks." The great attacks he calls epileptic fits, because he was said to suffer from epilepsy as a child. He was six years old when he awoke one night and found the whole town ablaze. After this he was subject to ' epileptic " fits. They occurred always at night. He was said to have uttered piercing screams on that occasion (Pavor nocturnus). He does not remember the exact details. These attacks lasted for three years.

[1] *Kurt Mendel* (" Die Wechseljahre des Mannes." Neurolog. Zentralbl., 1910, Nr. 20) traces anxiety neurosis in senium to the hypo-function of the seminal glands. This observation proves the contrary. The man had a slight hypertrophy of the prostate.

(He never used to wet the bed.) At fourteen he learned to masturbate, and continued the practice for many years. At twenty he began sexual intercourse and suffered even then from ejaculatio præcox.

At the age of twenty-nine he married and at first found intercourse somewhat easier. But during the last five or six years his sexual potency had perceptibly diminished.

His wife professes to be anæsthetic and always begs him to leave her in peace. For this reason coitus only takes place at intervals of six weeks. He finds, moreover, the performance of the sexual function distasteful because his wife uses a pessary. His sexual needs are, however, still very urgent and occasionally result in increased emissions. It is obvious that this is not a case of epilepsy but of pavor nocturnus persisting in later years. Analysis, however, reveals interesting details of the psycho-genesis of the attacks. Before the last so-called " epileptic " seizure he had been reading a book in which there was a description of an operation. A cataract was being removed from the eye of a blind man. *He is beside himself with fear*—goes to the doctor with great reluctance because he is afraid that he will learn something unpleasant. His heart begins to beat violently and his pulse increases to 140-160. The book had had a powerful affect on his nervous system.

He remembers a dream which he had just before the seizure. " He was condoling Mr. W., who had lost his son four weeks previously." This young man had been suddenly seized with appendicitis and had died in two days. This terrible death preyed on the patient's mind for a considerable time. He could not bear the mention of illness or death without becoming depressed and miserable.

The attacks were decidedly not of an epileptic character. (He was never unconscious for a moment—and merely experienced a tremendous sense of anxiety.) The symptoms corresponded with those of the attacks of pavor nocturnus to which he was subject as a child. They were the outcome of his perpetual dread of death, which again was a symptom of anxiety neurosis resulting from abstinence. He is moreover very easily irritated, and in a perpetual state of nervous anticipation, suffers from night sweats, palpitation and diarrhœa. His irritability is manifest in his behaviour to his wife. He makes the most violent scenes without any " apparent cause "—but in reality because she denies him sexual intercourse, which is so necessary for his happiness. His anxiety is free floating, due to the anxiety neurosis, hence available, and changed into hypochondriacal anxiety.

I instruct his wife accordingly. The husband is to be allowed perfect freedom of intercourse with her twice or three times a week. The wife is to simulate pleasure in the proceedings, which will satisfy him and strengthen his self-confidence.

The attacks disappear completely. His irritability subsides, and his anxiety diminished from day to day. Moreover, the relative impotence which was chiefly due to nervous apprehension and distaste for the pessary, is overcome. The marriage is transformed from an unhappy, unsatisfying one filled with hatred and strife, into one of happiness, peace and mutual concord.

Epicrisis.—Two years later. After a quarrel with his wife the attacks recommence. Analysis reveals a desire for his wife's death, and a decided liking for a relative. In the course of the first attack the husband of this relative was present in the room. The man was harbouring the unconscious idea of murdering his wife and the husband of the relative. The psychic mechanism of the attack was obvious. He dreams of the crime and awakes terrified at the evil demons in his breast. (Cp. the Chapter " The Psychic Treatment of Epilepsy.")

Here we have an example of the acute anxiety attack which apparently overtakes patients while in a state of quiescence. An attack which can be traced to psychical sources.

No. 11.—Miss J. K., aged twenty-four, while at her work, suddenly feels

C*

a pressure on her chest. She has to sit down, as she is seized with giddiness, is afraid of falling, and gasps for breath. She is possessed by an indescribable dread. This must be death—a pulmonary stroke. She begins to pant spasmodically. Her forehead is bathed in a cold sweat. After a few minutes the oppression gives way to a fit of weeping.[1]

Ever since this attack she suffers from a chronic lack of breath. She is obliged to take deep breaths, gasping for air, often ten times consecutively until she can get the " right " breath. She grows thin. She cannot eat much because food " weighs " in her stomach. Her sleep, hitherto tranquil and deep, becomes restless. She goes to sleep with difficulty and is troubled with uneasy dreams. She sees corpses, is attacked by burglers, somebody thrusts a knife into her stomach, she is pursued by raging dogs, wild bulls, and neighing horses. She awakes with palpitations and covered with perspiration, out of these (typical !) anxiety dreams. By day, also, she is tormented by groundless fears, palpitations, and giddiness. At times a fever seems to run through her veins.

The organs are perfectly sound. *But her young employer, with whom she is secretly in love, married a few weeks ago.* Her first attack took place a quarter of an hour later, within a neighbouring room, after she had surprised the young couple in a passionate embrace. On leaving the business there was a conspicuously rapid disappearance of all the symptoms described.

Epicrisis.—I had an opportunity of seeing her again three years later. She is again in a serious state of conflict and suffers from the same attacks. She has entered into a liaison with her employer and the attacks occur generally when she sees her rival, his wife. She admits that in dreams she has stabbed or shot her employer's wife. The attacks are manifestly fear of her own criminal thoughts.

Here we have an anxiety attack simulating " nervous asthma." In Case No. 8, it was indigestion : in Case No. 9, bladder trouble, as the most conspicuous symptom.

Anxiety can assume the most curious disguises. Sometimes the anxiety attack merely takes the form of violent restlessness and a desire to run away (an important root of the fugue). Janet gives a typical case in his well-known book, " Les Obsessions et la Psychasthenie," II, Paris, 1903, *Felix Alcan, p.* 88 :—

No. 12.—" A woman of thirty-eight runs excitedly about the room twelve times a day and upsets the furniture. She grows red in the face, gasps, and has violent palpitations, crying : ' Oh, my head hurts so, my temples throb—oh, my throat, my chest, my heart, my stomach—I shall never get well, I am sure to die.' Nothing is of any use to calm her agitation. Gradually she becomes quieter till the game begins afresh. This is the course of the attack in an anxiety neurosis. Janet and Reymond refer to the deflection of fear through excitation of the muscles, and pain. This patient exhibits another symptom which is very curious, and not at all rare. She talks incessantly throughout the attack. (Agitation intellectuelle, *Janet*).

No. 13.—A similar case of personal observation. It is that of an extremely strong man of forty-three, who suffers from such excessive weakness, that he feels little more than a fly. He is especially incapable of getting up in the mornings (aboulia), and every word he utters is preceded by a struggle for breath. He gets up, and feels he is about to collapse. The illness began

[1] Very often to be observed in anxiety neurosis.

suddenly fifteen years ago with a peculiar anxiety attack. He awoke one night, fought for breath, had no sensation throughout his body, and jumped out of bed. He dressed scantily, and went to a café to get something to eat. He then ran about for several hours as one possessed. Since that time he complains of great weakness (Adynamia) sensations of debility, headaches and a feeling as if the floor would sink beneath him if he speaks to anybody.

He masturbated regularly between the ages of thirteen and eighteen, then suddenly abstained. He has only practised coitus three times in his life, at a brothel. He could only effectuate an erection by evoking the image of a very beautiful woman of high standing, with whom he was acquainted.

We will not examine the psychic roots of this complicated case. The sudden acute appearauce of the neurosis is interesting. In this case we succeeded in afterwards reviving a dream he had had that night. The subject of it was incest with his sister-in-law. He had good reason to flee the house. His sister-in-law slept in the next room and his brother was away on that critical night. Our patient had every reason to fear his desire-phantasies. A further confirmation of the phrase, that all anxiety is fear of oneself.

No. 14.—Another case of acute masked anxiety attack is illustrated by the next example. A man, aged thirty-four, is seated reading at his writing table. Suddenly a knot seemed to form in his brain, as if there were a species of gathering in process. This is followed by a sensation of everything revolving. The thought crosses his mind : if this does not stop, you are done for. He becomes pale and begins to vomit. There is a singing in his ears, and his body grows cold ; he breaks into a violent perspiration, and is obliged to retire hastily to the lavatory where a copious motion takes place. After three hours the attack passes off and he feels perfectly well again, except for a not unpleasant languor in the whole body.

In view of a possible Meniére, the ear was examined—but the conditions are normal. This attack was several times repeated in one year, each time without any feeling of anxiety. Gradually, however, anxiety became the dominant factor in the malady, until he fell ill of agarophobia. He is afraid of having a similar attack in the street. The attack proves to be associated with the paper he has been reading, a fact which I had not previously realised. He had been reading of an act of violation.

Similar attacks occur after any event fraught with emotion.

This acute outbreak of an anxiety neurosis following a traumatic scene is very common and has led to the formation of the concept of a peculiar neurosis, the " Fright-neurosis " or " Traumatic neurosis." Our analyses have taught us that there was a tendency to indisposition before the attack. The patient already suffered, when experiencing the trauma, from latent anxiety neurosis. One is continually hearing of patients whose anxiety neuroses are attributable to some experience undergone.

In this connection a patient of *Janet* (Case No. 12) relates that during the birth of a third child the nurse suddenly cried out : " I think the child has stopped breathing, the child is dead ! " There was nothing the matter with the child, but the mother suddenly felt in a whirl and became like a changed being. This sudden fright is easily to be understood, but how explain the fact that after the woman had recovered, and the doctor asked the nurse to have a specimen of urine taken, she was seized with such an access of terror that she became seriously ill ? He merely said that he wished to ascertain whether there were any traces of albumen : " Ce mot qui lui rappellait vaguement la maladie d'une voisine produisit le même effet néfaste que la phrase de la bonne : douleurs de tête, trouble général, angoisses." She could scarcely get home and was again taken ill.

In this case there are secret associations which only psychanalysis can trace. We shall revert to this extremely interesting theme when discussing the various phobias. In anxiety neurosis the attack often simulates some traumatic experience. A patient complains of some heavy body passing over both legs—she feels as if she were being run over. Her anxiety-neurosis resulted from a railway accident. The sensation of being run over has nevertheless a symbolic significance, as will presently be apparent. The *anxiety equivalents* also are often of a symbolic nature.

Let us take another instance of anxiety attack with impaired respiration, from the works of *Janet* and *Reymond* (l.c.) *p.* 113 :—

No. 15.—The patient in question, a lady of thirty, is very tired one day and goes to bed in great need of rest. After a while she begins to doze, and in ten or fifteen minutes is fast asleep. " A ce moment elle se reveille en sursaut avec un sentiment de peur et une sensation d'étouffement." She grasps the bed instinctively, and tries in vain to recover her composure ; the feeling of suffocation increases however, and her heart beats wildly ; she feels her limbs contracting and begins to weep desperately. She strikes about her with feet and fists, her body writhes and she utters delirious, disconnected words, calls for help and accuses first one person and then another. The crisis is of short duration, and lasts only fifteen minutes. She begins to breathe quietly again and feels a desire to sip water, which sometimes mingles with a little blood. Completely exhausted, she lies down again, is overcome with drowsiness, and sleeps still more heavily than before. Then the same game is repeated all over again, and this goes on until morning. Towards dawn she has another attack, more violent than any of the preceding ones, after which she recovers, gets up and is not troubled for the rest of the day.

Here follows a case from my own experience :—

No. 16.—A man of forty-nine suffers from screaming fits, during which he struggles with an intense dread of death. The screaming fits last several hours and resemble partly a violent singultus and partly a paroxism of howling. During the attack, the patients' eyes markedly protrude. His whole body is bathed in perspiration. His face is noticeably flushed, the pulse feverish and rising to 140 degrees. Between the inarticulate screaming fits the patient calls for a doctor, takes leave of his relatives, assures them that he is about to succumb of heart failure as no man could long survive such suffering. The doctors can find no remedy ; an injection of morphia brings temporary relief.

I was present during one of the attacks and was able to help him by *an energetic conscious suggestion*. (The attack will pass in a minute, he must look me straight in the eyes and count calmly up to 20). The attack was overcome as if by magic. I now sent the family, who were standing anxiously round the sick bed, out of the room, and said to the patient :

" What have you on your conscience ? "

He looked at me rather startled for a moment, and then burst into tears. I let him weep for a few minutes and then advised him to confess everything to me and lighten his heart.

" You are the first doctor to ask me about my troubles—but I cannot speak now—I will come to you to-morrow."

After a few days I learn the psycho-genesis of the attacks. He had occupied a position of trust for over twenty-five years with a firm of business. His employer was fond of him and treated him as a friend.

He had begun, however, to speculate from time to time on the Stock Exchange, with a view to improving his children's position, but not to acquire wealth and luxury for himself. (He had always been a hard worker). He lost, and began to help himself to the funds entrusted to him. He had now lost a considerable sum (30,000 Kronen) and had no prospect of winning it back. He did not wish to speculate further for fear of precipitating his ruin.

The attacks were now accounted for. The inarticulate cries expressed what he dared not utter openly. He was afraid of going to the prison, for the audit of accounts was due next week on which he would be obliged to work and which he would have to falsify in order to postpone for a time the discovery of his theft.

I advised him first of all to confess to his wife. This he did, and the good woman not only succeeded in consoling him, but went with him to interview his employer who dealt so generously with the matter that our patient was able to retain his position. He was, however, relieved of the responsibilities of cashier.

The attacks did not recur after this interview, and when the unpleasant affair was settled. He was troubled by slight depression for some months, which is quite understandable.

This example proves that anxiety attacks may also occur as the result of psychic conflict and with no sexual foundation. Also the fear of ostracism as a " social death " may produce a serious attack. Anxiety is always of psychic origin, but the anxiety manifests itself in countless diverse forms.

CHAPTER V

CLINICAL PICTURE OF ANXIETY NEUROSIS: ANXIETY NEUROSIS WITH CARDIAC PHENOMENA

BEFORE we can diagnose a case as "nervous heart," all somatic sources of heart trouble must first be excluded. We will therefore turn our attention to this aspect of the question first.

A great many diseases are accompanied by "feelings of anxiety." The first stages of angina pectoris may manifest themselves by scarcely perceptible pain accompanied by extreme anxiety. How easily we may happen to diagnose a case as nervous anxiety, when arterio-sclerosis is already in process of formation. But curiously enough the contrary occurs much more frequently. Innumerable cases of heart trouble, which are regarded as "organic," are merely nervous, and are the result of psychic projections whereby the indefinite feelings of anxiety are transferred to some particular object, in these cases on to the heart.

For this reason the diagnosis, "nervous heart," calls for very great perspicacity on the part of the doctor. The symptoms of angina pectoris are well known—pain in the cardiac region extending especially to the left arm, fear of death, sense of oppression, palor, sweating, fainting, vaso-motor disturbances, and convulsions. *Leube*, however, points out that neurotic (psychogenic) forms of angina pectoris occur. (Spezielle Diagnose der inneren Krankheiten. Leipzig, 1902.)

An excellent description of differential diagnostic difficulties is afforded us in *Ortner's* "Klinischer Symptomalogie innerer Krankheiten." Vol. I, II part, Körperschmerzen (Pains in the Heart and Cardiac Region.) His investigations in this field of study provide abundant evidence of the difficulties of diagnosis which can often only be made from general impressions. I would draw special attention to the following extract from *Ortner*: "Angina pectoris nervosa seu hysterica" may be distinguished from coronary angina (in common with which it may also have considerable radiations in either one or both arms, and a feeling of oppression behind the sternum and in the throat) by the particular behaviour of the patient during the attack ; in coronary angina, the patient remains absolutely quiet ; in the nervous form he cries and groans, is extremely restless and evinces a marked tendency to move about." These symptoms, however, are not infallibly to be regarded as psychogenic. Romberg has observed cases of fatal angina in which grimacing and even arc de cercle were observable. Even combinations of organic and psychic maladies are frequently to be met with. A psychical super-structure over an organic disease is also quite common. A thorough analysis is often the only means of arriving at a clear conception of the case. Later on I will introduce a few of these cases in which heart troubles were taken for "angina pectoris," and which were nevertheless of simple neurotic origin without any somatic complications, since they were completely cured by psychic treatment and the sexually injurious conditions were removed.

But not only the sclerosis of the coronary arteries, but also the various diseases of the heart muscle and valves, aneurisms, especially fatty degeneration of the heart, myocarditis, pericarditis, and stenosis may cause anxiety of a very severe nature. But we may form some conception of the particular form of nervous heart by the mere description of the attack. That a careful examination is a condition *sine qua non* need scarcely be emphasized.

The "nervous heart" is the most common form of anxiety feelings. This is easily understandable. In ordinary fear the heart beats faster. The patients experience either a violent commotion in the heart which manifests itself in palpitation, or they complain of their heart "standing still." (I had a patient suffering from Adam Stokes' disease. The symptoms were either of an apoplectic character with loss of consciousness, the pulse decreasing to twenty beats, or there were violent attacks of anxiety in which the heart was said to "stand still"). The changing of the rythmical beats of the heart from rythmical to arythmical is also a common source of complaint. The heart is said to "flutter." Others say : "I feel a vibration as if I had no heart, a sense of void, as if there were a stone in its place ; there is a weight inside me, as if my heart were some foreign substance." Another lady says : "A vague feeling as if everything were too tight, as if my heart were trying to escape from my body. I feel a sense of oppression, of pulling, as if it was made of indiarubber." Some complain that the heart is not in order. It beats very fast, then intermits, and then begins to go slowly again. Something must be wrong.

The most frequent form of "nervous heart" is certainly palpitation and accelerated pulse which often reaches a remarkable degree. I have sometimes observed 180 pulse beats in cases of a purely neurotic nature. Neurotics are especially adapted to standing such an exceptional increase in the pulse rate.

Diagnosing an organic disease of the heart does not exclude the diagnosis "nervous heart" or "nervous stenocardia."

We must not lose sight of the fact that patients suffering from heart disease may also have neurotic tendencies. The positive diagnosis of mitral stenosis or an aorta insufficiency or of an arteriosclerosis is no proof that the attacks are attributable only to organic sources, as the following observations demonstrate :

No. 17 —I have been treating Mrs. H. F. for ten years for mitral stenosis. The vitium is not completely compensated. There are occasional slight œdemas around the ankles. Strophantus, cooling appliances to the heart, partial water applications, slight percussion treatment to the back, always bring about a temporary improvement. She decides on the advice of a friend to go to Elster to try a course of carbonic acid baths, now so popular. She is at first much better there. After the fifteenth bath, however, she awakes in the night in a violent state of agitation. Her heart beats to breaking point. The doctor is called. He orders digitalis in view of the low pulse. She remains in bed a few days and feels very ill. The carbonic acid baths are pronounced to be too stimulating and are discontinued. The patient returns home. Arrived there she complains of feeling infinitely worse. It is " all over with her." She must take digitalis and that's the last thing. She has no doubt about it ; she shows me her œdemas. She has an accurate knowledge of medical phraseology and knows her " Bilz " almost by heart.

It would take too long to give the analysis of this case in detail. I will merely mention that the first attack followed a dream in which she was attacked and violated by three men. On the day preceding the dream she was present at the Concert in the Kurkapelle, and saw three handsome men there. She has been a widow for two years and professes to have been always " anæsthetic." She cannot understand how such a " chilly " person as she should have had such a dream. Obviously because the day before, a young girl of her acquaintance had been attacked on the promenade and only escaped the violation of her honour by calling loudly for help. This occurrence had alarmed her very much. She was afraid to venture on the lonely roads unaccompanied for she was convinced that such an adventure would be the death of her. Her poor diseased heart would never survive it. The horror of this episode and the fear of experiencing a similar one had occasioned the " disgusting " dream.

Thus in this first example anxiety and repulsion appear as repressed sexual feelings. For it is obvious that it was the patient's desire to be violated. Rape plays an important part in hysterical phantasies. In Russia especially, where traumatic hysteria is artificially bred amongst the Jews, there are to-day large numbers of hysterical girls whose anxiety dreams are full of acts of violation. This dream is typical among sexually unsatisfied women. Sometimes burglars, robbers, strange black men climb in through the open window. We shall meet with this type of dream when dealing with anxiety-hysteria, in which it plays a great part.

We were inclined to diagnose the preceding case as one of anxiety neurosis resulting from prolonged abstinence. It is true that the patient professed to have a very cold temperament and to be thankful " to have done with the whole thing." She had only consented to cohabitation with her husband because he pleaded so fervently.

This shows how far we may rely on woman's reliability in sexual matters. Whoever is satisfied with this information might easily maintain that sexuality and neurosis are in no wise connected ; or it might equally be argued that in this case exciting phantasies were the result of heart disease.

Now, the art of the psycho-therapist consists in ignoring the patient's denials and conscientiously steering for his goal. In the present case my task was made easy for me. The patient was ignorant of the fact that a year before his death her husband had come to me in his heart's anguish to ask my advice on a very difficult matter. He complained that his wife was continually heaping unjust reproaches on him, engendered by her morbid jealousy. Not a day passed without her making a scene if he came home only a few minutes' late. The most painful part of the situation, however, was the fact that his wife was a hard " task-master " in the matter of cohabitation. She was quite immoderate in her demands. She wanted daily intercourse which he was unable to fulfil on account of his nerves. He wanted me to forbid all intercourse with his wife for a time. That very day she had reproached him with expending his strength on other women. " Two can play at that game," she had cried : " I also will go and pick up somebody from the streets." She had thereupon run hatless out of the house.

I of course prudently refrained from mentioning these facts to the lady, and endeavoured to enlighten her as to the meaning of her dream with the object of winning her confidence. She eventually admitted hesitatingly that she suffered a good deal from sexual excitement and that the attacks occurred regularly after a sexual dream (Orgasm !). We were therefore justified in assuming that the attacks had nothing to do with the heart. I allowed the patient to take two grs. Brom. for a few evenings before retiring, and reassured her as to the condition of her heart, prohibited the use of digitalis and strophanthus and prescribed six drops of validol daily. In addition to this I prescribed luke warm hip baths to counteract the twitching in the vagina. The attacks ceased after the first dose of Bromide and the first hip bath (24°C.). Erotic dreams still occurred of course. But having been enlightened as to the nature of her excitement the patient soon composed herself and went to sleep again. *It was a case of anxiety neurosis resulting from sexual abstinence.*

We see how difficult it may be to differentiate in our diagnoses between neurotic anxiety and somatic fear of death.

No. 18.—Muthmann (l.c.) reports on a similar case. It deals with a young woman who had been bedridden with heart trouble. Acute symptoms of groundless anxiety ensued causing the patient great suffering. This condition might well have been ascribed to organic disease.

Muthmann hypnotised the patient 'according to the fractional method of *Brodmann*. Scarcely had she reached the deeper stage of hypnotic trance when she awoke and complained of great apprehension. (Symptomatic of violent unconscious resistance against the betrayal of a secret.) The psychologist explained to her, however, that she must submit to being hypnotised for it was only through this means that the cause of her anxiety could be discovered. On falling asleep again, the patient began to weep bitterly and awoke and told something horrible that she now remembered. She had had to be examined when eighteen years of age by a doctor who was repulsive to her and was notorious owing to his dissolute life. He had also examined her gynæcologically in order to ascertain whether the menstrual blood could flow freely. During the examination she had experienced a curious sensation, hitherto unknown to her, in her sexual parts, she felt very frightened and ashamed ; at first she carefully kept the occurrence secret and soon forgot it (repression !). The anxiety she now felt during her illness exactly corresponded to that experienced during the examination referred to.

It is, then, a case of anxiety-neurosis, which appeared on the first apparent encounter with sexuality. Obviously a sexually hyperæsthetic lady, dominated by resolutely repressed sexual complexes. The anxiety with the doctor shows that she feared a repetition of the traumatic scene during hypnosis.

We shall have abundant opportunity of demonstrating how often neurotic symptoms of anxiety are regarded as the outcome of some organic trouble.

The following case related by *Strohmayer* (Beziehungen der Sexualität zu den Angstzuständen) is very characteristic :

No. 19.—Max V., a man of property, aged thirty-seven, masturbated frequently from the age of ten, seduced by friends. He suffered from bad palpitation of the heart at school, especially in the presence of strangers, *e.g.*, with the doctor. He continued to masturbate until about his eighteenth year. In the army he made his first attempts at sexual intercourse. " He was not very successful," because the palpitations were always too insistent. As he grew older libido and potency diminished. The attempts at coitus all ended in ejaculatio præcox. Two years ago he had the first attack of anxiety without apparent reason in the train : violent palpitations and the thought that he was going mad. Since then the patient has been permanently ill. He always complained of palpitations, heart weakness, asthma and anxiety. One diagnosis was " juvenile heart sclerosis of the coronary arteries " (!), another chronic nicotine poisoning. His condition became worse from month to month ; gradually the patient did not venture any more out of the house, even in a room he feared a heart attack. At the beginning of the treatment the patient was a typical example of anxiety-neurosis. He had an oppression at the back of his head ; he often lost the thread of conversation ; suffered from pressure on the chest and asthma, feelings of anxiety and perspiration. He feared to go out driving, to walk alone in the street, to sit in a restaurant or theatre. Even in his own room he was beset with uneasy premonitions: he had a feeling that something "fearful " was behind him and he would turn to look for it ; he was afraid of suddenly crying out or of entirely losing his reason. He worried a great deal over his condition, was irritable, depressed and over sensitive. At night he had vivid dreams and periods of increased emissions, during which he was more terrified than ever. Shortly before going to sleep and mostly before dinner when he lay down on the sofa " moving pictures," *i.e.*, a procession of insignificant figures, men, women, children, etc., passed through his mind and produced anxiety. There was no libido.

This observation by Strohmayer is very characteristic. We see how anxiety neurosis can be taken for "juvenile arteriosclerosis." What mischief has already been done through similar hasty diagnoses ! I know of severe, nearly incurable, anxiety conditions, chronic depression, attacks of despair with serious attempts at suicide, resulting from such superficial diagnoses.

It is in itself sheer cruelty to tell a patient he has heart disease. In most cases the fact can be evaded. But there seem to be many "unconscious" sadists amongst doctors ; otherwise I cannot explain the fact that patients come to me, saying that Doctor X or Prof. Y have told them they must take care of themselves as they have an injured heart. Or else they have "incipient calcination," which patients rightly look upon as a death sentence. And in most of these cases it is a matter of simple anxiety neurosis ! In many cases it is merely ignorance. It is especially easy for an inexperienced doctor, who is unacquainted with anxiety neurosis, when called to a case of anxiety attack with tachycardia to be misled by the tremendously accelerated pulse, a deathly palor, and trembling of the patient, to diagnose "Vitium," and come to the rescue with injections of ether and camphor ; whereas a few comforting words, some bromide and perhaps morphia or pantopon, would work wonders.

An attack of palpitations may sometimes be overcome by artificial respiration. Such patients evince the phenomenon of "Pulsus paradoxus." The pulse stops with a deep breath. That again is taken for arhythmia and extrasystole. The patients can bear a pulse rate of 200 beats without harm and manifest no change in the position of the heart. The work of Rudolf Beck, who X-rayed the heart during an attack, is proof of this. (Analyse eines Falles von paroxysmaler tachycardie. Med. Klinik, 1911.)

I repeat : innumerable people who go about having been diagnosed as suffering from " Organic Heart Disease," are victims of anxiety neurosis and clumsy diagnosis.

This is most frequently the case with sclerosis of the coronary arteries. I am convinced that a large percentage of patients suffering from "Angina Pectoris" are neurotics, and that their heart complaints could be traced to psychic causes. This is quite natural, since laymen seek the centre of life in the heart. The heart beats through joy and pain, it aches in affliction, it leaps for joy, it breaks in sorrow. Therefore psychic pain is so easily projected to the heart. Of the *young* people who complain of "pains in the heart," most of them, in fact, one may boldly say all of them, are anxiety neurotics, who are nurturing some great sorrow, some depressing obligation, some unhappy love affair, and with whom sexual disabilities are at the root of their trouble.

No. 20.—Miss E. Z. is introduced to me by her mother in their home. She suffers from constipation and violent pains in the heart. Both symptoms appeared only three months ago. Since then the girl, formerly so blooming and healthy, is becoming more and more run down. The pains in her heart are often so severe and torment her so much, that the poor girl cannot help crying convulsively. She is very irritable and ill-humoured and suffers much from anxiety dreams. Also by day, a sudden shock often causes her to wince palpably.

On careful examination the organs are found to be perfectly sound. The first glance convinces me that the trouble is of psychic origin. The girl gives a miserable, dejected impression. I comfort the agitated mother, promise an early improvement in the condition of her daughter, and make an appointment with the latter for the next day. Pretext : to give her galvanic treatment for the heart. I do this in the hope that she will come alone, and that is what happens. I go at once in *medias res.*

" I have examined you very thoroughly and find that your heart is perfectly normal. I assume that you have had some great sorrow of which your relatives know nothing, and perhaps you prefer them to know nothing. Will you confide openly in me so that I can help you ? "

My frankness immediately meets with a willing response. She tells me that for two years she has had a love affair with a young man, *without her mother's knowledge.* She firmly hoped he would marry her. Their relations had always remained within the bounds of propriety ; they only met in the streets. Once only—shortly before her illness—they had made an excursion together, when he had asked her to give herself to him completely ; she refused, saying that a respectable girl could only be won by marriage. He also tried to gain his ends forcibly, but she prevented this by screaming. The next day her lover failed to appear at the usual rendezvous, and she received a long letter from him, stating that in view of his poor material circumstances, he had been forced to marry a rich girl. He would never forget her, etc.

These experiences were followed by the acute pains in the heart, constipation, and the nightly attacks of anxiety. The attempted violation alone would be capable of producing anxiety neurosis.[1] We are dealing here also with a case of violent affect, which could not find the usual reactive outlet in weeping, resentment, outcries and raging. Breur and Freud[2] call this a " constricted affect," " eingeklemmten Affekt," which should be given the opportunity to discharge by means of speech. Herein lay the first task of the original psycho-therapy (cathartic method), which worked from the idea that the constricted affect acted as psychic trauma and recognised the cure in the dissolving of the affect. (The significance of this psychic trauma was greatly over-rated when these things first became known, as also the importance of the " constricted affect." We now speak simply of psychic " repressions," of psychic conflicts and call the method after Freud the " analytical method.") The girl had nobody to whom she could speak of the saddest experience of her life. She had also come to know the whole crude brutality of sex at this time. She had a so-called " ideal " nature, *i.e.,* one that suppresses its natural instincts and which transforms sensuous into super-sensuous strength. She suddenly became conscious of the sex life in all its crudeness. Her mother knew as little of the affair as her sisters, with whom she was not on the best of terms. She possessed no friend, and did not want to confide in " so-called " friends. There was nothing else for her to do but to face the facts alone. At first the sensations of anxiety troubled her, followed by constipation. *It is almost incredible how often psychic conditions are the cause of the most obstinate cases of constipation ! Serious cares, heavy sorrow, especially money troubles,* the tormenting knowledge that something is not right, general mental depression manifest, themselves in stubborn constipation,

[1] Cp. the Chapter " Das sexuelle Trauma der Erwachsenen," Vol. III.
[2] Studien über Hysterie. (Wien, 1895).

because in any case these feelings produce a certain lowering of the vitality and metabolism. The dream analyses show us how closely associated are *money* and fæces, as well as innumerable tales and myths—as *e.g.*, the fairy tale of the little man who could produce ducats per anum.

In this case frank confession had a wonderful effect. The stubborn constipation yielded at once, the cardiac pains diminished. I had a few more interviews with the girl, in which I confined myself to consoling her and to convincing her that a pretty girl of nineteen had no reason to despair. An unsuccessful love affair was better than an unhappy marriage. In short—she was able to discuss the painful subject quite freely. After a week, her heart troubles, weeping fits (and constipation) had disappeared. The only symptoms that still worried her were anxiety dreams and wincing. These, too, gradually began to leave her.

It would therefore be wise always to seek psychic reasons for cardiac pains. Even if there is a developed arterio-sclerosis one should at least consider the possibility of a complicating anxiety neurosis before giving the distressing diagnosis, " Angina Pectoris." The Case, I. D., already published by me elsewhere, drastically proves this.

No. 22.—Mr. I. D., fifty-one years old, by profession a musician, born of healthy parentage, a man of herculean proportions, who until now has never known a day's illness, wakes up one night with the feeling as if he was being strangled. He fights laboriously for breath, groans, and is assailed by the horrible thought that his last hour has come. The attack soon passes off and he attributes it to an over-sumptuous repast of the night before. The alarming episode is however repeated a few nights later, and thenceforward with increasing frequency, occurring by day as well. Mr. D. is a philosopher, and not easily alarmed, but thinks it prudent to ascertain the nature of his condition. He therefore pays a visit to a Professor, with whom he is on friendly terms, with a view to asking his advice.

" I have important matters to attend to," he says to his friend, " before I die. Tell me frankly and without reserve—for you know me—how long I have to live. As you know well, death has no terrors for me. You need not hesitate, therefore, to tell me the name and nature of my complaint.

The Professor examines the patient and diagnoses incipient arterio-sclerosis. He informs him that with care he may live two years still. The consequences of this information are terrible. The patient enters a sanatorium on the advice of his friend, from which he actually runs away and goes on a sea voyage. While on board ship he realises that he feels remarkably fit and is troubled by no feelings of anxiety whatever. But on land he feels very bad indeed. The anxiety attacks are now coupled with the presentment of his approaching death. He becomes more and more dejected until he eventually comes to me for treatment.

It now transpires that these remarkable attacks, despite the existing symptoms of arterio-sclerosis are not indicative of angina pectoris, but are a purely neurotic symptom. The man is under the dominion of a severe psychic conflict. He had lost the woman he loved (and with whom he has had a liaison for five years, although the union was perforce without issue)—through the betrayal of his best friend, to whom he had confidingly introduced her. For weeks he has been wrestling with the thought : " You must rob this scoundrel of his prey and strangle him." And one day, as surrogate for these repressed ideas, the above mentioned symptoms make their appearance. This is a process which we term " conversion." This originated with Freud, to whom we are indebted for the discovery of this interesting phenomenon. Hysterics are capable of banishing from consciousness a thought which is painful to them and of relegating it to the unconscious. The painful idea can be converted into a physical symptom, (as in the case of the musician), which we then call conversion; or it may take another form less painful to the conscious mind, whereupon some phobia results. We are dealing, in the present instance, with an admixture of conversion and phobia. I will merely mention that the attacks entirely ceased after a successful psychanalysis and the patient is now, many years since the gloomy prognostication of his friend, enjoying perfect health, and taking pleasure in his work.

But the case proves very clearly how difficult it is to differentiate between neurotic and organic diseases, and that it is equally important for the physician to consider one cause as the other.

Epicrisis.—I had an opportunity of seeing the man after ten years. He is perfectly well, happily married and at the height of his creative powers.

Ortner (1. c. *p.* 11) is of opinion that a paroxysmal tachycardia may in this way lead to overstrain of the heart muscle and cause excessive pain. The cardiacal pain is of a very violent, burning, oppressive, overwhelming nature, and is distinguished by its peculiar intensity.

It is not impossible for the symptoms of anxiety neurosis to be combined with those of arterio-sclerosis. Such cases have come under my notice. It is advisable in any case, when dealing with serious cases, to bear the psychic components in mind, and to seek for sexually injurious complications. The regulation of sexual intercourse often works wonders. But on the other hand, the experienced practitioner will guard against *undervaluing* the importance of organic disorders. This question is often of the greatest importance in dealing with any form of anxiety neurosis of the senium in which the arterio-sclerosis is practically of physiological character.

The patients ask the doctor frankly whether sexual intercourse is injurious to them or not. They are afraid that it may be conducive to a stroke ; others go in terror of an attack of angina pectoris, or of a fainting fit attacking them when with a puella publica, and of the resultant scandal. This question always requires very careful consideration. On the whole I regard the anxiety neurosis as the worse of the two evils. I have often witnessed the complete suspension of the anginary symptoms in elderly persons after coitus and have never observed any injurious effect on the arterio-sclerosis. In such cases it requires great tact and still greater foresight taking the individuality into consideration, before we can arrive at a solution.

The following circumstances must be borne in mind : Sexual intercourse in marriage, and especially in marriages of long standing, seldom produces a high level of excitement and an increase of blood pressure. Nor is the stimulation immoderate. (All cases of ruptured uterus after violent congressus which we meet with in literature occurred in illegal unions.) Elderly persons are advised to form a permanent attachment, if they are not married, and if circumstances permit.

The attacks of palpitation and " paroxysmal tachycardia " which in most cases are merely equivalents of a severe anxiety attack, deserve a brief consideration. Patients suffering therefrom are intensely nervous. In fact it has been discussed whether anxiety or tachycardia is the primary trouble. According to my experience anxiety is always primary. But it is often so disguised that it almost retires into the background. Here and there we meet with a case of tachycardia unaccompanied by anxiety. We then regard the tachycardia as a completely adequate anxiety equivalent. The most frequent case of tachycardia is a " psychic caffein," *i.e.*, some violent affect.

During the war I had opportunities of observing and diagnosing innumerable cases of functional tachycardia. I have at the same time learned the sources from which they arise.

Many private patients confess to me that they can psychically produce before an examination such an excitement that their pulse increases from 70 to 140 beats.

Observations made during sleep have convinced me that the psychic factor is the only decisive one. Patients whose pulse when awake was 120 beats, showed a perfectly normal pulse rate during sleep. In hypnotism it was also possible to produce by suggestions of excitement an increase in the pulse rate, and to reduce a very agitated heart to normal activity again.

No. 22.—A masseuse of about thirty-five, was suddenly attacked by tachycardia. She experienced no anxiety but became pale, and her skin cold to the touch ; slight outbreak of perspiration. She did not drink, smoke, or indulge in excessive tea or coffee drinking. On the other hand she had had a love affair for three years, resulting in frustrated excitement through fear of consequences. Rapid and spontaneous cure on relinquishing the liaison. The liaison was contrary to her morality. She had a chaste, pious temperament, and preferred abstinence to the qualms of conscience.

We shall deal with further cases of " nervous " heart troubles when considering the phobias.

These few examples will suffice to illustrate how important is the intimate knowledge of anxiety neuroses for the practitioner. It is a safeguard against the danger of serious misconceptions and mistakes in the diagnosis of heart affections.

I will conclude with an observation of my own with regard to cardiac pains which is very instructive and contains, in some respects, particular points of interest.

No. 25.—Mr. I. Ch., a city clerk, complained of a peculiar stabbing pain in the region of the heart, which was so unbearable that he could not sleep. Sometimes he felt *as if a weight were pressing on him*. The pain alternated with feelings of anxiety, especially fear of a stroke. He had an indefinite *anxiety of being responsible for some crime*, and yet he had committed none ! He felt very low and depressed, was unfit for work, and suffered from chronic constipation. He also complained of a peculiar twitching and jumping in the muscles, especially in the thigh and forearm. He occasionally experienced a passing vertigo, a sense of upheaval—but he used to pull himself together and the symptom passed over. He had bad dreams, of *falling down a bottomless abyss*, or of his body being lacerated, or of *sitting for a difficult examination* for which he was not prepared. He localised the cardiac pain in the apex of the heart (about 2 cm.). He had been married eighteen years. One child was sixteen, the other eight. Except during periods of pregnancy he practised coitus interruptus with his wife. This patient was ordered a course of carbonic acid baths by his doctor. *Difficile est non satiram scribere.* If we consult a doctor nowadays in a case of heart trouble, no matter of what form, we may be certain of leaving the surgery with the prescription : " Carbonic acid baths." In this instance, the first bath resulted in a decided aggravation of the symptoms. This is a fact frequently to be observed in cases of anxiety neurosis. *Carbonic acid baths do not agree with patients of this type.* They tend to increase the libido by stimulating the skin, and to increase the palpitation of the heart. Some patients are altogether unable to remain in the bath.

Our patient was suffering from a typical anxiety neurosis. But whoever is satisfied with this diagnosis has overlooked the most important factor in this case. There are a variety of symptoms indicative of psychic conflict. I asked him whether he was happy in his marriage.—" Yes, I am happy now that we are alone." " Were you not formerly alone ? " " No, we lived with my wife's parents and there were always disputes."

It would take too long to give the whole conversation. I will merely mention the result. He had been hoping and longing the whole time for the old people to die ; then there would be peace in the house. There was also the question of a small inheritance. After the death of his parents-in-law, he began to reproach himself with not having done all that lay in his power to save them. He was a very pious man. This remorse was the moral, religious reaction against his death-wishes.

The pains and perplexities of the patient are now explained. There was something weighing on his conscience. What is this else but a realisation of guilt ? He was responsible for a crime. He was accountable to God for his criminal death-wishes. His dreams reveal the religious and criminal complex to the initiated. The fall is the fall of sin, the descent into hell. The examination is the trial on the judgment day before the Seat of God. (We will here overlook other determinants.)

This case clearly proves the genesis of the diseased heart and cardiac pains, for the man was involved in an unhappy love affair into the bargain, and was possessed with the same death wishes against his wife as against her parents. His greatest sin was the thought : " *If only my wife were to die now* (and two of my wishes have already been fulfilled !) *then I should be a free man and could marry the other woman.*

In this case it was his guilty conscience that was at the root of his heart neurosis. Neither abstinence nor the preceding coitus interruptus were the cause of the neurosis, but the dire conflict which the man was going through with his conscience. The experiences of the Great War have taught us that sexual etiology of heart neurosis cannot be universally applied. The danger of every science is its one-sidedness. We must be prepared to acknowledge previous errors, and to learn anew. I have dealt fully with the tremendous influence of unhappy love in cases of heart neurosis in my paper " Das nervöse Herz " (The Nervous Heart), published by *Paul Knepler*, Vienna. I wish to emphasize here the fact that other conflicts also may be conducive to heart neurosis. I have met many an " old soldier " whose " heart neurosis " has been self-engendered, and who now goes in terror of the " real thing."

No. 26.—Mr. I. F., a man of herculean proportions, had made the most of his vagotony in order to secure a certificate for heart disease, and obtain a position at the base. Some of the doctors even thought they could detect a murmur, so that the diagnosis alternated between " heart neurosis " and " vitium." That of " heart neurosis " was eventually confirmed at the Depôt for heart diseases. Before joining the army the man had never given his heart a thought. He had contrived, at the instigation of a comrade, to produce symptoms of heart trouble by excessive smoking and drinking coffee. After his breakdown he began to suffer in reality from his heart, from palpitations and pain in the cardiac zone. He was now a prey to doubts, thinking to himself that, after all, so many clever doctors could not have been mistaken and that there must be something really wrong with his heart. The pain soon increased ; there were heart attacks and premonitions of death ; doctors were sent for hurriedly and diagnosed serious heart-weakness ; he was " pulled through " with caffein and ether injections, underwent the usual treatment, until at last he came to me. I came to the conclusion, on witnessing an attack, that it was a case of Air-Hunger, that he was an " air swallower " (aerophagist) and that the attacks were engendered by the unconscious inhalation of deep breaths of air. He evinced an exceptionally high degree of pneumotosis. The abdomen in the region of the stomach was considerably distended, the heart was undersized and pushed up, the diaphragm high, the respiratory movements were convulsive, and interrupted by deep inspirations and gasps ; the pulse, feeble, scarcely perceptible and irregular, the heart beats hollow and almost inaudible, the frequency 128, face pale, pre-inspiratory distention of the nostrils, slight cyanosis, pupils enlarged, cold sweat on the brow. After psychic tranquilisation the attack rapidly passed off. The patient had a few respiratory spasms, and then seemed relieved.

I enlightened him as to the nature of the air swallowing and advised him to keep a watch over himself ; his hypochondriacal phantasies were explained as auto-suggestion, and work and distraction prescribed. The cure was remarkably rapid.

In this instance there were no sexual complications, but an obvious tendency to self-observation and hypochondria. The patient's self-love increased the death anxiety, which may be the forerunner of innumerable neuroses, as we have witnessed by the thousand during the war.

In heart attacks we must note that by aerophagy the psychic condition leads to actual and serious organic sensations. The significance of pneumatosis is not sufficiently realised by the medical profession. Its connection with heart neurosis has also been insufficiently recognised by science.

The following case provides an interesting clinical illustration :

No. 27.—Mr. Z. I., a twenty-four year old engineer suffered from shortness of breath and pains in the heart. He had a three years' military service behind him, in which a heart neurosis enabled him to avoid the more arduous obligations of warfare. One day he had a sudden attack of anxiety in the street, and a violent stabbing pain in his side reminded him of his heart ; he began to inhale deeply, he was obliged to slacken his pace and sit down on a bench ; he thought it must be all over with him. Strong coffee, or a dose of brandy succeeded in pulling him round.

His former doctor diagnosed neurasthenia, which diagnosis was confirmed by a specialist who was called into consultation. He was ordered bromide, a hydropathic " cure," from which he obtained no relief whatever. As the attacks increased, he was recommended to come to me by his brother-in-law, who is a doctor and suspected psychic complications in the malady.

Analysis elicited the following facts :—His was an exceptionally happy family in which ancient, patriarchal customs were still observed. The children were all accustomed to obey the dictates of the father, who insisted on his sons being at home at nine o'clock every evening, and who continually preached the doctrine of a virtuous and industrious mode of life, of which he was himself a shining example. Our patient was so attached to his family that he made himself quite ill with home-sickness when separated from them for a few months during the war.

His sexual life was in no way abnormal. He had masturbated very little, and had had regular sexual intercourse since his sixteenth year. Since he was twenty he had always kept a mistress, since prostitutes were repugnant to him. His latest love affair had already lasted a year. These liaisons were discovered by the father; but although the latter soon put a stop to the previous affairs, in this instance he contented himself with warning the boy against excess, and getting too deeply involved.

He is thoroughly aware that the girl may only be regarded as an episode in his life. He has tried to break with her. His reason tells him that it would be better to give her up. It is true, she is strikingly beautiful and very charming, but she comes of a frivolous family, is fond of finery, lazy, will not settle down to learn anything, and only lives for pleasure. Moreover, she has a frivolous sister, half actress, half cocotte, who is bent on inducing her sister to join her mode of life. He is continually having rows with the girl, but cannot summon the courage to break with her. Analysis reveals the fact that he is madly jealous, but will not admit it. In dreams he discovers her in an act of infidelity, shoots her and his rival, and quarrels violently with her family. Such dreams are followed by attacks, as are also the scenes with his sweetheart, which, aggravated by his habit of air swallowing, attain serious dimensions. He is an exceptionally great aerophagist.

The air swallowing takes the form partly of sighing and partly of swallowing motions, by which the air is drawn in through the nostrils and wind pipes.

Enlightenment and instruction as to the nature of his condition result in a speedy diminution of the attacks. The psychic conflict, however, demands a solution which it does not seem possible to arrive at for the present. He loves the girl—is jealous, forbids her to leave the house, and cannot contemplate life without her. Yet he knows that he cannot marry her—knows her too well to consider marriage. He also dreads the conflict with the family, and his reason bids him make an end of the affair. The quarrels certainly form a pretext for separation, but they are ineffectual, in as much as they always end in reconciliation, and the resumption of intimate relations, for they are physically well mated. The orgasm he experiences with her is exceptionally intense, such as he has hitherto not known. He cannot forego this pleasure.

He is advised to undertake a long journey, which is of great financial importance to him, but which he has always postponed on account of the girl. The heart attacks vanish, and the conflict stands revealed to his inmost soul. During the attacks he had plunged a knife into her heart. Thence the severe stabbing pains which he had felt in his own heart.

We see illustrated in this case the characteristics presented by all types of neurasthenia when examined in the light of psychology. Freud attributes neurasthenia to the effects of onanism and regards it as an actual neurosis. But I have sought neurasthenia for twenty years and I have never found it. I can find again and again nothing but anxiety neurosis in which the anxiety is partly apparent and partly disguised. In the foregoing case we have a man whose sexual instincts are fully gratified. But it is this very gratification which brings him into conflict with the family and himself. Sexual gratification is at the root of the neurosis, but he is no longer able to exist without the intense pleasure which it affords him, in fact he finds life not worth living without it.

Doctors would be well advised to take the trouble to investigate the psychic life of their neurasthenic patients, and not confine themselves solely to the physical phenomena of their reflexes, to vagotony, sympatheticatonia, dermagraphism, eye blinking.

A neurotic cannot be dealt with in a quarter of an hour. We must talk with him, ascertain the circumstances of his life, learn to know his hopes and disappointments, before we can judge of his condition. Investigation invariably reveals a psychic conflict.

Every " neurasthenia " presents the same picture :—Severe psychic conflict and the well known phenomenon of the anxiety neurosis. In other words :—There is no such thing as neurasthenia or psychasthenia. There are only diseases of the soul which in predisposed individuals (by heredity, milieu, education, disturbances of the inner secretions, etc.) cause various somatic disorders.

These psychic diseases we will henceforth designate as " Parapathias."

CHAPTER VI

CLINICAL PICTURE OF ANXIETY NEUROSIS: ANXIOUS FEELING REFERRED TO THE CHEST AND OTHER DISORDERS OF THE RESPIRATORY SYSTEM.

BESIDES cardiac diseases we must consider disorders of the respiratory organs (lungs) as causes of anxiety phenomena. Cases of impaired nasal breathing (polypi, deviations of the septum, hypertrophied nasal turbinates, adenoids, acute and chronic colds) are often characterised by a feeling of oppression and anxiety, especially at night. There is, moreover, a variety of organic diseases of the lungs invariably accompanied by intense anxiety. Usually it is air hunger manifesting itself in fear of suffocation. It is therefore not surprising that patients suffering from severe exudations of the pleura should complain of feelings of oppression, air hunger and breast anxiety. Strange to say, we may frequently meet with cases of lung disease accompanied by objective symptoms of a serious dyspnœa, without the patients complaining of shortness of breath. We find cases of pneumonia in which the number of respirations amount to 40-50 per minute. The patients are extremely cyanotic, they have rattling in the throat, the pulse is feeble, scarcely perceptible, and yet the air hunger produces in them no feeling of anxiety.

The most characteristic symptom of nervous breast anxiety is this very disparity between the objective conditions and the subjective disorders. In no disease is this disparity so clearly apparent as in the so-called nervous form of asthma. I say, " so-called nervous form of asthma " because it is very questionable whether other forms really exist. We differentiate at present between cardial asthma and bronchial asthma, calling such asthma cardial which we considered traceable to mutations of the heart, and bronchial asthma that which we had observed in countless objective maladies of the lungs (emphysema, various murmurs, etc.). But it has occurred to more recent investigators that both these forms are frequently to be met with in the same case, that on the one hand the quality of the pulse in bronchial asthma grew markedly worse, and on the other, the cardial asthma was combined with pulmonary symptoms. It was believed for a time that the presence of Charcot's crystals and Curschmann's spirals was sufficient foundation for diagnosis. But as *Leyden* points out both symptoms are not necessarily characteristic of asthma. They should be regarded rather as catarrhal in character, and, as we shall learn presently, this catarrh is of a secondary nature, a species of bi-product of asthma.

In a large number of cases asthma is merely a manifestation of some particular form of anxiety neurosis. The anxiety is, to a certain extent, disguised under the mask of air hunger. It is transferred, as I have repeatedly demonstrated, from the psychic to the organic. *Brügelmann*, the great authority on asthma, years ago expressed the opinion, contrary to that of Freud, that the primary factor of the asthma attack is invariably anxiety, and that air hunger and the various bronchial phenomena are merely second-ary symptoms. This theory was in a certain sense, *i.e.*, partially, accepted long ago by eminent physicians. The connection between nervous conditions and asthma was so conspicuous that an entire group of asthma were distinguished as nervous asthma or reflex asthma. To avoid misapprehension let me hasten to emphasize the fact that by the term asthma we do not mean that air hunger which torments the emphysematic (an aggravated form of catarrh) but that well-known respiratory disorder characterised by shortness of breath, which suddenly attacks patients who are otherwise healthy, is of short duration, and sometimes, but not always, accompanied by catarrh of the bronchials, and then either rapidly or gradually subsides. It was then observed that a large number of asthmatic patients evinced other nervous symptoms, and it was believed, therefore, that asthma was a complication of neuras-thenia. Nasal specialists refer to the connection between changes in the nose and asthma. It was found possible to effect a temporary or a permanent cure of asthmatic attacks by the removal or cauteris-ing of hypotrophies, or of specially sensitive portions of the mucous skin, or by the removal of polypi. This connection is not surprising when we have realised that asthma is a particular form of anxiety neurosis. We know that the nose, as irrefutably proved by *Fliess*[1] forms a centre for the nervous tissue which serves the sexual organs. The connection between the genitalia and the nose has been proved by so many reliable observations, that we are inclined to attribute the success of nasal treatment in cases of nervous asthma to the influence of the genital zones. *Leyden* maintains that the nerves of the uterus may be responsible in producing asthma, because of the regular occurrence of some attacks at the menstrual period, thus incidentally proving the connection between sex life and asthma. We have already dealt (I believe thoroughly and con-vincingly) with the relation between anxiety neurosis and sexuality. But why the seat of the anxiety should be sometimes in the heart and sometimes in the lungs still remains a mystery. It is possible that hypochondriacal apprehensions to which even normal people are subject, are contributing factors of this variability. Anyone

[1] Beziehungen zwischen Nase und weiblichen Geschlechtsorganen. Franz Deuticke. Vienna and Leipzig.

who is firmly convinced that his heart is not in order will be more easily susceptible to cardiac disorders in the course of an anxiety neurosis, and on the other hand one who is constitutionally disposed to air hunger, who suffers, for example, from chronic bronchial catarrh (locus minoris resistentiæ) is very liable to experience this attack in the form of asthma, as anxiety frequently falls into the background during an attack of asthma. Since, moreover, the other phenomena of anxiety neurosis are completely obscured by the marked symptom of air hunger, it is no matter for wonder that it has taken years to unmask the asthma attack as an anxiety equivalent. It seems now, however, to be universally acknowledged that bronchial asthma is of anxiety origin. *Goldschneider* also ("Ueber Asthma bronchiale," Zeitung für ärztliche Fortbildung, 1907, Nr. 23) maintains that the presence of asthmatic crystals and spirals are not necessarily symptomatic of asthma. "It is possible," he says, "that the catarrh may be due to the forced respiratory movements." This theory is borne out by experiments made independently by *Talma* and *Strübing*, and which showed *that healthy people who simulated asthmatic respiratory movements were susceptible, under certain conditions, to coughs and catarrh.*

The production of the asthma attack by psychic movements is analogous to certain expressive movements of the affects, and owes its origin to associations of correlated feelings and moods. The asthma attacks are combined with anxiety and dread of suffocation ; psychic emotions such as fright, anxiety, etc., may be responsible for the concomitant affective movements of the asthma in consequence of the affinity of the emotions.

It has now become the fashion to speak of diatheses. The French, and especially *Janet*, often talk of "arthritic diathesis." *Czerny* has recently evolved the novel theory of "exudative diathesis," and draws attention to the connection between infantile maladies such as eczema, strophulus infantum, urticaria and the later forms of asthma, and *Strumpell* attaches great importance to these connections. This may, however, be attributed to the fact that the patients in question are neurotics who have evinced neurotic symptoms from childhood. These symptoms naturally manifest themselves in such a way as to betray the constitutional weakness. The various forms of asthma merely bear a strong likeness to respiratory disturbances which are peculiar to *all* neurotics, and which are so characteristic of the anxiety attack. We must never lose sight of the fact, however, that anxiety is the primary, and respiratory disturbances the secondary, factor. *Janet* (Les névroses, *p.* 221) holds the mistaken doctrine that "many conditions of anxiety of the psychasthenic are merely respiratory disorders." On the contrary, the impaired breathing is a manifestation of anxiety neurosis. In a subsequent passage *Janet* very justly remarks : "all phobias are attended by a sensation of oppression on the chest : the patients feel as if their breath were giving out, that they are suffocating, as if there were no movement in the chest, and it seems to them as if other people too have ceased to breathe,—that is the end of the world—everybody dying of suffocation. If we examine the respiratory curves in such cases we find all manner of irregularities, sakkadiertes respiration, very peculiar tremors of the stomach, polypnœa and sighing cramp.''

These disturbances affect not only the lungs, but also the nose and throat. Many cases of persistent colds which defy all treatment are cases of anxiety neurosis. I know patients who get heavy colds after any great excitement, but especially after frustrated sexual pleasures. These colds may last for weeks and are sometimes attended by all kinds of unpleasant complications. The secretions are exceptionally copious, so that one may be justified in speaking of nervous hydrorhœa (*Bosworth*). *Janet* observed a case of rhinorhœa in which 600 ccm. of fluid were passed in one day. In a case of my own, psychanalysis effected a cure without any further intervention on my part. The case in question was one of severe phobia and the rhinorhœa was on the one hand a protective measure (the patient fell ill whenever he proposed to visit a strange woman !) and on the other, was the result of identification with his governess who suffered from a chronic cold.

Hay fever is likewise a neurosis, as *Morton Prince* has demonstrated (Journal of Abnormal Psychology). Other forms of anxiety neurosis are : a hacking (barking) cough—choking in the throat, and irritation of the Adam's apple.

The following case is recorded by Janet :

No. 28.—A woman of thirty-four wrote to the author : " I have no other trouble but an insufferable dread of ' crises,' the sense of impending suffering. Sometimes it comes to nothing, but I feel it hanging over me. The apprehension, the fear that the crisis is coming on." She describes this " crisis " as a " squeezing together of the breast," " an iron band about the chest and loins," a feeling of suffocation, with violent palpitation of the heart. Her chest feels like " a bottle that is being shaken up.'' Nausea, desire to vomit, giddiness, singing in the ears and excessive salivation, complete the picture. The illness dated back to childhood. She had a similar attack as a child when frightened at the sight of workmen on the roof of the boarding school. She is unhappily married and dreads being alone, because a " crisis " would come on. It is not very difficult to interpret the " iron belt " and the " squeezing together " of the chest as the phantasy of an embrace, the libido of which takes the form of anxiety, as the result of repression. The image of the shaken bottle is significant. We cannot overestimate the importance of symbolic forms of expression used by patients. They reveal everything.

The connection between sexual excitement and anxiety is not so easily demonstrable in any other example as in the case of asthma. But we must keep our eyes open.

If we turn over the leaves of the publications of other doctors on the subject of asthma, we shall seek in vain for those decisive moments at which, according to our experience, an anxiety neurosis is called into being. If we question asthmatic patients, in the course of our practice, as to such determining moments we invariably discover the presence of other symptoms of anxiety neurosis, and that the sexual etiological moment is also not lacking. I will illustrate this by an example from my own experience which conclusively proves the connection between asthma and anxiety neurosis.

No. 29.—Mr. O. N., suffered from asthma for twelve years. He attributed the attacks, which always occurred unexpectedly at night, to a chill, an unheated room, the hot restaurant, etc. Various cures which he underwent at Reichenhall, Davos, etc., were without result. Nasal treatment, the removal of hypotrophies, a crista septi, brought temporary relief, but were unable to effect a permanent cure. There were periods, sometimes of nearly a year, during which no attack was experienced. He always attributed this to some specific circumstance, to the beneficial effects of a summer resort by the sea, to a dry house, to regular digestion, etc. The following facts transpired from his sex life :—The man had been married eighteen years. For the first four years of the marriage he did not suffer from asthma. The sexual function was at that time performed normally. In the fourth year, however, his wife nearly lost her life in giving birth to a child, and he decided to be content with the one child, and coitus interruptus was the course in future adopted. Two years later he began to suffer from asthma. The attacks increased, but ceased again after a " cure " in Reichenhall. Incidentally, it may be mentioned, his wife had again become enceinte despite coitus interruptus and he had been able to resume normal intercourse for eight months. It is therefore obvious that the history of his illness synchronised with the regulation of his sex life. He also evinced symptoms of anxiety neurosis. He suffered from excessive perspiration, was very irritable, nervous, and had attacks of bulimia, diarrhœa and migrane.

No. 30.—The second case is equally interesting. Mrs. B. G., a woman of forty-two, suffered for six years from asthma. The attacks occurred not only at night, but in the daytime as well, especially after any violent excitement. I had an opportunity of examining her during one of these attacks and discovered to my astonishment that there was nothing objectively wrong with the lungs. I essayed a sudden suggestion, and said sharply, " Don't get so excited," and ordered her to imitate my own tranquil breathing. And lo and behold ! the attack, which usually lasted several hours, was over in a few minutes. This lady had been practising coitus interruptus for six years, and had been for the last year or two, sexually anæsthetic, which is a provision of the organism to protect itself against frustrated excitement. She, too, exhibited many other symptoms of anxiety neurosis. She was subject to fainting fits, heart weakness, deadening of one finger, goose-flesh, attacks of vertigo and morbid anxiety. She had typical anxiety dreams in which she was trampled on by wild horses, was pursued by wild steers, saw ghosts and corpses and often awoke with an attack of asthma, generally attended by violent pain in the region of the heart. Rapid cure after regulation of sexual intercourse (pessary !).

Stegmann (Ergebnisse der psychischen Behandlung einiger Fälle von Asthma. Zentral bl. für Psychoanalyse, Vol. I, *p.* 377) relates of a patient who always has an attack of asthma when her husband, with whom she is not on good terms, goes into town and leaves her alone. The same psychic mechanism as in case No. 28. That lady was also taken ill when left alone. Phantasies of assault and violation, too, come into play and beget an anxiety which is, at root, a desire. It is almost incredible what an important part is played among women by violation phantasies. All women who are afraid of being alone are afraid of their own weakness and of the superior strength of the aggressive male. Violation is therefore an ardent desire and an unconscious ideal. For it brings within the realms of possibility a condition which all neurotics long for and which I have described as "*Pleasure without guilt.*" (Lust ohne Schuld). In further analyses we shall meet with a number of such cases.

The second case which *Stegmann* mentions concerns a lady of forty-five who suffered for twenty-one years from severe asthma; this lady traced her sufferings to emotional excitements. "After she had done that for some time," so *Stegmann* tells us, "she declared one day quite spontaneously that she found, when following the associations, that every time sexual themes appeared these could be traced as immediately prior to the asthma attacks. The more she revived her earlier memories in this way the more serious attacks diminished, while slight feelings of oppression continued till now nearly every night."

The well-known phenomenon of glottis cramp also comes within this province. In adults this is generally of psychogenic origin, but we also meet with it in children as a very useful means of opposition. Many patients lose their voices during violent emotion and sound as if they are crowing. I have repeatedly met with instances of anxiety attacks attended by slight or serious cramp of the glottis combined with a feeling as of some strange hand strangling the patient. *Grünwald* regards this phenomenon as "Disturbance of the automatic function through the intervention of attention."[1]

Included in the same chapter are the well-known sensations of a foreign body in the throat, a feeling as of "something sticking" in the trachea. (The well-known globus hystericus).

The asthma attacks are the extreme form of lung anxiety or breast anxiety. From these extreme forms there runs a species of descending scale to the light forms, in which the patient merely yawns or sighs deeply. *Yawning is a very frequent symptom of anxiety neurosis.* There are forms of air hunger which pass off in a few seconds. Breast anxiety usually manifests itself by a dull sense of oppression (the patient has a choking sensation and gasps for air). This gasping is well recognised by the medical profession as nervous asthma. It occurs most frequently at night. The patients awake out of an anxiety dream, take a deep breath, and the attack is over.

Sometimes, however, this habit remains also in the day-time and they then repeatedly have to stand still, take a deep breath, gasp or heave a sigh, after which they feel perfectly well. Most of these patients acquire the very frequent and annoying habit of swallowing air. They then have to exhale the air again as an unpleasant sensation of anxiety and oppression is produced by the distention of the stomach. Nearly all sighing neurotics are

[1] (Über psychisch bedingte Erscheinungen im Bereiche der oberen Luftwege. Münchener med. Wochenschrift, 1909. Nr. 33).

D

air consumers. (Very important for the medical profession. Cp. Chapter VIII.) Sighing is mostly the accompanying symptom of a neurosis. But this symptom need not necessarily be nervous. It also frequently appears in organic diseases, especially in light forms of pleurisy. I remember that the pleurisy I suffered from years ago began in this way. I awoke at night inhaling deeply, as if I were going to be suffocated and had to fight for air ; this lasted for some seconds, after which I turned round and went to sleep again. By day I also felt at times an acute pain in the front left thorax in the vicinity of the third rib. An examination made by a distinguished practitioner produced a negative result. Other colleagues also examined me and did not hesitate to diagnose " nervous " asthma and " nervous " pain. Exsudatory formation only appeared after a week. This breast anxiety had by this time, curiously enough, completely disappeared and only recommenced at the period of convalescence.

Since this personal experience I have paid great attention to this " premonitory symptom," and have in fact discovered it in some cases of *pleurisy*. I should rather say that it had drawn my attention to an existing pleuritis sicca or the beginning of a pleuritis exsudativa.

One should therefore not be too ready to diagnose " nervous asthma." Slight pleuritic exsudations, an acute pneumothorax, certain ambulatory forms of pneumonia can be accompanied by severe anxiety sensations of oppression and air hunger. The following case is of diagnostic interest :

No. 31.—Mr. J. D. has for some days complained of oppression in the chest, which was considered to be " nervous asthma," by his panel doctor. At the Polyclinic he is advised to undergo a mild cold water treatment. On the fourth day he is obliged to come back from the stairs owing to severe pains in his chest and extreme shortness of breath. Being the nearest doctor I am called in and pronounce it to be an extended pneumothorax. As the lungs were otherwise quite sound, the existence of a traumatic cause had to be considered, and this proved to be a fact. The patient rode a bicycle. One day before the commencement of his " nervous asthma " he was trying to avoid a motor car and ran into a lamp post. He does not remember having felt any pain at the time. But evidently the tissue of the lungs and the pleura must have been rent at one spot in consequence of the deep, convulsive inhalation which takes place at such sudden frights, and the patient began to pump air into himself as though through a ventilating valve. Strümpell reports a pneumothorax which began while hanging out laundry, and another while in the act of rowing. The pneumothorax was completely cured in six weeks. During the last week frequent sighing and nightly oppression still troubled the patient.

These cases are, however, comparatively rare. The various forms of breast anxiety might much oftener be taken for symptoms of an organic disease. This would especially apply to the severe forms of breast anxiety which are manifested by symptoms of an acute dyspnœa. We have already spoken of the general characteristics of asthma ; there still remains something to be said of the psychic mechanism of an attack of dyspnœa.

The heart plays a large part in these forms, as the shortness of breath seems to be connected with palpitations. Short attacks of dyspnœa, where no trace can be found objectively in the lungs, are very suspicious and betray their origin to the expert physician. We know a physiological act which causes dyspnœa and palpitations. This is coitus. Such attacks of anxiety betray their sexual etiology by the exact imitation of coitus. In an attack of hysteria this resemblance is often complete, even to a correct copy of the abdominal movements. But slight nightly attacks of dyspnœa may also be the result of a sexual phantasy or the outbreak of unconscious forces through the inhibitions of the conscious mind.

No. 32.—Mrs. A. S. complained of harassing nightly attacks of asthma. She usually awoke after midnight with a suffocating sensation. She breathed' as fast as possible. After several minutes she felt curiously languid and fell asleep again. *Several times she wetted the bed on these occasions.* A doctor took the attacks to be reflex asthma of the nose. A specialist removed the hypertrophied nasal turbinates. A slight temporary improvement took place after the operation. Then the old conditions reappeared with renewed violence. After a further period of two months the attacks had completely ceased. These peculiar vacillations are very easily explained. Her husband had to undertake a fairly long sea voyage. He remained away for over a year. During this period of complete sexual abstinence the nightly anxiety attacks appeared in the form of dyspnœa. She is therefore a typical anxiety neurotic. She was operated on by the specialist before her husband came home. The improvement in her state of health is therefore attributable to the anticipated resumption of marital relations. She had never felt so well in her life. It is well known that as a rule after such a long wait and a hard separation the sexual need seems to be completely satisfied. The renewed set-back is connected with the journey to a watering-place which she had to undertake to please her children. A second interesting symptom of this anxiety neurosis—almost daily sickness—should be mentioned. She is often nauseated in the presence of her husband. He has a *foetor ex ore.* Her attacks of asthma introduce erotic dreams, in which she is unfaithful to her husband. If, on one day she makes the acquaintance of a man who pleases her, on the following night she will immediately dream of some intimate scene with him, followed by an attack of asthma.

This observation is a proof that many cases of "nervous asthma" and reflex "asthma" have their origin in sexual disturbances, and that it is incumbent on us to think of an anxiety neurosis in every case of asthma. I can only corroborate the words of M. Saenger (Uber Asthma und seine Behandlung. Berlin. S. Karger, 1910) : "*Asthma is caused by mental influences, it is a traumatic neurosis arising from a psychic trauma.*" But I should like to add : In most cases it is a matter of a sexual Trauma—and asthma is only a particular form of anxiety.

The little known forms of asthma which can be traced to a so-called womb-phantasy are of great interest. There are neurotics who continually dwell in the fancy of being born. They often wake at night with shortness of breath. Their dreams mostly contain a symbolic representation of birth. (They force themselves through narrow chimneys, they crawl along a passage, the walls of which threaten to crush them, growing narrower and narrower, forcing the chest and head together.) The dream, which often disappears from consciousness, is succeeded by an attack of asthma. These people often show fear of narrow rooms and of any kind of a crowd.[1]

The asthmatical attacks of these patients mostly date back to their childhood, and serve to evoke the sympathy of the family, to attract the attention of those surrounding them and to become the centre of universal interest. The neurotic then responds to every humiliation and degradation with his attack of asthma, which symbolically represents a flight into the past and the wish for regeneration. (Phantasy of a new life). From this point of view the following case offers very instructive information :

No. 33.—Mr. U. R., a railway official, aged thirty-six, has suffered since his childhood from asthma, which often attacks him at night. He takes atropin-drops and smokes stramonium cigarettes for the asthma. After a chronic tripper which is followed by a lengthy Prostatitis his condition grows much worse.[2] A slight improvement sets in after prostatic massage. During the last six months he is much worse again. His promotion to a higher rank was overlooked and he cannot conquer this mortification. He now uses the asthma as an excuse to become exempt from service and to attain a long leave. He asks me for a certificate for a year's leave. As I know from experience that such holidays only serve to stabilize the illness, I refuse to write out the certificate and recommend an analytic treatment. He agrees to my proposal. During the analysis it transpires that in his attacks he always goes through the process of birth and that all his dreams contain womb phantasies. He admits that he is otherwise interested in the subject of regeneration, and that also when he is awake he occasionally experiences the phantasy of a birth, without ever having realised its connection with his attacks.

It is little known to practitioners that there exist purely psychogenic forms of bronchitis. I know people who get bronchitis at every suitable opportunity. They always take refuge in the disease with the aid of their bronchial muscles, which are easily irritated. If they have experienced some official slight, or they wish to avoid some unpleasantness, or obtain extra leave, they produce (often unconsciously) their bronchitis. I know women who always keep their husbands away in this manner, who are sent to undergo fresh air cures and are even mistakenly treated for catarrh of the apis pulmonis of a specific nature, although the existence of a tubercular bacillus had never been proved. A careful investigation of the various sanatoria for pulmonary diseases will bring to light many a neurotic catarrh of the lungs, which points to the shirking of work or of the duties of life. An attack of influenza is often concentrated in the tips of the lungs and manifests both clinically and through X-rays the symptoms of pulmonary catarrh, although tubercular bacilli are never found. They are mostly the wives and sons of

[1] Cp. in my book, " Die Sprache des Traumes " (The Language of Dreams) the Chapter headed " Womb-dreams."

[2] Cp. the important work of Max Mareuse, " Ueber Atonie der Prostata." Med. Kl., 1912. No. 45, in which the connection between Neurosis and Prostatitis is referred to. Cp. page 45.

rich men who repeatedly retire to their castles of sickness when they do not feel able to cope with life and are too lazy to work.

I have observed many women who suddenly get "their usual bronchitis" after a matrimonial dispute, in order to punish their husbands, and then just as suddenly recover if they have to undertake a journey or go to some festival.

The success of psycho-therapeutics has enabled us to recognise that it was a case of purely mental suffering. I know of no other complaint in which the triumph of psycho-therapeutics is so pronounced as in asthma bronchiale, which is always asthma nervosum. I should like to mention two cases of my late practice in which I employed hypnotism in order to effect a rapid cure.

No. 34.—F. H., twenty-three years old, a medical student, who is obliged to earn his living with the aid of his musical and theatrical gifts. He is to accept an engagement in a cinema but is prevented by a severe attack of asthma. It attacks him quite unexpectedly, but especially if he plays the violin for long at a time. He now fears an interruption in his new employment which is very remunerative and practical. He can study medicine by day and earn his living in the evenings. He begs me to hypnotize him. He is very easily hypnotized, falls asleep in a few seconds through my method of seizing him unawares and receives the suggestion : " You will play quite calmly for the next three evenings without suffering from asthma." This suggestion helps him through the first three days and then I become bolder and suggest : " One week without the slightest attack." The result is excellent. Hypnotic treatment is reduced to once a week, later on once a fortnight, and is stopped altogether after a period of three months. In a year's time my colleague comes to me again. He is to take the chief part in an operetta and has violent tremor. Before going on to the stage he is hypnotized and given the suggestion that he shall play his part without the slightest agitation, in certainty and self-confidence. The hypnotic treatment was again extremely successful.

The asthma has entirely disappeared since this hypnotic treatment.

It stands to reason that a neurosis cannot be permanently cured by hypnotism. It only cures the symptoms and is of temporary help. But it is just with asthma that hypnotic treatment sometimes works miracles in desperate cases. The following case is a striking proof of this :

No. 35.—My colleague, Dr. Th. W., brings me a peasant of about fifty, who has been suffering most severely from asthma for a year and a half. All medicines have hitherto been tried in vain, with the exception of asthma cigarettes which gave slight relief and injections of Adrenalin which help to overcome the attack. The patient is now already in need of two or three injections daily, and sometimes also at night ; he is quite incapable of work. He has a bad attack while he is with me. Objectively the well-known symptoms of a severe asthma bronchiale are present. Individual consulting specialists surmised the trouble to be of organic origin. Judging from the history of the illness I believed it to be a psychogenic asthma, and suggested hypnotic treatment to my colleague. I at once hypnotized the patient during the attack and achieved complete tranquility. I explained to Dr. W. the method of hypnotism and recommended him to try hypnotic treatment daily—with corresponding suggestion—instead of the Adrenalin injections, and later on less frequently, using the method that he had seen me use. The following report shows how easily hypnotism can be learnt and what an important weapon it can be in the hands of an experienced doctor. Dr. W. writes on February 2nd, 1920 :

" I hope you will allow me to give you a short report on the asthmatic patient whom I brought to you on January 7th, 1920. Our return home in an open carriage in a snowstorm was not pleasant and on our arrival he had another attack which was so severe that I could hardly get him into bed. He was given five injections that day. On the following morning I hypnotized him and he slept well ; I then sent him to sleep every other day, followed by a pause of three days, so that *after a week* I was able to register *a sudden and most striking improvement* in his condition through the treatment recommended by you. The patient falls asleep immediately. I hypnotize him at eight o'clock at night so that the trance is at once followed by his night's rest. I gave him about five injections during the whole month, whereas in December I gave him about eighty. Now he would like hypnotic treatment daily. But I cannot make further progress, the charm only works for two or three days. How can that period be drawn out ? Last night he sent for me for the first time again. It was a slight attack, but he was afraid. I do not know whether I do it correctly or not. I begin as I learnt from you. He promptly falls asleep and I then convey the suggestion that he will have three good nights, that he can go out and do some light work (rubbing maize) specified by me. I let him sleep for ten minutes. Is that enough ? Even if he coughs occasionally he does not wake up until I call him. Then we have a short conversation, followed by his night's rest. He is already undressed and in bed. I frankly admit that I came to you an unbelieving Saul, but the success has been so conspicuous that I have now become a Paul."

The report ends here. So far I have not heard any more as regards the destiny of this patient. The psychogenesis of the disease is proved by the startling success of hypnotic treatment. A return of the trouble is probable. Only an analysis could of course effect a complete and certain cure. But this cannot be taught in one interview.

It will be readily understood after this experience that in cases of chronic colds, bronchitis and even inflammation of the throat, psychic treatment will effect a cure when other therapeutics are powerless. There are certain catarrhs of a most tormenting kind where the patient has always to clear his throat and feels a dry phlegm in it ; he is generally a frequent visitor to the throat specialists, who give temporary relief by painting the throat.

In the case of many an actor or teacher (professional diseases !) resistance to the unpleasantnesses of the vocation declares itself in the form of a chronic catarrh of the throat, or the trachea, or in temporary hoarseness which can eventually grow into dread of catarrhs. These patients tremble at every change of temperature ; a falling temperature is to them a phantom of horror ; they avoid smoke and dust, they cover their mouths with cloths, wear scarves round their necks and succumb at every suitable and unsuitable opportunity. Their cure requires not only analysis but also psychopedagogics, which represents the most satisfactory and at the same time the most arduous task of the practitioner.

A very curious manifestation of an attack of anxiety, in which the respiratory organs are primarily concerned, will form a conclusion to the accounts of these diseases :

No. 36.—A delicate woman of twenty-nine falls a victim to an illness characterised by slight ill-humour, general weakness and headaches, very similar to hay fever. Her eyelids become red and swollen, the conjunctivæ are conspicuously red and discharge a thin mucus ; the eyes water badly.

The nose, hitherto pale, reddens intensely and looks inflamed. Sometimes, but not always, the nasal passages are obstructed as a result of the swollen corpus cavernosum. She has an unpleasant sensation in her throat, as if she were being strangled. Severe anxiety accompanies these symptoms. The pulse dwindles until it is almost imperceptible. She speaks in a low voice : " I am going to die. Let me see the child before my death. Give me your hand, that I can press it once more," etc. I am called to an attack of this sort. In half an hour, by kindly and, at the same time, forcible encouragement, I succeed in completely appeasing the patient. There is no sign of the convulsions that otherwise followed such an attack.

It transpires that she does not love her husband. During coitus she is entirely anæsthetic. Now and then she produces an orgasm by imagining that she is being embraced by a man who is married to a friend of hers.

The attack imitates the act of dying and the changes resultant from violent weeping which she had observed in her mother after the father's death. It is a curious fact that these changes (reddened eyelids and nose) precede the weeping convulsions in this case.

No. 37.—A man of about thirty gets violent hay fever as soon as he smells violets. This idiosyncrasy is so pronounced that even violet perfume brings on an attack. It begins with an unpleasant irritation and burning in the nose, then the eyelids redden and the nose commences to discharge profusely, a liquid as clear as water. An attack of this kind, which is mostly complicated by coughing and slight fever, lasts from several days to a week. The patient once went to a prostitute and got hay fever afterwards. He went again and forbade her to use violent scent. She assured him that she had never used it. After a prolonged stay he again noticed the pernicious odour of violets, following her micturition. The girl had taken turpentine capsules on the advice of a doctor in order to disguise the odour. It is well known that turpentine causes the urine to smell strongly of violets.

The protracted analysis revealed a peculiar reason for this idiosyncracy. His governess had always powdered him with a kind of violet powder if an unpleasant smell remained after he had defæcated. The memory of various pleasurable scatalogic occurrences of his youth had been completely repressed. The scent of violets had by association brought back to him everything that occurred between him and his brother in the lavatory.

This same governess had a bad habit. She used to lift him up and press him against her breast so violently that it took his breath away. His attacks of hay fever, for which he had in vain used " Pollenserum," alternated with various respiratory troubles, which were in reality nothing but the memory of his governess's games, to which he had stubbornly clung, half in pleasure and half in fear.

In a very instructive article (Ueber das Asthma bronchiale und seine Beziehungen zur sogenannten exsudativen Diathese. Med. Klinik, 1910, Nr. 23) *Strümpell* has drawn attention to the fact, that asthmatic patients manifest a psychopathic constitution and an exsudative past. He points out that these patients also suffer from colica mucosa (peritoneal asthma), œdema, flow of saliva, inflammation of the sinews and intermittent pains in the joints. They were nervous already in their childhood and were afflicted with urtikaria, strophulus and excema. Those interested in the question of " neurotic selection " will often realise that neurosis makes use of the inferior organs in order to carry out its secret designs. Neuroses mostly begin in childhood.

All observation points to the fact that psychic influences play an enormous part in asthma and similar diseases. In many cases it is necessary to extend the investigations back to the days of childhood, if permanent success is to be obtained. Behind the disguise of the asthmatic attack is concealed the anxiety attack of the anxiety neurosis so well known to us.

CHAPTER VII

CLINICAL PICTURE OF ANXIETY NEUROSIS: DIGESTIVE DISTURBANCES

THE accompanying symptoms of anxiety as manifested by the digestive organs are also well known to the layman. Anxiety diarrhœa is so popular a symptom that it is even used for satire by modern comic papers. Also the other symptoms: stomach-ache, sickness, active, noisy peristaltic movements, heart-burn and choking as accompaniments to an attack of anxiety and symptoms of an anxiety neurosis are not difficult to explain when they are accompanied by distinct sensations of anxiety. With most anxiety neurotics we find that disturbances of the digestive organs, loss of appetite, sickness, constipation, cardialgia, bulimia, diarrhœa, spasms, can occur simultaneously with the other characteristic symptoms of anxiety neurosis and it then depends on clinical observation to decide between organic trouble and the result of the anxiety neurosis.

The masked anxiety conditions of the digestive organs are much more difficult to diagnose.

No. 38.—Mr. N. V. suffers from an obstinate stomach trouble that perferably declares itself in the form of violent stomach-ache. He gets irritable, depressed, loses his appetite and looks wretched. The pains are independent of his meals. He often awakens at night from an anxiety dream, with tormenting stomach-ache. During such times he is exceedingly agitated and also suffers from palpitations and perspirations. He was then having relations with a woman whose husband was dying. For ethical reasons, out of consideration for her husband's condition, the woman refused him intercourse with her. Mr. N. V. who did not wish to be unfaithful to her practised total abstinence during this time. The pains in the stomach were equivalent to an attack of anxiety. His illness was an anxiety neurosis. For as soon as he resumed regular intercourse with her, after the death of her husband, all the symptoms, including the pains, speedily disappeared. The patient remained in Vienna during the following summer, while the lady of his heart was obliged to remove to her parents on a country estate. As a result of renewed abstinence the pains in the stomach recurred in all their former violence. At the resumption of his intimate relationship with the lady in the autumn there was sanatio completa. This phenomenon recurred in the second, third and fourth summers, when the lady married. The patient followed her example and since then is perfectly well.

A very distinct and strictly circumscribed form of anxiety neurosis is represented by that species of nervous diseases of the stomach which perferably declares itself in hypochondriacal apprehensions of a faulty diet. A large number of these nervous stomach troubles already present the character of a phobia and will be specially mentioned later on in the study of hypochondria. Others, however, which show no hysterical features, have their origin in anxiety neurosis. We have repeatedly emphasized the fact that the anxiety due to anxiety neurosis is very often imputed to organic causes, *i.e.*, the anxiety, being unattached, clings to some object, and after the heart and the lungs, the stomach seems to be especially adapted thereto. Such patients manifest a unique form of apprehension. They are afraid of a faulty diet, they suffer from all kinds of disorders such as a nasty taste in the mouth, loss of appetite, cardialgia, sickness, ærophagia, for which they consult all sorts of doctors, go to Carlsbad, Kissingen, Marienbad, have massage, electric treatment, and cold water cures. The most important thing for them is, however, diet ; the stricter the better. As the disorders must however be ascribed to far different causes, there is no kind of diet which secures them a painless existence. But they have the habit of attributing their troubles to the last food they may have eaten, with the result that the choice of dishes that suit them becomes more and more limited. At first oily, savoury dishes seem to be the only harmful ones, then follows fruit, later on vegetables, alcohol, coffee, tea and red meat ; in the end they find milk injurious, they try vegetarianism and in short go so far as only to live on a few chosen foods. In consequence of this they of course lose weight considerably, grow more and more enfeebled and in fact give the impression of being seriously ill. As they thoroughly spoil their stomachs they are soon unable to digest the heavier dishes, feel an unpleasant oppression in the stomach after every meal, often put their fingers in their mouths, in order to vomit, bring up a little water or phlegm, and then feel much better. It is frequently to be remarked that the pains felt by these patients arise from nothing but hunger. It is possible in such cases to attain extraordinary results by correcting the origin of the anxiety neurosis, the abnormal vitus sexualis. I will relate the following very characteristic case as an illustration of this fact ; it is not the only one in which I gained brilliant results through such energetic procedure :

No. 39.—Four years ago a little, weak man stood before me, a merchant from W . . ., Mr. T. W. His eyes lay in deep hollows, and were dull and dry ; his pale hands trembled and oscillated delicately with every movement. His voice sounded hoarse and toneless. He gave the impression of a patient languishing from an incurable disease, whose days were numbered. The cruel wit of man would call him a candidate for death.

The man told me a long tale of woe. He had suffered from stomach troubles and digestive disorders for years. He had consulted all kinds of doctors and had several times vainly tried a cure at Carsbad for " excessive uric acid."

" Although I keep to the strictest diet," complained the man, " I have terrible pains, tormenting heart-burn, and complete lack of appetite. I am daily getting weaker and can hardly get through my work as a merchant. My diet is evidently not strict enough, or not suitable. Will you please prescribe one that will be accurate and appropriate."

I realized at the first glance that the poor man was obviously starving. His pains were probably due to a very common sensation—that of hunger. A thorough examination confirmed my opinion. For once I wished to make a bold experiment. The man had no appetite at all, as he said. Perhaps this was only because he always eat the same dull food, which already repulsed him?

"Will you promise me to follow out my directions accurately?"

"Naturally. I always follow the doctor's orders scrupulously."

"Good. Your hand upon it!"

"Yes. Here is my hand!"

"First of all answer me one question. What sort of food have you avoided for years? What do you long for most? And what would tempt you?"

"Good Heavens! What is the use of talking and making my mouth water, if I am not allowed to eat these things?"

"Please tell me what they are."

"Well, then, if I must: meat pies, stew with dumplings, plum pudding, those are my favourite dishes. Also a young gosling, a duck, a hare—are not to be despised."

"Good! Then go to the nearest restaurant and order a few of these dishes. And for the next few weeks eat just what you have a fancy for, without troubling about any kind of diet."

"No! For Heaven's sake, no! I cannot do it! That would be certain death for me. I should not be able to bear the pains."

"On the contrary, you are now courting certain death with your diet. And as for the pains, are you entirely free from pain when you diet yourself so severely?"

"What an idea! I have the most terrible pains all day long."

"So you see it would be much better in that case to eat as much as you want. You have pains in any case. Then why chastise yourself so mercilessly, when nothing is gained by it?"

That seemed to appeal to the patient. He promised me to make the attempt and to live for a fortnight as though there were nothing wrong with his stomach.

My surprise and joy may be imagined when the same man introduced himself to me four weeks later and at first I did not even recognise him. He now looked absolutely flourishing, with full cheeks and moist shining eyes, flashing with the joy of life. He had become a different man, in the true sense of the word. The very day after our interview he had, to the despair of his acquaintances, ordered the most piquant, indigestible dishes, which he devoured voraciously. He thought that this would be his last meal and had the sensations of a man condemned to death, who is allowed to choose what food he likes for the last time.

After this first meal he immediately felt a slight relief. He anxiously awaited the severe pains which used to accompany the process of digestion. They were absent. He could not grasp the idea that he should eat "everything." But having gathered courage from his first successful attempt, he gaily commenced to eat and drink whatever he fancied. And his strength and self-confidence increased daily. His appearance also improved daily, until at last the startling fact dawned upon him that he was now completely cured and that on the whole there was nothing the matter with him. Since he had eaten sensibly and everything that he wanted, all pain and disorder had disappeared.

Other patients stop eating because they are afraid of appendicitis. These cases can also be traced to psychic grounds; it might be a matter of a phobia. The patients are then very fastidious as to their diet and very anxious in the observance of their stool. Now there is no better means of disturbing the normal course of the vegetative functions than self-observation. As soon as people begin to enquire into the nature of their sleep, their digestive processes and excretory functions, the sleep will assuredly grow disturbed, the digestion impaired and the stool arrested.

A great deal of anxiety that craves to discharge itself is accumulated in everybody through the anxiety neurosis, because a man would far rather endure the most terrible anxiety if he can change it into fear, *i.e.*, if he ascribes it to a particular object ; while the true anxiety, the anxiety of the unknown, the uncertain, is simply intolerable to him. For this reason anxiety takes certain fashionable forms in which to express itself ; in our times they are : fear of brain diseases, lunacy, uric acid, and not least, appendicitis.

No. 40.—Mr. E. V. introduces himself to me as one afflicted with chronic appendicitis ; he is on the point of undergoing an operation. He is as thin as a skeleton, and has the most dreadful pains, especially after rather a larger meal than usual. Consequently he has lately eaten as little as possible. Every time he feels the pain he thinks : Now I am suffering from appendicitis and shall soon be operated on, etc. He has never had an attack with fever ! In spite of this the surgeons advise him to have the appendix removed. But his fear of the operation is as great as his fear of the disease. This patient made a pitiful impression. I have never seen anybody so excessively emaciated. I thought his was a case of a neoplasm or of tuberculosis.—Objectively, however, there was nothing to prove it. I assumed it to be an anxiety neurosis and made enquiries as to his sexual life. For three years he had had an affair with a girl whom he was not allowed to impregnate and with whom he satisfied himself by all kinds of thwarted excitation. I now advised him to put an end to this state of affairs entirely, and either to marry the girl or not to have any relations with her until he should be in a position to marry her. Meanwhile he might practise normal coitus with contraceptives. Besides this I prescribed three tablespoons of olive oil daily, for the pains, and oil enemas for constipation, and assured him that he would now day by day be able to eat more. The pains were of no consequence and were nothing but the manifestation of hunger and nervous excitement. If appendicitis really should make its appearance under the influence of food, it would be better to have the illness once and for all and to undergo an operation, rather than go about in everlasting apprehension. The patient saw the point of this. In the first week he gained 1 kg. in weight, and 15kg. in the course of three months, and it was only after this that he began to look normal and human. Hitherto he had only weighed 50 kg., with a height of 175cm., and was therefore 25 kg. below the normal weight. The pains entirely disappeared. He married soon after and since then—three years ago—he is in perfect health. In the meantime he has put on more weight and is now a strong, powerful man weighing 80kg.

The associations between loss of appetite and the libido can be inferred from the following observation. Many patients who complain of a lack of appetite have lost sexual desire and suffer from unconscious conceptions of repugnance. The patient whom I am about to introduce also manifests a characteristic respiratory disorder and forms a connecting link with the observations of the previous chapter.

No. 41.—Mr. D. B., a master cabinet-maker, of forty-eight, complains of loss of appetite and respiratory troubles. Also of excessive bodily weakness which hinders him in his work. He suffers from painful attacks. He seems fairly well, then suddenly feels a cardiac weakness and great breathlessness and has to sit down at once, in case he should fall. He opens his mouth wide and the breathing becomes spasmodic and irregular. The condition grows worse and sensations of anxiety appear, so that he is obliged to lie down. He feels chilly internally, he is cold, then he gets hot and breaks out into a violent perspiration ; the attack is then over. He had four such attacks within six months. The doctor diagnosed a weak heart and prescribed strophantus. Then the patient went to the South, where he felt slightly better.

When he returned home he had completely lost his appetite. He fears lung trouble, as he had already had catarrh of the apis pulmonis as a boy.

To my question as to whether he had intercourse with his wife, he replied : " No, since I have lost my appetite I feel too weak. I am also completely impotent now."

" Do you suffer from emissions ? "

The patient reddened. He answers hesitatingly, almost stammeringly, " Yes—no—now and then."

" Can you remember the dream that accompanies the emission ? "

For I surmised that his sexual desires had been transferred from the elderly wife to some younger woman. My inference was correct, for Mr. B. said angrily :

" I entreat you—surely one is not responsible for one's dreams ! One dreams all kinds of stupid nonsense ! "

" Then tell me about the stupid nonsense."

" Well, if you insist on hearing it, I dreamed last night that I was having intercourse with my wife's niece. Such nonsense ! I would not even dream of her ! "

" You are giving yourself the lie. You have thought of her in your dreams !—"

On my first visit I had already been struck by a charming, shy girl who had been in the house for six months in order to relieve the wife. Unconscious feelings of desire were directed towards this young creature and his wife had lost all charm for him. He lost the appetite for his wife and with it the appetite for his meals !

The progress he made in the South was due to absence from this permanent psychic conflict. Desire for the death of his good, faithful wife, which is inevitable in such a case, completed the conflict and formed the deeper root of the attacks of anxiety. Perhaps criminal thoughts also had a part in it. I could not probe so far in my analysis of this simple man.

The cure was very easy. In spite of violent opposition on his part I advised him to send the girl away from his house. He would not consent to that. But the girl soon found an admirer in the large town. Her uncle came upon her unawares at a rendezvous and chased her out of the house. After a few months he regained his appetite and strength and could again enter into marital relations with his wife. He ascribes the success of his cure to an advertised remedy that he took in defiance of the wicked doctors.

But not all cases are simple and easily solved. Digestive disturbances play an important part and anxiety about food takes the most peculiar forms. It goes without saying that it is the complicated, hysterical disorders for which many months of analysis are required.

I know patients who eat very little owing to fear of pain. It is often very difficult to distinguish it from an organic disease of the stomach.[1] Certainly if a woman patient whom one

---

[1] Pick (l.c.) draws attention to the fact that in organic diseases of the stomach the Boas' pressure point is easily verifiable (on the *left* of the eleventh and twelfth rib). In neurotic disorders of the stomach great pressure sensitivity is to be found *between* the shoulder-blades and on the spinous-process itself.

suspects of having ulcer can stand solid food without any trouble and complains of pains after liquids, the diagnosis will not be difficult. The absurdity of many an anxiety idea will also betray its neurotic origin. One mostly finds that the pains are not so bad and only serve to " rationalize " the various idiosyncracies. Some patients are afraid that what they eat will stick in their throats ; they go through a regular ceremonial at meal-times ; others avoid food that causes flatulency. Some only eat cold things, others only warm food ; some can eat no meat, others no vegetables. One would really have to write a whole book in order to do justice to this host of neurotic troubles and variations.

Dietetic' disorders are exceedingly frequent amongst neurotics. Almost every nervous subject has his special idiosyncracies. One cannot endure the skin of milk, a second cannot bear any kind of fat sauce, a third retches if he has to eat a raw beefsteak, a fourth can only eat liquid foods, a fifth only solids, a sixth must eat a small mouthful of something every hour of the night, a seventh is attacked by bulimia at certain hours. These disorders can always be explained by analysis. It is evident that with these neurotics the mouth is an " erogenous zone " ; such people have been suck-a-thumbs, are still addicted to sucking, or are gourmets. They have mostly repressed some kind or other of sexual impulse (fellatio, cunnilingus, cannibalism, necrophilia, vampirism). The repressed phantasy becomes associated with the act of eating and the inhibition transfers itself from the sex act, which is morally vetoed, to the act of feeding, which then falls under the same ban. The importance of guarding against a one-sided conception is shown by the following observation :

No. 42.—A man of thirty-two years of age comes to see me with the complaint that he has suffered from severe dietetic disorders for ten years. He can only eat liquid substances and then only at certain times. He eats his principal meal in the mornings. During the day he can only take liquids and often in the evenings he succeeds in eating a few mouthfuls of solid food. His trouble consists in the fact that he is conscious of the whole process of swallowing and is tormented by the fear of choking if something were to stick in his throat. He has the greatest difficulty when eating meat or very nourishing food, while dry (stale) bread often slips down surprisingly well. He also suffers from the fear of food going down " the wrong way " (trachea).

The objective examination with sounds and Röntgen rays repeatedly undertaken, revealed perfectly normal conditions.

One is inclined to suspect the presence a priori in such cases of a fellatio phantasy. The patient's sexual record was however a perfectly normal one. He had masturbated very little, commenced sexual intercourse at the age of fifteen, had a liaison with a dressmaker for some considerable time and was now living with a nurse whom he hoped to marry soon. His sexual potency was satisfactory, he betrayed no unhealthy tendencies to perversion, had no homosexual experiences in childhood and his inclinations did not deviate in any way from the normal path.

He exhibits no neurotic symptoms other than the digestive one, is very capable and industrious and managed during the war, despite the altered conditions, to secure a good position. He became very run down while on active service on account of the digestive disorders and was given light work at the base.

On our enquiring when the disorder first made its appearance, the following incident transpired. Ten years previously, in time of peace, he was serving as a volunteer at S. They had just been through a strenuous drill and he returned to the canteen with an enormous appetite and found one of his comrades devouring some roast veal. He called out " Waiter, bring me some of that, too." As he was very hungry he fell to and swallowed large portions of the meat. But a piece of it stuck in his throat so that he was obliged to spit it out and could eat no more. From that time onward the digestive disturbance developed, growing systematically worse by wrong treatment, until the present condition was reached.

On the first day of the treatment he was able to give the following account of a dream :—

I found myself in a passage open on one side which overlooked a terrible abyss. I clung to the right hand wall and came to a little door through which I slipped, and the situation in which I found myself was indeed a precarious one, for I was on a roof, still in danger of falling. There I saw a small, pale, very thin little boy. He was walking up and down along the roof. I was surprised that he was not afraid and asked him how he could wander about so fearlessly. He said : " Oh, that is nothing to me ! My mother has made me an angel ! " and then I saw that he had wings. He rose, looked at me very seriously and sadly and suddenly flew away. I felt as if I had been abandoned, awoke in a fright with my heart throbbing and could not go to sleep again.

The passage reminded him of a court of law where he was once the clerk of a barrister. He also had a dim remembrance of having been accused of something against which he had to defend himself. The accusation appeared to be an unjust one.

The boy reminded him of no boy in particular.

Now the story of his life had made me acquainted with the fact that he had lost a child. I made him go over the history of this event again in detail. When he was eighteen he had begun a liaison with a dressmaker, to whose support he also contributed somewhat as he belonged to a wealthy family. The affair lasted six years. During this time his mistress bore him three children. The first two children died very early. The third was still living. The dressmaker had married a shoemaker who had adopted the child as his own and brought it up. The first two children were boarded out and died of under nourishment during the first year.

They had been given into the care of an angel-maker !

This was the name given to women who made a profession of starving illegitimate children for mothers who wished to be rid of them.

This explained the dream. It was his own child whom he saw on the roof and whose mother had made him an " angel." The legal proceedings were the summons before the court of his own conscience. He had let two children starve and left the third to a strange, and probably rough man. Is there not such a thing as retributive justice ?

His whole life had been passed on the edge of a terrible precipice. He was a criminal—an infanticide—for he was morally responsible for the death of his children.

This explains the origin of the digestive trouble. He had eaten very little on that particular day and had rushed to the restaurant in a state of ravenous hunger. It then occurred to him : This is how my children must have felt—and the food stuck in his throat.

The drill took place in the vicinity of a cemetery. During a pause he sat in the shade of the cemetery and saw some children's graves. This impression must have diverted his unconscious thoughts to his own dead children.

His digestive disorder was that of a *diseased conscience*. At every meal he was confronted with the vision of a starving child. " Something " always whispered to him : You are a criminal ! You have let two children starve, and you have not the right to eat your fill.

His neurosis was the Pœna Talionis. His punishment was self-determined. The analysis of further dreams justified this interpretation. The children were continually appearing in one form or another. In one dream he saw the living child in the street of the metropolis selling newspapers, in rags and tatters, and his heart was heavy within him at seeing his own flesh and blood in such a condition.

Before the analysis he paid no attention to his dreams and in fact maintained that he hardly dreamed at all. It was all quite clear to him now. According to the account of his mistress he often moaned and cried out in his dreams. He used to wake in the night with violent air hunger, fighting for breath. His sufferings were aggravated by aerophagia.

He was now able to eat again and learnt to know himself. But we recognise that his neurosis represents a moral process of purification. He had also begun a frivolous relationship with the nurse. But he was now resolved to put an end to this frivolous existence. His treatment of the dressmaker was atoned for by his honourable action towards his new mistress. He led her to the altar, and his erotic escapades were relinquished once and for all. He made substantial provision for his child and his digestive troubles soon disappeared.

It is of the greatest importance for the practitioner to realise that certain neuroses take the form of severe ulcus ventriculi. The diagnosis is a very difficult one and can only be arrived at with the aid of all the most modern methods of treatment. The next observation is a proof of this :

No. 43.—Mr. Y. M., a man of forty-six, suffered for some years from severe pains in the stomach. The pains occurred after eating and after excitement. He was treated by a very eminent specialist, Dr. X. A special diet was accordingly prescribed together with Belladonna to be taken internally. The pains only became the more acute and unbearable. The careful doctor warned the patient that he was suffering from erosions, or perhaps even from a tumour, which necessitated a four weeks' rest in bed and a strict diet of milk food. The patient followed this advice implicitly. But the pains only increased in severity. Every night he writhed in pain and kept the whole household awake. Hot fomentations, thermophor and morphia had no effect.

At this juncture I was summoned to the patient, whose family I had treated for many years. He himself had consulted only professors and specialists for his stomachic troubles.

The whole stomach was very tender —the tongue thickly furred.

In this connection the following diagnostic process may be appropriately mentioned. Neurotics almost invariably project their stomachic pains on to the navel, the middle line, or else they are diffused over the whole region of the stomach. In ulcer one particular spot is always found to be extremely sensitive and tender.

The patient protested that he would commit suicide if this state of things continued. It had already lasted some years and was growing steadily worse and he was getting more and more pulled down.

I was confirmed in my suspicion that it was an anxiety neurosis by the presence of other symptoms. He suffered from attacks of shivering and night-sweats ; he worried about the future of the family and had practised coitus interruptus for the last ten years.

I recognised hunger in these nightly attacks. I can only repeat : *With those who adhere to a strict diet many pains are a sign of hunger.* As our patient had never vomited blood, I was certain that it was a case of stomach neurosis which had escaped the notice of the experienced internist. With many diagnoses a decision is formed by the first impression, the diagnostic flaire. I also had the stool examined : no blood was present. An X-ray examination with bismuth afforded no evidence of the existence of a tumour in the stomach,

I prescribed an adequate meal for the next night : a minced beef-steak.

stewed fruit (pulped) and three well masticated rolls. Also a glass of Pilsner beer which the patient used to drink with gusto, but which he had been forbidden to take. And lo! he had a better night. Emboldened by this success, I proceeded straight to an ordinary diet without a transition stage. The patient was to have stopped in bed for another three weeks. I let him get up and advised him to go to the office. I explained to him that it was a matter of nervous fear of diet. He should now eat a substantial supper: Black bread with butter, cheese, some roast joint, etc. *After three days the pains had completely disappeared!* Since once having had my attention drawn to this, I have had many similar experiences.

I recommend all those suffering from stomach troubles to be thoroughly examined with a view to an anxiety neurosis and to look for the fear of food. I am convinced that over half, perhaps even two-thirds of such patients, suffer from anxiety neurosis.

Just as with the heart, organic diseases (enlargement of the heart after paroxysmal tachycardia, and heart disease after mental traumata) may now and then be formed, it sometimes happens that an ulcer may have a neurotic origin. I have observed patients who have suffered for years from a stomach neurosis, who showed all kinds of dietetic disturbances of a hysterical nature and eventually went to pieces from a carcinoma ventriculi. Westphal, Katsch[1] and Bergmann[2] have drawn attention to these associations, and Strauss also recommends caution and more discriminating diagnostic examinations. But I must emphasize the fact that in difficult cases all diagnostic remedies are useless, whereas a careful psychotherapeutic treatment will have excellent results. But he who practises psychotherapeutics must guard especially against a partial view. Nobody should become a neurologist without first having studied internal medicine and tested it by practise. Practise alone can perfect the internist. I look upon the years I spent as a practitioner as the best introduction to my profession. Wenckebach, who has also eaten the bread of the practitioner for some years, once expressed the same opinion.

Doctors do not yet realise that psychic forces can eventually take the form of organic trouble. Hans Dörfler points out in a lecture, "Nervöse Magenkrankheiten" (Münch, Med. W. 1920) that nervous irritation of the vagus can declare itself in an organic form and in the end actually leads to organic disease.

I have also observed severe intestinal neuroses which eventually led to ulcers or cancer, though only after a period of twenty or thirty years. Intestinal diseases often begin with ordinary cramp or diaphragm neuroses, then improve, recede, reappear, and the serious symptoms only declare themselves in course of time. *It is*

[1] K. Westphal and G. Katsch, Das neurotische Ulcus duodeni. (Mitteilungen aus den Grenzgebieten der Medizin und Chirurgie 1913, Bd. 26, H. 3, S. 405.)

[2] Cp. especially Bergmann, Das spasmogene Ulcus pepticum (M.m. W. 1913, Nr. 4.) ; Ulcus duodeni und vegetatives Nervensystem (B. kl. W. 1913, Nr. 51) ; Zur Pathogenese des chronischen Ulcus pepticum (B. kl. W., 1918, Nr. 22 und 23).

always the anxiety which creates those diseases of which one is afraid.

The most obstinate form of this species are the so-called stool hypochondriacs, who anxiously count every flatus, almost measure their daily motions, take the most expensive purgatives for constipation which does not exist at all, and stop eating, etc., for fear of an accumulation of fæces.

The simple forms have their origin in an anxiety neurosis. It is the same game that I have previously described in detail in the case of diseases of the stomach. The patients begin to fear that the stool is inadequate. The apprehension of course arises from other sources and is transferred to the functions of the stool. Certain symbolic associations, to which we shall have to refer later, have their part in this. The painful observation of the waste products of the digestive system now commences, as also the experiments with different forms of diet, laxatives, massage. In most cases of this kind " spastic constipation " is diagnosed. For the constipation is not the result of weakness of the intestinal muscles, but rather of excitation of the intestines.

Patients of this sort are so numerous that I may be spared the illustrative history of a case in point.

" Nervous diarrhœa " is also no more than a special manifestation of anxiety neurosis.

One form of diarrhœa in particular, the so-called " *colica mucosa,*" is an accompanying symptom of anxiety neurosis. Sometimes enormous quantities of mucus are excreted with pleasurable feelings. Diarrhœa is in such cases the actual equivalent of an emission, where the libido is either openly manifest, or operates in the form of anxiety.

By differential diagnostic we find according to *Ewald* and *Zweig* (Diagnose und Therapie der Magen-und Darmkrankheiten) that in the case of the nervous " colica mucosa " no mucus can be traced in the rectum between the attacks, whereas in colitis mebranacea signs of inflammatory redness and abundant phlegm are to be found objectively at all times. *Foges* (Zum Wesen der Colica mucosa. Wien. klin. Wochenschrift., 1918, Nr. 49) even maintains that he found the mucous membrane in colica mucosa conspicuously pale and free from mucus during the intervals. Foges emphasizes the sexual character of the disease, without reference to my remarks (II. Ed. : *p.* 75) which evidently escaped his notice.

The following observation by *Foges* is interesting :

" It is a case of a girl of seventeen, who stated that about a week before her menstrual periods she often had colic pains in the left hand region of the stomach. The pains disappeared on the excretion of skin-like, grey-white quantities of phlegm. There were at the same time vaginal emissions. The periods themselves passed off with little pain and lasted two or three days. The genital examination per rectum of this pale girl showed a small uterus in the middle, the ovaries not enlarged but perceptibly behind the uterus. Touching them caused discomfort.

" I examined this girl rectoscopically at different intervals so that I was able to observe the mucous membrane of the intestines before and after the attacks. I now noticed that the mucous membrane appeared pale and *dry* some time *after* the attack of pain and the excretion of mucus. By chance I was twice able to conduct a rectoscopic examination *before* an attack, and then the mucous membrane of the rectum and the lowest part of the flexure appeared *hyperoemic* and *swollen*.

" This fact of the reddening and swelling of the intestinal mucous membrane before the attack naturally suggested to my mind, as gynæcologist, that in the colica mucosa it might be a matter of an occurrence that called forth analogous changes in the intestinal mucous membrane, just like the endometrium in menstruation ; *i.e.*, that the colica mucosa represents a reaction of the intestinal mucous membrane to the inner secretion of the ovaries. There was abundant evidence that it was a case of a pathological phenomenon of the intestine, which only appears in the female sex."

The author's second observation is also significant.

A woman of forty-one, who had been undergoing X-ray treatment for severe, irregular hæmorrhage resulting from myomatosis uteri told me a year after all hæmorrhage had ceased, that the frequent attacks of mucous colic she had had since her youth had now completely vanished. This case seems to prove that the cessation of the ovarian functions can suffice to account for the disappearance of colica mucosa ; Ewald has to a certain extent intimated this, when he speaks of the presence of colica mucosa during the climacteric years and its disappearance when this stage has been passed.

For the present I must only support my hypothesis upon actually related cases, for those that give the true impression of colica mucosa very rarely come under observation at the proper time, as they have already in many cases developed into an inflammatory colitis, which seems to blot out the nature of the original picture. The reason for this probably lies in the fact that individuals suffering from colica mucosa react much more vehemently to an acute intestinal catarrh. The too frequent use of purgatives and enemas for constipation, which mostly accompanies colica mucosa with nervous girls, may also induce continual irritation in the mucous membrane of the large intestine ; sometimes I was also able to verify the fact that colica mucosa only developed into colitis of an inflammatory nature through local therapeutics ; tannin and lapis enemas are prescribed on account of the presence of mucus and in this way the sensitiveness of the mucous membrane is gradually increased and its condition grows permanently catarrhal.

Lastly we come to the case of Regelsberger, who mentions nasal menstruation. I have repeatedly heard of homosexuals who suffer from monthly nose-bleeding and regard these as their periods. Hirschfeld also mentions various equivalents to menstruation in men (Die Homosexualität, 1914. Verlag Luis Marcus, Berlin. S 130). According to Hirschfeld menstruation in men can take place from the mouth, nose and anus. Regelsberger's case may terminate these observations :

A certain man of a sensitive and irritable disposition suffered from regularly recurring intestinal hæmorrhage. Besides hæmorrhoids of moderate size, 8 c.m., I found rectoscopically mucous membrane above the sphincter which was extremely swollen and very actively injected with blood-vessels, and that looked like a bleeding sponge. The patient himself regards these hæmorrhages as his periods. At intervals of about three weeks he has typical premenstrual disturbances ; he gets restless, uneasy and irritable, like a nervous woman at the corresponding periods, and feels mentally relieved as soon as the bleeding begins. In connection with this case and another of a very hysterical woman suffering from colica mucosa with an inclination to hæmorrhage, Regelsberger remarks that the periodicity of the hæmorrhage is unexplained and adds :—" Possibly it has a purely psychic origin ; possibly, too, the influence of glands with an inner secretion plays a part in it."

The following observation made by me proves the truth of Foges's statement that originally functional diseases (colica mucosa) can develop into an organic disease (colitis ulcerosa) :

No. 43.—A woman of thirty consulted me about various nervous disturbances which were traceable to sexual causes. Her husband was only slightly potent and was moreover unfaithful and very seldom had intercourse with her, which did not suit her passionate nature. As she was very moral she controlled herself and declined all the well-meant proposals of other men. She complained of pains in the stomach, bulimia, sleeplessness and mucous diarrhœa, which had been treated by all the specialists as colica mucosa. Rectoscopically nothing was to be found. Her condition improved temporarily as the relations with her husband improved and he induced an orgasm in her by means of cunninlingus. But there was soon a recurrence of marital discord. The husband got a divorce. She then suffered from bleeding diarrhœa and the doctors pronounced it to be colitis ulcerosa, which was completely cured after two months' treatment at a sanatorium.

The associations between anxiety and the intestinal functions do not call for a more detailed discussion. Even fear felt by little children can by a sudden agitation of the vagus overcome the power of the sphincter ani. But similar things have also happened to adults under the influence of fear, terror or anxiety. Frequently there are involuntary stools, which escape the notice of the patient in his excitement. In most cases the feeling of anxiety is only accompanied by diarrhœa. Various obscure cases of "nervous intestinal catarrh" or "nervous dyspepsia" can be explained quite simply in this way. The following observation throws some light on this point :

No. 44.—Mr. F. O. had for many years suffered from "nervous" diarrhœa. All dietetic cures were powerless against it. A cure at Carlsbad, whither his wife accompanied him, increased the disease to such an extent that his agitation grew correspondingly and he had to relieve himself oftener than ever. He was mostly awakened in the mornings by an attack of diarrhœa[1] (very characteristic in cases of nervous diarrhœa !) and this was followed by three or four more during the day. A cold water cure at a home afforded slight improvement. But even afterwards he still had from two to four attacks daily, and never a solid stool. But the fact that he was completely free from these attacks when travelling, although he did not adhere so strictly to his diet as he did at home, is curious. He was, on the contrary, obliged to eat dishes of a very questionable quality at the various inns and restaurant cars. From time to time this man also suffered from attacks of giddiness, which in the same way refrained from appearing on his travels. The psychic investigations of the patient elicited some interesting facts. He was highly erotic and very polygamously inclined. His wife, who was his senior by a few years, had long lost all attraction for him. He forced himself to perform the act of coitus by picturing another woman. In order to satisfy his wife he postponed the ejaculation by desperately repeating his tables or his A B C a few times, thus transferring the psychic attention from the coitus to another conception and deferring the reflex act. Every beautiful woman he saw during the day roused erotic phantasies in him. He always pictured himself possessing her, how she undressed herself, etc. These

[1] Such morning attacks of diarrhœa are always traceable to an anxiety dream. The dream hardly crosses the threshold of consciousness.

phantasies recurred at night in his dreams, interrupted by the fear that his wife might catch him at it. Even in dreams the neurotic is not happy. His erotism ends with an anxiety affect. The attack of diarrhœa that woke him in the morning and forced him to hurry away, was a " rudimentary " attack of anxiety or an accompanying symptom of an anxiety dream. On his travels he used to play the so-called " gay dog," enjoy himself with the chambermaids of the various hotels and make the cheap conquests that flattered his vanity and satisfied his erotic needs. It was for this reason that his anxiety neurosis improved when travelling and his attacks of diarrhœa disappeared.

It is a characteristic circumstance of this nervous diarrhœa that the patients can look flourishing, whereas in a real intestinal catarrh they are very much pulled down.

The neuroses grow more complicated when patients suffer from the dread of anxiety, *i.e.,* in this case the *fear* of diarrhœa. The poor things dare not go into society, to a theatre, or into a train, if they are not sure of a lavatory close at hand to which they can resort. These phobias necessitate a fairly long psychanalytic treatment.

Patients sometimes transfer the seat of anxiety to the stomach. The attack resembles stenocardia, but the patients localize the pain in the centre of the stomach. We must, however, exercise great circumspection when diagnosing the " neurotic stomachaches " of elderly people as anxiety equivalents or accompanying symptoms. We have only of late years become acquainted with the various forms of arteriosclerosis of the abdominal arteries. The work of the Viennese school of Schnitzler and Ortner, has rendered this diagnosis possible. We have found a valuable diagnostic remedy in theobrominum natriosalicylicum (Diuretin). Nothnagel and his pupil Breuer have afforded proof, by means of clinical experiments, that the pains resulting from arteriosclerosis of the arteries diminish rapidly after the administration of large doses of diuretin or agurin, both of which have a similar action. Strophantus can also be applied for the purposes of differential diagnosis. Convulsive abdominal or cardiac pains which are relieved or cured on the administration of diuretin or strophantus are almost certainly indicative of arteriosclerotic pains in the stomach or of angina pectoris. Bromide, on the other hand, has a specific action in cases of nervous pains. When pains in the stomach vanish as if by magic after 10-15 drops tinct. valerian, or when after a dose of from 2-3 gr. bromnatrium taken in the evening, the night is passed without pain, we may fairly safely attribute the pains to neurotic sources.

We must, however, bear in mind the existence of certain composite forms in which the symptoms of two diseases are mingled. Some patients feel " *as if there were something sticking in the stomach.*" Great attention should be paid to the expressions used by patients. There are some people who actually have "somebody in their stomachs "[1] (*e.g.,* a husband who is repugnant to his wife).

[1] Im Magen liegen.

Flatulency plays an important part in anxiety neurosis, as does also the fear of flatulency. Flatulency is a frequent equivalent of anxiety.

Two anxiety equivalents having a certain diagnostic significance have only been cursorily mentioned here : *vomiting* and *bulimia*. Some patients are attacked at an unwonted hour in the street by ravenous hunger. I have an unpleasant recollection of the first patient who presented himself to me with this symptom because I was over hasty in my diagnosis and, coming into frequent contact with the patient in question, I am perpetually reminded of my carelessness.

No. 46.—Mr. J. R., fifty-four years of age, complained of a sudden attack of bulimia—especially at mid-day. Whether in the street or engaged on some business matter (it also happened in trams, buses, or in his bath), he was suddenly seized with such ravenous hunger that he was obliged to hurry to the nearest restaurant and get something to eat. The sensation of hunger did not confine itself to any particular hour. It occurred most frequently in the morning, even though he had just had a substantial breakfast. He endeavoured to avert this unpleasant feeling by partaking of an early lunch. In vain. After an interval of one to one-and-a-half hours he was again attacked by bulimia. It is characteristic of this condition that even the consumption of a substantial meal fails to satisfy the hunger. The attack never occurred in the afternoon, but was sometimes experienced at night, so that the patient never went to sleep without having provided himself with some rolls, fruit or biscuits on the bed-table.

Diabetes suggested itself to me and I examined him as to the usual well-known symptoms of thirst, polyuria, dryness in the throat, itchings, etc. The replies indicated diabetes. The thirst was occasionally as tormenting as the bulimia. During the morning he was sometimes compelled to drink four mugs of Pilsner beer in order to still the hunger and thirst. He was obliged to get up three or four times in the night to urinate and also suffered in the daytime from a positively torturing desire to micturate. He urinated every half-hour and the act always appeared to him to fall short of completion. A peculiar twitching and irritation in the urethra would then produce the desire to urinate. Dryness of the throat, soreness of the gullet and slight pruritus were also evinced. Examination of the urine revealed the undoubted presence of nylander. I therefore diagnosed diabetes and prescribed the diet accordingly. After a week I found not a trace of sugar and I was disposed to attribute the improvement to my diet. Nor did I hesitate to impart this opinion to the patient. My surprise may be imagined when he informed me that he had not changed his diet by a single iota. A friend had advised him to have his urine analysed in a " chemical laboratory " and no " trace " of sugar had been found there.

It then transpired for the first time that on the night before I examined him he had partaken of a large quantity of sweets. It was a case of " alimentary glycosuria." But my prognostication that this condition might well be symptomatic of incipient diabetes did not find favour with the patient. He was not going to allow such theories to interfere with his pleasure in good living. And strange to say, he was right. Six years later I again examined his urine ; during that period the patient would not hear of analysis, and I found no trace of reducing substances. This case proves how careful one should be in diagnosing and prognosticating. Nor is a *single* sugar test ever sufficient. The urethra may have contained other reducing substances (uric acid) in considerable quantities.

The nature of this bulimia and polyuria was made clear to me in later years after I had acquired a deeper understanding of neurotic symptoms through similar cases and by studying the works of Freud. Mr. J. R. was suffering from anxiety neurosis which I had simply failed to recognise. He had just separated from his wife after many disputes and was living alone with his aged mother. The suddenly enforced abstinence was very irksome to him. He suffered from frequent erections. He was afraid of venereal disease and could not bring himself to frequent a brothel. It was at this period of psychic conflict between libido and anxiety phantasies that the bulimia and symptoms of irritation of the uro-genital tract commenced. The poor tormented creature, who had not enough means to satisfy his erotic instincts, then took refuge in the practice which he had found beneficial in his youth. He began to masturbate; whereupon the various symptoms of anxiety neurosis disappeared. He was obviously incapable of enduring abstinence and the masturbation was the lesser evil for his organism. Some years later he looked me up to consult me about writer's cramp. With the exception of slight irritability, a disposition to weep, pressure on the head (neurasthenia), and the aforesaid writer's cramp, which yielded rapidly to psychic treatment, he felt perfectly well. During the psychic treatment of the writer's cramp, which was easily interpreted as "distaste for work," I learnt the details of his malady above related. He admitted that he was still obliged to masturbate once or twice a week.

The following is a similar case :—

No. 47.—Mr. H. H., a man of thirty-six, born of healthy parents, who was married and had several healthy children, the youngest of whom was five years old, had suffered for the past four-and-a-half years from various stomach troubles. He mostly felt a " pressure and twitching " in the stomach all day long. Between ten and eleven a.m., he used to get tormenting attacks of bulimia. Between five and six p.m. the other attacks would appear (giddiness, faintness, sickness and perspirations). He fell asleep with great difficulty and was then obliged to breathe very deeply as if he were being suffocated. He always wore his trousers very loosely round his body, as the stomach was always so distended. At night the flatulence became most tiresome. He also had to get up continually to urinate. On falling asleep he would have the most unpleasant thoughts: " I shall soon die and leave my family unprovided for." Or: " I shall lose my post through my illness and may have to go begging." His head always felt constricted as if he were wearing a helmet. The stool was slightly obstructed. The tongue slightly furred. The size of the stomach normal. (Also intestinal rumbling ! A frequent symptom of anxiety neurosis. Atonia of the stomach is often of sexual origin !)

The symptoms were traceable to a very characteristic form of aerophagia. By taking deep breaths he pumped great quantities of air into the stomach, which then caused a variety of sensations.

For the past five years he had practised coitus interruptus.

Therapeutic treatment : A pessary and appropriate counsel regarding the ill habit of aerophagia. At the end of a few weeks his condition showed a striking improvement and after a few months he was perfectly well.

This sudden attack of bulimia, as is the case with hunger in general, has a very interesting relationship to the libido. A violent desire can manifest itself in the form of tormenting hunger. It is the well known hunger for love. The fact that the attacks always took place between ten and eleven in the morning had in this case a special reason. At this hour his housemaid was alone in the house as his wife went shopping. The man, whose marriage left him unsatisfied owing to the practise of coitus interruptus, turned his images of desire to another object. The bulimia really said : Go home and satisfy yourself with the housemaid. This idea did not come into his conscious mind, as he was highly moral.

The bulimia appeared as a substitute for this. I know of many similar cases. The desire for life and love declares itself in a marked increase of appetite, while loss of appetite often points merely to the lack or the relinquishment of sexual desires. We must in all cases remember this psychic interpretation of bulimia. Sudden attacks of bulimia, especially when they are accompanied by giddiness, paræsthesias, congestions, flatulency, and diarrhœa always give rise to the assumption that they are symptoms of an anxiety neurosis or masked anxiety attacks. The clinical picture grows much more distinct when the attacks of bulimia or " emptiness of the stomach " are accompanied by a sensation of anxiety. Air hunger is often used to produce organic symptoms (tympanism, food-repeating, passing of wind, raising of the diaphragm).

The following lines from Prof. Dr. Jagic's essay " Ueber Neurosen der Respirations—und Verdauungsorgane," (Wien, med. Wochenschr., 1919, Nr. 40) prove how little is known of the malady of air hunger :—

" In rare cases nervous disturbances of the intestinal movements lead to a curious condition that has been repeatedly observed during recent years. The chief symptom of this condition is an inflated stomach. An organic cause for the peculiar meteorism could not be found in these cases, even with the most careful examination. Such cases then suggested the idea of a neurosis. In the majority of cases the meteorism abated after a dose of atropin. For further symptoms of a vagus-neurosis, hypersecretion, slackening of the pulse, eosinophilia, were either found in such cases simultaneously or each of these signs of an increased vagustonus was found separately in various groupings. In individual cases the X-ray examination showed local spasms in various intestinal sections, with a strong accumulation of gases. It appears that vasomotor disturbances in the intestinal wall in such cases also hinder the reabsorption of gas. This condition was called tympanismus vagotonicus. The exclusion of an organic contraction of the intestines and an intestinal trouble already past, namely, typhus and dysentery, is important for the diagnosis of this condition."

I, too, have also seen a few cases of " tympanismus vagotonicus " (pneumatose) in the hospital. It was always the case of an aerophagist who in the absence of the doctor was able to pump air into himself by sighing and cleverly taking breath. Hysterical tympanismus, the various appearances of swellings in the stomach, are also caused by swallowing air. The neurotic can in this ingenious manner create organic substrata for his parapathias. The mechanism of air hunger explains those to us who eternally suffer from fear of flatus and who can produce flatulency by the hour.[1] They can naturally go to no party or theatre in case this misfortune should happen to them. This excessive generation of gases is due to no digestive trouble, but is only the result of eating air.

The success of the therapy often determines the diagnosis. A regulation of sexual disharmonies, a solution of the psychic conflicts

---

[1] Zola depicted such a " Bombardeur " in " La Terre."

and the relief caused by a free expression of thought, produce a speedy improvement. But not always. In many cases another psychic component has to be reckoned with. There are " compulsion neuroses " and " hysteria of every-day life " for which the most important thing is relief and freedom from *repressed* thoughts.

The soul-doctor must always seek the " *psychic conflict* " that manifests itself in stomach or intestinal troubles. He will often come upon sexual causes, but also at times they will be the results of a bad conscience, as proved by the interesting case of dietary disturbance (No. 42). I should be trespassing beyond the limits of this treatise were I to point to the correlation between religion and diseases of the stomach. I have given a detailed account of these associations in my pamphlet, " Der Nervöse Magen." [1] The next chapter will give us still further insight into the psychology of dietary troubles and will show the practitioner how complicated and concealed can be the psychic associations which manifest themselves in the form of " nervous vomiting " or " nervous dyspepsia."

[1] Verlag, Paul Knepler. Wien, 1917.

CHAPTER VIII

CLINICAL PICTURE OF ANXIETY NEUROSIS: NAUSEA AND HYPEREMESIS GRAVIDARUM.

CHOKING, hiccoughs, belching, retching and even chronic sickness can also be symptoms of an anxiety neurosis or of an anxiety hysteria, combined or alternating with feelings of anxiety. This is an obscure province where much has still to be accomplished. The cases of so-called " nervous sickness " are much more frequent than one would believe. They are usually cases of repressed phantasies linked with affects of disgust. The sensations of disgust are transmuted in a very roundabout way into a tendency to vomit and into actual sickness. Many a case of enigmatical sickness is solved most strikingly by the psychanalytic method.

Our feelings of pleasure and displeasure oscillate between the two poles of desire and aversion.[1]

Aversion is the fear of contact: desire is the wish for it. Experience of daily life shows us that the thought of things that are repulsive to people only produces a feeling of nausea if a sensation of contact is combined with this thought. We can calmly watch somebody else eat certain food that seems to us disgusting ; but if we are asked to share it, the idea of contact immediately manifests itself and we experience a feeling of disgust, and the attempt to overcome this can eventually reach the pitch of the most acute defensive reaction of the organism, the act of vomiting. Vomiting is the mechanical response expressed by the fear of contact in a coarse manner.

Feelings of shame and nausea must first be inculcated into the child and they are the first sensations that he has to express to the outside world, against his innermost convictions. Both thus gain the disguised and concealed character that distinguishes all sexual sensations. In this way the feeling of nausea is first emphasized as a sex feeling and it is this emphasis that constitutes its deepest significance. Nausea is a sex feeling par excellence, or, more accurately expressed : it is the faithful accompaniment to all sexual feelings. In the child the daily digestive functions belong to the sexual feeling ; a child does not differentiate so exactly as the adult : whatever happens in the erogenous zone, belongs to sexuality. Defecation and micturition in the child are connected with sex feelings. Having learnt from his surroundings that these conceptions are disgusting, he now connects the idea of what is

[1] The remarks on aversion are partly taken from a larger work, " Der Ekel." (Die Wage, 1903.)

disgusting with the idea of sex for the rest of his life. These conceptions of the relations of defecation, etc., to sex, disappear in the adult except for obscure remainders, but not completely and not with everybody. In some people this erogenous zone is fixed for their whole lives and we designate a morbid fixation of this kind as a paraphilia. *It is well known that all paraphilias are fixations of the first sexual feelings.* If this morbid fixation is very marked, deeds can be committed which would cause violent repugnance in a normal being. The child puts every óbject into his mouth. The mouth of the child is equally an erogenous zone. The act of sucking is for mother and child a sexual act. Havelock Ellis (" The Sex-feeling," a biological study, Würzburg, 1903) speaking of the interpretation of the sex impulse, appropriately remarks :

" There is a similar connection between infants and nursing-mothers.* The mother derives the pleasant sensation of relieving her full breasts from the child, and although, on a higher mental plane, intellectual factors force this side of natural alimentation into the background, in primitive relationships and among animals the desire for this relief forms a genuine bond between the mother and her offspring (in a sense, a detumescent instinct). The analogy is, in fact, a very close one. The erect nipples correspond to the erect penis, the greedy, watering mouth of the infant, to the moist, throbbing vulva, the life-giving albuminous milk, to the life-generating albuminous semen. The complete mutual physical and psychical satisfaction derived from the transmission of a valuable organic fluid which takes place by the process of sucking is the only real physiological analogy between man and woman at the culmination of sexual intercourse."

Ellis further refers to the Spanish sociologist *Salilas*, who has proved that the Spanish popular tongue has given clear expression to this analogy.

The taking of nourishment is therefore the child's first sexual act. We shall now understand why all sex feelings are associated with feelings of disgust. We shall be able to grasp the radical meaning of the connections between the digestive processes and sexuality, the primeval co-operation of hunger and love. Only by starting out from these assumptions shall we be able to understand those repulsive phenomena known to the psychopathologist as sexual coprolagnia and urolagnia, *i.e.*, " those forms of perversion which connect the acts and products of the final metabolic excreta with the libido sexualis and procure from them sexual gratification." (*Iwan Bloch*, Beiträge zur Pathologie der Psychologia sexualis, Dresden, Verlag von H. Dorn, 1903.) This writer explains very strikingly that he has, after a thorough study of the question, become convinced that these are not cases of morbid phenomena, since the most diverse investigators, among others Tarnowski and he himself, were able to observe similar inclinations in people of perfect mental health.

An association of ideas was formed from infancy—as we have already stated—between sexual acts and the large and small cloacas. He says : " It cannot therefore be asserted that the disgust of themselves and of the act just perpetrated, which befalls the coprolagnist and the urolagnist after the completed sex act, arises from the fact that those acts were committed while in an irresponsible condition." This moral " Katzenjammer " made its appearance after all sexual acts. He quotes *Eulenburg :* " Just as every great physical and psychical pleasure is inevitably followed by a bitter after-taste of reaction and disappointment, a stage of physical and moral wretchedness,—so is also sexual gratification, the most passionate and the most arduously obtained joy, followed by a feeling of revulsion and disgust." This feeling of aversion could therefore not be regarded as a standard for health and disease. A list of factors were united to prove this. As already the haut goût of certain gourmets is allied to this feeling, so did similar bridges lead from conceptions of aversion to sexuality.

As I have previously demonstrated, the feeling of nausea is acquired by children and is not inborn : it is much more likely to have been a feeling of surprise and of strangeness, which certainly bears a resemblance to repulsion and would account for the fact that we find almost every new, unaccustomed article of food more or less distasteful and can only bring ourselves to partake of it after a certain amount of resistance has been overcome. *Darwin* seems likewise to have realised this for he writes : " This was all the stranger, for I doubt whether the child really felt any repulsion, since its eyes and brow expressed great surprise and thoughtfulness. The protrusion of the tongue in the expulsion of some unpleasant matter from the mouth may serve to account for the origin of the protrusion of the tongue as a symbol of contempt and hate." This explanation, if not to be entirely rejected, does not seem to exhaust the significance of this symbolic action. Just as spitting is intended to convey to the person spat upon that he is an object of repulsion to us, so may the protrusion of the tongue serve, in part, to indicate this feeling.

The well known French psychologist *Richet* (" Les Causes de Dégout," 1887) maintains that aversion is aroused by things dangerous and useless. As the digestive and sexual excreta were either useless or according to far-reaching primitive ideas even highly dangerous, the genital-anal region became the general centre of repugnance. The untenableness of this hypothesis is easily proved. As in childhood the anal region belongs to the erogenous zones, it is natural that the genital-anal feeling should be preserved in all sexual feelings, and of such are shame and aversion. In spite of this there are many useless things which arouse absolutely no nausea at all in people. Some, for example, eat oysters with equanimity, while others feel the greatest repugnance for them. What is useless alone does not explain this disgust ; it has far deeper sexual roots, as we shall show later. Neither does the element of danger call forth disgust, for there are numberless poisonous foods which are highly dangerous and can be enjoyed without the slightest feeling of repugnance. A woman, too, can appear repugnant to us without being dangerous or useless. In support of this hypothesis *Havelock Ellis* refers to the fact that the Esquimos preserve the urine as a highly valued liquid and that to urinate at table is not considered in the least disgusting or shameless. According to *Burke* it is often incumbent upon the daughter of the house to look after the needs of the guests at meal times.

But this only proves that the Esquimos have in this respect remained in an infantile state. As little as the urinal excreta of her child, with which she is soiled several times a day, disgust the mother, as little as the children themselves feel any kind of aversion for it, and have, on the contrary, to be taught to regard these things as " dirty," just as little has the association between urine and disgust been formed in these tribes. There has simply been no sexual repression in this respect. *Children are all passionate coprophiliacs.* I do not think one can err in assuming an individual scatalogic tendency, which manifests itself as mysophilia in a direct form and as purity mania and disgust after repression.

A search amongst a number of people for objects which arouse their aversion will principally always bring to light certain sex symbols. A lady of my acquaintance stated that mice, snails and worms were repugnant to her. Now the mouse is a sex symbol that needs no further explanation. The lady in question vigorously denied that the snail should be a sex symbol, but already on the following day she related a dream in which snails were served up in a chambre séparée and a closer analysis proved that by snails she understood the vagina. I have had similar experiences with worms, snakes, oysters and all foods that are greasy, sticky and slippery. On the other hand repugnant foods can also be those to which we are unaccustomed. Where the firmly united association between food and hunger is lacking, a feeling of aversion can appear very easily. Thus the Jew finds food that is in itself appetizing, but is not ritually prepared and therefore in his opinion unclean, disgusting. These are already transitions leading to the symbolized feelings of aversion—aversion for a certain form of art, aversion for corrupted political conditions, aversion for one's profession.

We can say on the whole : *The unaccustomed is repugnant to us ;* a clean food, if it is associated with certain unpleasant conceptions, seems to us disgusting. I cannot eat soft cheese because in my youth I heard that it contained worms and this idea rouses a feeling of disgust. If I had eaten it from my youth, this association would belong to the feelings of disgust which have been overcome by habit. Many find kidneys repugnant because they think that the urine washes over them ; others cannot eat brains because it makes them think of human brains.[1] These associations can however

[1] A *cannibalistic* root of aversion is often found in neurotics.

in time be forced into the background, the aversion then disappears. Habit can therefore repress disgust.

The contrary also manifests itself on the other hand—habit generates disgust. A dish that has been partaken of many times will become thoroughly repugnant. It is the monotonous repetition of the same stimuli which drives the organism, always hungry for stimulation, into reaction. And this proves that disgust is an important regulative biological factor. Without disgust—the reaction from pleasures—that undulating motion would not arise, the alternation between the waves' rise and fall which is indispensable for our lives.

I count aversion among those psychic inhibitive feelings which, like the anchor in the working of a clock, guarantee its correct movement. Before coitus the inhibitive conceptions of the individual are overcome by desire ; after the sex act the inhibitions are set free ; the unrestrained outbreak of the sex impulse without inhibitive feelings would be dangerous to the individual. On the other hand it is possible for these inhibitive feelings to suppress the feelings of desire and the doctor has frequently the opportunity of observing that such inhibitions are the causes of great psychic impotence. As an instinctive feeling disgust plays an enormous part. It helps, like desire, to ennoble the race by natural selection and provides, like the instinct of self-preservation, for the safety of the individual.

We now come to the psychological explanation of a phenomenon, hitherto obscure, and defying every treatment. This is the well known *sickness of pregnant women.* The female desire is, we know, at the outset accompanied by two powerful feelings of displeasure—anxiety and disgust. Both must be overcome by the power of instinct. But the stronger the feelings of displeasure, the greater is the female resistance to coition. If pregnancy results and is for some reason or other undesired, the wish may arise in the woman's soul that her resistance had at the time been greater ; in other words : that anxiety and disgust had kept better watch. And just as the civilized woman compensates herself for the (unsuccessful) choice of her husband by a dreadful uncertainty in all her decisions relating to every-day life, in the same way are the succeeding acts of vomiting supposed to form the psychic substitute for the great aversion that failed before coition.

I know a case that seems to me to justify this view. A woman who was not impregnated by her husband, but by a lover, was so tormented by sickness that it was thought an abortion would be necessary. In her second pregnancy, caused by her husband, there was an entire absence of vomiting. It seems as if the bad conscience and the self-reproach of this woman, perhaps even the feeling of disgust for her own offence, had been transmuted into the physical act of vomiting. Nervous women therefore tend much more to vomit in this condition than those with strong nerves and a robust conscience. I do not doubt that many of the disorders

of pregnancy can be explained in this way. *The morbid cravings of pregnant women are also psychic equivalents of an unconscious sexual desire characterised as morbid.*
The vomiting of pregnant women has hitherto been an obscure puzzle to us. What hypotheses were not invented in order to explain these symptoms ; Since I have taken the psychological factor into consideration as well, it has become clear to me why some vomit and not others. Just this symptom shows the correctness of my assumption that in an anxiety neurosis *two* factors must work in unison in order to bring about the disease : the toxæmia and the psychic conflict !
Even the ordinary menstrual disturbances are often conditioned by nervous influences. Menstruation actually fails to put in an appearance from the very fear that it will not do so, and arrives late, as I could prove by numberless observations in my practice. How often have not women and girls come to me and confessed that they had good reasons to fear pregnancy. They had awaited the day of their periods in nervous suspense and to their horror they never appeared. In many cases this disturbance is caused by psychic influences and here tranquilisation works wonders. Gynæcologists underestimate the influence of the psyche and *Rudolf Denker* is right when he says : " Gynæcologists only know woman from the outside ; her inner being not even God knows, who is supposed to have created her."
Pregnancy facilitates the development of a severe anxiety neurosis.
The phenomena during pregnancy are well known. They correspond strikingly to the symptoms of the anxiety neurosis. The best known symptom is the change of taste as regards food. The symptom of pregnant women being unable to digest *meat* is especially frequent. Many evince such disgust for meat that they cannot swallow a mouthful. (Symbolic expression of sexual rejection !) In some parts this symptom determines the diagnosis of pregnancy. Sickness is just as frequent and sometimes becomes so insistent that pregnancy has to be artificially interrupted. Others have peculiar cravings which recall the desires of hysterics and chlorotics. A tendency to faint, palpitations, asthma, diarrhœa and constipation, salivation, spasms, shivering fits, complete the picture.
In the foreground of the neurosis, however, is the anxiety that is naturally connected with birth and is transformed into objective fear. The pregnant are filled with bad forebodings. They know for a fact that they will die this time, etc. Melancholy depression and a tendency to weep are often aggravated to the pitch of a real melancholia ; and it is altogether worthy of note that a large percentage of all female suicidal attempts is either made during menstruation or pregnancy.
The following case will prove to us how closely sickness is associated with psychic events :—

No. 47.—Mrs. P. K., aged thirty-three, suffered during her third pregnancy from severe vomiting, fainting fits, anxiety sensations and irritability. All attempts of the family doctor to assuage the sickness proved futile. Some days she was obliged to vomit as often as thirty times and was terribly run down. Finally, she developed the most peculiar attacks of cramp of the tongue, during which she moved her tongue rhythmically to and fro, but could speak no word. These attacks also took place when she tried to eat. Because of this trouble she sought my advice. A conspicuous point in the analysis was the fact that she had lost all libido and had since her last pregnancy refused to have sexual intercourse with her husband. When he came near her she cried : " *Don't touch me—don't touch me—because—.*" After a similar occurrence the first attack of dumbness set in.

Now it immediately occurred to me that the continuation of the sentence, " Don't touch me, because—" must solve the enigma of this case.

" Can you not tell me what you wished, or were obliged, to conceal from your husband ? Because . . . "

" I do not know. I think—because I am ill or unattractive. A pregnant woman is unattractive, don't you think so ? "

" I should not like to assert that. But I have another suggestion. Did you not want to say : ' Don't touch me, because I am unclean ? ' "

Now the woman wanted to answer and had an attack of this cramp. At first she put her tongue right out and quickly drew it in again. Then she rolled it up and wedged it between her teeth. Finally she rolled it and moved it quickly to and fro in the mouth. The attack, which at the end was a distinct image of an orgasm, culminated with a deep sigh and she became slightly pale and turned her eyes upwards.

Only then was she able to speak. I learned that she had had a love affair with a batchelor friend of her husband. She was quite convinced that the child was not her husband's. In this affair the seducer had understood how to initiate the woman in all kinds of perversions. Love-making *per os* was also diligently favoured, as the movements of her tongue had already revealed to me. She had felt very well during the first month of pregnancy. Then she heard that her lover had become engaged, whereupon the vomiting started and she felt the need of confessing everything to her husband. The attacks of the cramp in the tongue saved her from this, though they revealed just as much to the expert as the woman wanted to conceal.

After several long interviews the condition improved, and disappeared altogether on the birth of a dead (syphilitic !) child.

The sickness of pregnant women is comprehensible when we consider that there are many women who are obliged to vomit after every cohabitation with their husbands.

I am convinced that (except for rare cases of organic disease) the psychanalytic examination of women with hyperemesis gravidarum will confirm my investigations. Disgust plays the most important part in this symptom.

The best illustration of the above is afforded by a recent observation (1920) :—

No. 48.—A fairly strong woman of twenty-three, who had been married eight months and had been pregnant for six weeks, suffered from incurable sickness. She was taken to a sanatorium where the internists and gynæcologists suggested an abortion as an *ultima ratio*. They first made an attempt with artificial feeding. She only had iced milk and iced tea. In addition to this they gave her nutritive enemas which she was, however, just as unable to retain as the other food, as she vomited every five or ten minutes. She was very much run down and they feared for her life.

This was the report of the family doctor, whom the husband had begged to make another attempt in conjunction with a psychotherapist. The family doctor was acquainted with the fact—from my work on " Conditions of Nervous Anxiety,"—that I upheld the opinion that hyperemesis was always of a psychic nature and that ᵀ inferred an (unconscious) resistance to pregnancy. But my colleague (Dr. A. E. Mohr) did not fail to add that in this case he could not believe in a psychogenic disorder and was much more inclined to assume a toxæmia of the placenta. He had been confirmed in this belief by his consultations with Prof. K. and Doz. L. The urine was normal, except for slight traces of albumen.

During my discussion with the patient's highly intelligent husband, whose mother I had once cured of a heart neurosis, I learned the interesting fact that the patient had already once consented to an abortion on account of hyperemesis. She longed for a child and was inconsolable because an abortion (excochleatia) was to be carried out again on the following day. I enquired about differences in their married life and received the stereotyped reply that it was the happiest of marriages. Made shrewd by experience, I then enquired about the relations between the two families. The husband had to admit hesitatingly that his parents were against this marriage and that they had even broken off relations. His mother especially was so irreconcilable and hated his wife so much that he had not visited her for many months. He had only gone to see her again a few weeks ago—His wife had herself sent him to his mother, as he had just taken his doctor's degree and wanted to tell her this. He now remembered that his wife had not vomited this time at the beginning of her pregnancy and that the vomiting had only grown so violent about two-and-a-half weeks ago. I assumed some connection with his visit to his mother. (Hysterical people often express similar wishes, which give them an appearance of heroic generosity, whereas they secretly hope that the husband will be firm and not fulfil their wishes.) He had to corroborate the statement that the trouble had only acquired its menacing character since that visit, without his having any idea as to the connection between the two.

I continued my anamnesic investigations and heard that the patient had repeatedly informed him that she would not bind him, he could get a separation from her any day, she would always set him free. That kind of statement always contains a germ of truth. I enquired whether she had had any other relations before her marriage and learned that she had previously been engaged to a doctor and had broken it off. The assumption that the patient still loved her first fiancé was made probable by the fact that she was nearly always completely anæsthetic during coitus and only showed signs of feeling before the second pregnancy.

(*This anaesthesia with a hyperemesis is an important symptom and shows an inward resistance and an inner inhibition against pregnancy, also a dislike for the man who has caused it.*)

I was then taken to the patient who was lying in bed in a darkened room, holding a spittoon and giving the impression of being seriously ill. I dismissed the mother and nurse, vigorously assured the patient that she would not be able to vomit even if she wanted to, and began to tell her at once that I understood the misfortune of her marriage. Although she loved her husband, the thought that she was not recognized by his family was unbearable to her. She immediately responded with animation to this theme. The colour returned to her pale cheeks and her eyes shone. She laid stress on the fact that she belonged to a distinguished family and that her husband lived on *her* means, had done good business with the help of her brothers and had consequently been able to get his doctor's degree. She would not hold or bind her husband and had repeatedly set him free to return to his mother.

In the course of conversation she also confirmed the fact that she had not yet forgotten her first fiancé, although he had been a " devil-may-care." Neither did she hesitate to give me information regarding her anæsthesia. She had thought to herself : " This occurrence is the cause of numberless tragedies ! On account of a so-called pleasure, women desert their husbands !" She would rather her husband left her in peace.

E

Then I tried to explain to her the psychic mechanism of her sickness. " You do not want to have a child, because it would bind you to your husband for ever. You still want to preserve the freedom of your future decisions." She admitted this. Such thoughts had come to her, but her love for her husband had been stronger . . .

After further explanations I summoned the doctors and gave the following instructions. The patient was to leave the sanatorium that very day. She needed no nurse. The sickness would cease after hypnotic treatment and if it recurred now and then, it would not hurt her. She could eat what she fancied. There was no question of performing an abortion. As a transition to ordinary diet she should that day have minced meat and stewed fruit. (She had an aversion to milk !) I then hypnotized her, according to my method of catching the patient unawares, in a few seconds and gave her the suggestion not to vomit any more that morning and to welcome the thought that she would bear her child.

This met with startling success. She only vomited after two hours ; she was able to eat and then only vomited a little mucus and not food. The next day she returned home. After three days I found her at home in bed. I confirmed the impression by hypnotizing her a second time, in which she received the order to get up on the following day, take up her domestic duties and go for frequent walks.

After a few weeks had passed I learned from the family doctor that the patient was extremely well. She went out, worked in the house, went to the theatre and vomited only very little ; she ate a great deal, but developed a curious taste in food. On the third day she had already asked her husband for quite unusual delicacies, which he, however, always found means to procure. She thus explained in the organic language of the soul that her wishes pointed to something difficult of attainment.

This case proves the importance of psychotherapy. How much harm could be avoided if doctors would also consider psychic causes. How necessary would the instruction of doctors appear to be, through the medium of a psychotherapeutic college !

The sickness of pregnant women manifests an unconscious setting of hate for the new-born child. This element can persist after its birth. In most cases the hatred is transformed into an exaggerated love. The phenomenon of the " exaggerated reaction formation " will frequently demand our attention. It is just those women who harbour hostile feelings for the child during pregnancy that become exaggeratedly fond mothers.

CHAPTER IX

CLINICAL PICTURE OF ANXIETY NEUROSIS:
VOMITING

A S we learned in the preceding chapter, disgust, like shame, is a sexual feeling with a negative sign. It is a product of repression. In psychanalysis there is no province of deeper interest or one promising greater reward. Cases of cardialgia accompanied by feelings of aversion occur very frequently with an anxiety neurosis. Sometimes considerable differential diagnostic difficulties can arise, especially when the actual anxiety feelings are absent and vomiting appears as an equivalent of anxiety. That is chiefly the case when sexual aversion conquers the sex impulse. The psychic conflict, from which most neurotics suffer, is, as we know, a violent struggle between the sex impulse surging up from the unconscious, and sexual aversion laden with conscious inhibitory ideas. Wherever this sexual aversion carries a very high value, there is " nervous " sickness. The three cases of sickness, the analysis of which is dealt with in this chapter, bring us to the complicated psychic mechanisms and call for tests in similar situations.

No. 49.—Mr. Z. K., aged thirty-six, came to me on account of a peculiar malady. Every day after his dinner he was attacked by violent pains, which did not abate until he had put his finger in his mouth and brought up the whole meal. Sometimes he also vomited spontaneously. He had consulted nearly all the distinguished doctors and professors of Vienna in the matter. A pile of prescriptions (rheum, belladonna, natr. bicarbonic, menthol, argentum, intricam, cocaine, morphia, anæsthesin) proved that he had already tried everything that is usually applied with success in such cases. Most of the doctors diagnosed " nervous stomach trouble." A cold water treatment and a severe milk treatment were unavailing. What he ate was immaterial. He brought up everything. He was best when he went entirely without his mid-day meal, and this he often did.

It should be added by way of anamnesis that the sickness first occurred after a severe attack of migraine about four years previously and that the patient had been obliged, six years ago, to consult a doctor on account of obstinate headaches ; a highly developed syphilitic exanthem over the whole body was discovered, and also a concealed primary affect.

Objectively there was absolutely nothing perceptible in the patient, not even a sensitive spot. I got him to describe the course of the attack once more—was the pain very severe ? The patient now depicted the attack quite differently. In reality it was not a distinct pain, but rather a tormenting pressure. It frightened him. Then the pressure and the oppression harassed him so much that he would bring on the sickness. I asked if he had the pressure after other meals. " Only after the mid-day meal." I questioned further :

" Have you never yet vomited after your evening meal ? "

" No."

" Do you eat less in the evening ? "

" I cannot say that I do. As I often only drink a cup of coffee at mid-day, or else bring up everything, I frequently eat much more at night. But I soon fall asleep and no unpleasant feelings occur."

" Have you never tried to get in a little doze after lunch in order to overcome the pressure ? "

" That is impossible. I never lunch at home."

" What—you never lunch at home ? But you have been married for three years ? "

" Yes—but I always have business outside the house and then lunch wherever it is convenient."

I found that very suspicious. The marriage was evidently an unhappy one. For otherwise the husband would, like many other men, be glad to come home, if only to enjoy the advantages of home fare.

I therefore carefully probed further in this direction and learned that the man actually was unhappily married. I could not discover more on the first day. After two days he returned and was much more willing to be cross-questioned. I understood that he had several times caught his wife leading an improper life. He had found letters which proved it. He had moerover surer proofs—the admission of two lovers. He was a traveller. The thought that always pursued him here and on his travels was : While you work here your wife is deceiving you.

" Now I see why you do not wish to lunch at home. But I do not understand how you can live with your wife at all."

" I did chase her away about three months ago, when I discovered the last love affair. But she stood outside the door crying and begged me to let her in. She promised to improve. So out of pity I took her in."

" Is it not possible for her actually to improve ? "

" Inconceivable. I am certain that I shall soon catch her again. I shall tell her that I am off on my travels and shall then return secretly."

" I hope your wife will have learnt something from the experiences of the last three months and that you will have no further cause to be angry with her."

" Oh—no—I shall certainly catch her at it. She is too stupid and too sensual."

It was now clear to me that the sickness must have had some connection with his marriage, that it was a case of repressed ideas and sexual symptoms of defence. In this case it could only be *repugnance* for his own wife. There were still a few points in his married life to be cleared up.

Our consultation was continued :

" How do you live with your wife *now* ? "

" I do not look at her. She always wants to be affectionate with me and kiss me. I do not let her touch me and shout ' Don't touch me. You disgust me. You are a harlot ! ' "

" Have you had sexual intercourse with her during these three months ? "

The patient was obviously embarrassed and hesitated for a moment before answering. His pale face reddened slightly.

" I am obliged to tell you the truth in all things. I have almost daily intercourse with her."

" Who takes the initiative ? "

" My wife, of course. I have a bad habit : *When my stomach is satisfied I become sensual and want a woman.* But in the evenings I go straight to bed. My wife comes to me and begins to make love to me. But I hold her severely off . . . and go to sleep. In the mornings when I awake I always find myself next to my wife."

" Did you also cohabit in the afternoons formerly, when you were newly married ? "

" Yes—it has sometimes occurred. After a large meal. I am a very sensual man and cannot live without women. What am I to do now ? Am I to go to strange girls and even pay them for it ? I never kiss my wife during our sexual intercourse. I do it as if I were at a brothel. Often I say to her afterwards : ' After all you are only a low woman ! ' "

This obscure sickness was now much more comprehensible. A further analysis of the case brought the following facts to light : The patient was one of those with whom a replete stomach causes a violent libido. The alcohol which he drank at meals had also to be taken into account. He had urgent need of intercourse with a woman. He did not want to go to a stranger. He had an aversion to his own wife. " She lay on his stomach." (The symptom of pressure and pain in the stomach explains the conversion of this idea.) What was he to do in the matter ? He subconsciously remembered the monthly attacks of migraine that used to get better after he had vomited. The mechanism of the relief of pain by sickness was probably known to him. What did he do ? He tried to get rid of the food that had awakened his sexual feelings. The aversion he felt to his wife transmuted itself into a disgust of food. He put his finger into his mouth and forced himself to vomit. Or else the repugnant conceptions grew to such a pitch that he vomited involuntarily. At night he did not vomit because the sexual aversion was overcome, because his libido was greater than his disgust. I still conjectured that there was some perversion (fellatio) at the bottom of it. Otherwise the man would really have chased his wife away. But she seemed to practise a form of sexual gratification (fellatio ?) which he could not get with any strange girl and could not pay for out of his modest income. We shall later on study a similar case in detail amongst the analyses of complicated phobias. This case also bears the stamp of hysteria and is worthy of the practitioner's attention. The condition improved after psychanalysis. Pains and vomiting occurred much less frequently and seemed to dwindle.

I afterwards learned that I was right in my conjecture : they practised fellatio only. As a syphilitic he feared diseased descendants.

In all cases of nervous sickness we must seek psychic causes. We shall always hit upon sexual disharmonies, violent repressions and unconscious ideas of disgust. The poison-complex often plays a part and sometimes the warding off of coprophilic and cannibalistic impulses. Every case of vomiting that arises from no apparent cause calls for a certain analysis, of course only after all organic reasons have been excluded. The diagnosis is frequently attained by intuition rather than established with certainty. A fine diagnostic flaire is essential for the study of vomiting.

I should like here to publish a second, quite classic case, and will endeavour to depict the genesis of the psychanalysis as accurately as possible :—

No. 50.—One night I was called to a patient who was seriously ill. An old woman stood in an ante-room weeping. Her daughter was dangerously ill and she was convinced that her last hour had come. She had vomited all night and complained of terrible pains in the stomach. It was no longer to be borne. Would I, in Heaven's name, come as quickly as possible ? I hurried to the patient as fast as I could. I found a delicate, somewhat exhausted looking girl of twenty-two, whose clear blue eyes did not at all give the impression of a serious illness. This was not the first attack of sickness that she had had. She must have a tumour in the stomach, or cancer. She had had stomach trouble for about three years and lately she had vomited nearly every morning, but it had never been so violent as that night, and these terrible pains ! " Birth " pains could not be worse. She also had similar pains during her " periods." She begged me to relieve and help her as soon as possible.

The objective result did not in any way tally with the subjective statements. I asked her if she had lately been through many psychic struggles or excitements. This she denied. " Not more than usual." I told her that it was a case of nervous stomach trouble and that some kind of " repugnant " idea must have been the cause of the sickness and the pains. She could think of nothing like that. I prescribed cherry-laurel drops and a little morphia and promised to return on the following day.

The next day I found her much calmer and more controlled. She wished to speak to me alone and I then catechized her sharply. I learned the following facts : She had been engaged for three years and was having sexual intercourse with her fiancé, although, as I discovered later, they did not practise coitus. She was still *demi-vierge*. Unsurmountable obstacles stood in the way of marriage. The father was a strict Catholic, a Christian Socialist, and the lover was a Jew. This led to continual friction at home and left her not a moment's peace.

That of course did not explain the sickness.

" Have you had no repugnant idea which has dominated you ? " I asked. " Not that I know of. Oh yes, I remember. As I went to school yesterday— I am a teacher—I did not feel very well. I met many people whose faces were so repulsive to me that I was nearly sick--I had to look away when I saw any of them." " What did these people look like ? In what way did they differ from others ? " " I cannot say. They were repulsive to me." " Why ? " " I do not know." " You see, some other repugnant conception must have been associated with it, another component of your psychic life, a component that corresponded to the aversion to your liaison." " Not that I know of. I am very fond of my fiancé." " But perhaps because he is a Jew ? " " No," she answered. " Ever since my youth I have had a great liking for Jews and have liked associating with them best. But it has just occurred to me : I had a friend who worked in the same office with me—I was then a clerk—and I was very fond of her. We were in complete accord with each other. Now I have *broken* with her." " Why ? " " My attention was drawn to her true character." " What is her true character ? " " Do you know, Doctor, she has certain bad qualities characteristic of the Jewesses of Leopoldstadt ? " " On what occasion did you break with her ? " " On the Feast of Purim she went to another parish dressed in men's clothes. I told her that this was not proper for a respectable girl. Since then we have not met." " Was there otherwise no conflict ? " " No." " And your fiancé has never seen your friend ? " " Yes, he told me he could not understand how I could associate with a person of her stamp. It was he who opened my eyes to it." " What did your friend say about your fiancé ? " " She liked him very much and said : ' Do you know, I could straightway fall in love with that man. I could marry him at once.' " " So jealousy, and not your fiancé, opened your eyes. You evidently feared that by associating further with her, he might often meet her." She was silent. After a time she continued : " Now I remember a gentleman who always comes to see us and who wants to marry me." " Also a Jew ? " " No. He loved me so much that he told me he would shoot himself if I did not marry him, whereupon I replied : ' And if I had to marry you, I should shoot myself on the day of the wedding. So somebody's life has to be sacrificed and you will understand that my own life is of the greater value to me.' " " Was this gentleman with you recently ? " " Yes, he was here three days ago in order to congratulate me, and my father hinted how nice it would be if I would marry him now."

She was again silent for a time : " This gentleman has a brother who has lived with us for years as a lodger." " How do you stand with him ? " " I dislike him extremely." " What sort of men are they that you dislike so intensely ? " " Sensual natures." The strong emotional stress laid on this utterance made me very suspicious. Wherever such passionate repugnance existed, there must also certainly have been a marked tendency to a strong attraction. After a pause she said : " Now I remember something that greatly disgusted me. The day before yesterday my sister brought some Christian sausages home and I did not want to eat them. I said I would get some ' Jewish ' ones for myself. No sooner said than done. I fetched a couple of sausages from the Jewish stores. As I ate them my sister said all kinds of disgusting things to turn me against them : ' Doesn't it repel you to eat such sausages ? Don't you know what filth the people put into them ? They spit into them,' she said, and she added worse things which I cannot repeat."

" *You see, that was the conception of disgust that you wanted to withhold from your conscious mind and that was the cause of your alleged stomach trouble, of the vomiting and of the pains in the stomach.* In your unconscious mind you thought : Perhaps there is some truth in it, perhaps they do really spit into the sausages ; and it was this unconscious idea that caused that uncontrollable sickness. I will also hazard the statement that the conflict reaches still further. *Your fiancé sticks in your stomach.* You would rather *break* with him and take the other one if you had not already given yourself to him. In other words : You would now prefer to eat your sister's sausages, if you had not already the Jewish ones inside you. And the sickness is nothing more than the symbolic endeavour to liberate yourself from this situation."[1]

On the following day she came to see me. The patient who was seriously ill, who had received me with the diagnosis of a " tumour in the stomach," had got up soon after my departure and could already teach the next day. She had not vomited once more.

What had remained, however, was a feeling of pressure on the stomach, an indescribable feeling of anxiety that something " terrible " was going to happen to her.

Further investigations proved that all her troubles were due to her liaison, in which the fear of pregnancy only permitted frustrated excitement. She tried to make herself believe in a love that no longer existed. Finally, I explained these circumstances to her. She contested it all with great affect and I then brought my chief argument to bear :

" Why do you not marry the man if you love him so intensely ? Is he in a position to support a wife ? "

" Certainly. At first he was not. But now he has become independent and is materially very well off."

" Well, even the opposition of your father will hardly stand firm against a good match. All obscure relations are injurious to such a trouble as you are suffering from. Try and persuade him to solicit your hand."

She promised to follow my advice.

After a week she came to me again. " You see, Doctor, everything has happened just as I said it would. My fiancé has proved himself to be a man of honour. He at once wrote to my father and solemnly asked for my hand."

" And your father ? "

" — declared that he would hear nothing of this marriage. Perhaps he would have given in in spite of this, as mother was on my side. But my sister, who is terribly anti-semitic, announced decidedly that the moment I married a Jew she would commit suicide."

" Then what is your decision in this matter ? "

" You must admit, Doctor, that I cannot be the cause of my sister's death ? I am having a dreadful struggle. I do not know what to do. Advise me, help me ! "

I drew the patient's attention to the answer she gave her rejected suitor who threatened to shoot himself : " One of us must die. Must I be the one ? " I assured her that her sister's threat should not be taken seriously. She would certainly not shoot herself.

The girl vigorously contested this : " She certainly will shoot herself. You do not know my sister. If she says so, she will do it."

[1] Another reason for this vomiting is found in the idea of fellatio (sausages are phallic symbols !).

" And have you no fear that your fiancé will commit suicide, if you now desert him ? "

" I don't think about it. I cannot live without him. But I believe he would soon console himself."

Now I realised that her opposition to this alliance was just as strong, if not stronger, than her fondness for the man. I proved to her that her love could not be very great and that a woman in love leaves her father and mother and even her sister (with whom, by the way, she always quarrelled) to follow the man she loves. She vehemently denied this and could only repeat the refrain : " She could not have her sister's death on her conscience." She demanded definite advice.

Now he who is experienced in psychotherapy will take good care not to take sides in the struggle of contradictory feelings, if it is not absolutely necessary. He only transfers the conflict from the unconscious to the conscious mind. I did likewise. I analysed her feelings and left the decision to her.

After three months I met her in the street. She looked flourishing and was hardly recognizable.

" How are you ? "

" Very well.—I have gained eight kilos."

" Are you married ? "

" Oh, no. After full consideration I wrote to my fiancé declining to marry him. Oh—I am so happy ; for I feel physically so well. I have a good appetite, sleep peacefully and am happier and more contented than ever before."

Only a few days ago—two years after the last conversation—she came to see me again. She is still very happy, as if she had escaped from some danger. The anxiety neurosis is completely cured.

I need not dwell upon what would have happened to the patien t in this case if she had not been treated psychotherapeutically. In any case she would have been unnecessarily tormented, on account of an organic stomach trouble, with all the weapons of the modern pharmacopœia, as in the case of No. 41. Every case of sickness which manifests a certain amount of anxiety at the very least raises the suspicion that it might be a neurosis. I am fortunate enough to be able to recount another interesting case of nervous sickness. In this case, too, feelings of anxiety and aversion were mingled in a curious manner. This is worthy of note in consideration of the fact that I succeeded in curing the obstinate vomiting at *one* sitting, whereas various specialists had already tried their luck in vain for a fortnight.

No. 51.—I found Mrs. L. K. in bed. Her absolutely flourishing appearance contrasted curiously with her complaint that she had not been able to eat anything for a fortnight. She brought up all that she ate. She felt an unpleasant sensation of disgust, a vague anxiety, followed immediately by such violent sickness that she had no time to put out her hand for the basin. (She had already been treated unavailingly by doctors with galvanization, Carlsbad Waters, tincture of iodine, creosote, alkaloid, etc.)

I gave the lady, who was very intelligent, to understand that it was probably a case of repressed ideas, caused by some kind of phantasy or real experience. Would she care to be psychanalysed ? She consented and I began. I told her to close her eyes and tell me what she was thinking of. She of course replied, like most patients, " Nothing. There is absolutely nothing in my mind." Opposition to the revelation of the unconscious secret is in such cases so strong that weeks and often months pass before it can be overcome. Countless ways and means are used in order to break the resistance and create a breach in this stubborn negation. One of the best means is through dreams. After a successful dream analysis which convinced the patient, her resistance quickly yielded.

I enquired whether she were troubled by vivid dreams, to which she replied in the affirmative. Almost every night she awoke from a horrid dream. Mostly they were dreams of dead people, murderers, thieves or wild beasts. " What did you dream last night ? "

" I have already forgotten that. No, wait—I have just remembered. *I dreamed that I was in the ' Diana ' baths and had bathed with my little boy. Suddenly I ducked him. I repeated this several times until he was almost drowned.* Then I awoke, bathed in perspiration, and happy that it was only a dream."

The anxiety dreams of neurotics have typical characteristics. We shall discuss these typical anxiety dreams in detail later. Now I shall only reveal the fact that this bathing dream was typical. Young girls dream it when they play with the desire to surrender themselves to a man. It is the child, the result of these love-joys, that they drown. Young women who are not satisfied with their marriages and who prefer another man who happens to be courting their favour, also dream the same thing. The child is the hindrance to a new marriage. They put it out of the way. (The child is drowned in the waters!) For an anxiety neurotic is incredibly cruel in his dreams. The dream becomes an anxiety dream because the suppressed desire is the weaker. Whenever two desires of a conflicting nature struggle for mastery, the weaker, submissive, suppressed one is manifested as anxiety. Here, in this case, the wish : Oh, if I could be childless ! was the weaker. The wish : Oh, may the child be spared to me ! was the stronger. The dream, the domain of the unconscious, fulfils one of the wishes. But this fulfilment contrasts vividly with the desires of the conscious mind. They awake with all the somatic signs of anxiety (palpitations—perspiration—trembling).

I took good care not to reveal this interpretation to the patient. I did not wish to impute any meaning to the dream. She was to interpret it herself so that there should be no more escaping. I therefore questioned further as to whether she had been alone at the " Diana " baths.

" No, a friend was with me. Of course—she was so repulsive in my dream. She had several sores and they wanted to turn her out. But a gentleman intervened and said : ' I know that rash. It is not infectious.' "

" What comes to your mind in connection with your friend ? "

" She is a student at the conservatoire. She has singing lessons from the same professor as I do. The other day she complained of pains and showed me a sore on her leg. That was really disgusting."

" You see, there we have a repressed idea. But go on. Who was the gentleman in your dream who intervened ? "

The patient reddened and hesitated for some moments. Then she replied quickly and carelessly : " That is quite an indifferent personage who has nothing to do with me."

" Please tell me all you know about this gentleman. There are no indifferent people in dreams. I have an idea that you are concealing something from me."

" Why should I ? I have no reason to do so. The gentleman is also a singer and often goes to the house of my friend of whom I dreamed."

" What sort of a man is he ? "

" A strikingly tall, handsome man, who courts every woman."

" You, too ? "

" Unfortunately—"

" Why do you say unfortunately ? "

" Because it is no honour to be courted by Mr. X. Besides he is not healthy."

" No ? What is the matter with him ? "

" May I tell you ? You will not betray the things I speak to you about, to anybody ? "

E*

" That is my duty."

" He h́as been infected. He is syphilitic."

" When did you hear that ? "

" Two weeks ago I went to see my friend. I noticed a disgusting smell of iodine. Mr. X lives, by the way, in the room next door belonging to her mother. I asked what that horrible smell was. Would you believe it, my friend told me that X. had got into a nice mess. He had been infected. She was so terrified lest she herself should have caught it too. At this juncture she showed me the sore on her leg. But that was only a harmless carbuncle."

" So that was two weeks ago. Had you seen Mr. X. often before this ? "

" Of course ; he courted me, like all women."

" Did you like him ? "

" Well—yes—he is a very handsome man, *although I attach importance to such things.*"

" Although you attach importance to such things ? "

" That was a slip of the tongue. I meant to say : Although I attach *no* importance to such things."

Slips of the tongue belong to those symptomatic acts by whose analysis Freud[1] has gained everlasting merit. It reveals the truth from the unconscious mind, a truth that has won through against the will power and the control of the conscious mind.

There was no further resistance in this case. I drove the patient into a corner, until she admitted that her husband excited but never satisfied her. (He suffered from ejaculatio præcox.) Mr. X. had wooed her passionately. A fortnight ago she had gone straight to him to discuss a rendezvous. When she learned the truth she ran away and returned home in a state of incredible excitement. Then she ate some pork that was too fat and thoroughly upset her digestion.

" Well, the pork is certainly not the cause of the sickness. You felt a sense of disgust with Mr. X. You repented of your weakness and thought : If I had gone to him two days earlier, I too should now have been infected. This " unconscious disgusting idea " the fear of infection, was the cause of the sickness. And you still love the man. Your dream last night signifies a fulfilment of the wish : The child is put out of the way, my friend's rash is not infectious."

The patient stared at me in amazement. " I myself thought of something similar on the first night. And you believe that was really the cause of the sickness ? "

" We shall see—"

The following day the lady was up to receive me. She did not allow me to speak :

" Doctor, you must first look at my boy to-day. His cough worries me."

" And how are you ? The sickness ?—"

" Is gone. Oh, I must take a back seat to-day. Please do look at the boy."

She was cured at one sitting. The matter was disposed of. It was painful to her to return to these unpleasant things.

When anxiety neuroses, especially in women, are accompanied by sickness, one will never do wrong in seeking an emotionally coloured sexual repudiation or, in other words, *disgust.*

Such patients are frequently sexually anæsthetic.

Those idiosyncrasies, which are very often psychically conditioned, are of particular analytical interest. There also exists a " psychic anaphylaxia." The sensitiveness of patients against certain foods grows to such a pitch that grave organic symptoms make their

[1] The Psychopathology of Every-day Life.

appearance, which almost put one in mind of a toxæmia. As soon as we enquire into the earliest symptoms we find that they were at first quite trifling and increased in the course of time. Then, quite reflexly, an organic reaction against certain food is manifested. (Conditioned reflex of Pawlow.) There are, for example, people who cannot bear the " skin on milk," and have to vomit if they chance to swallow some. In some cases I was successful in proving a reaction against repressed cannibalism. Other neurotics cannot eat blood food (black pudding, raw beefsteak, etc.) and are obliged to vomit if they only eat a mouthful of them. This is a symptom of repressed sadism (vanhirism) and calls for an analysis that goes back to childhood, in which these atavistic instincts are very highly developed.

In most cases an apprehension of the results of having eaten certain foods is formed. Even the thought of the food rouses defensive reactions of nausea. Frequently they are only superficial associations with the blood complex. (Carrots, all red foods, red ices, raspberries, strawberries.) The organic idiosyncrasy can nearly always be analysed as a " psychic anaphylaxia." Other conceptions of anxiety belong to the province of the phobias. Some people tremble with fear that the soup may contain a hair or a pin. Others believe they might swallow small animals. The far-reaching hypochondriacal fear of poisonous foods is also proved to be psychic, determined by the poison complex which plays a large part in the phantasies of all neurotics.

One should never fail to examine psychologically every case of sickness that appears to be the result of eating certain kinds of food. I have only been able to give a few examples in these chapters. The exhaustive work on nervous diseases of the stomach has not yet been written. But the practitioner should bear in mind that most chronic stomach troubles are of psychic origin or have at least a psychic superstructure. The central point of all the symptoms is, then, the fear of injurious results. And how many stomach troubles, especially cases of sickness, do not evince associations with a bad conscience, and are themselves punishments dictated by the neurotic to himself! No other sphere awaits a more exact, systematic investigation and offers at the same time such possibilities of startling success. Sexuality finds such variety of expression in the organic language of the stomach, for which there is no rule. Every fresh case is a novum and requires the doctor's sharpest intuiti n.

CHAPTER X

CLINICAL PICTURE OF ANXIETY NEUROSIS:
CONGESTIONS, FAINTING, VERTIGO

A SPECIAL form of anxiety is that known as head anxiety. It either appears in connection with a feeling of anxiety or as an anxiety equivalent. Patients complain of " Congestions." All the blood goes to the head, the face burns, there is singing in the ears and quivering before the eyes. Or else it is as if a curtain were falling before them. Their faces redden and they have the sensation of anxiety that they are going to have a " stroke." Sometimes the symptoms of head anxiety are associated with slight vertigo. Vertigo can be associated with sickness and violent perspiration, so that the malady resembles a menière. Symptoms connected with the lungs and heart are combined with it. Patients are obliged to take a deep, convulsive breath, or else the attack culminates in a violent tachycardia. One of my patients had to yawn for a considerable time before the attack was over.

No. 52.—Mr, J. V., a herculean man of forty-six, with sound organs and soft arteries, complained of having had congestions and vertigo for three years. Suddenly the blood would rise to his head and he would feel as if his last hour had come and that he was going to have a stroke. He was obliged to lie down at once and have cold compresses on his head for some time. Only when he gave way to uncontrolled flatulency at the end of the attack, did he feel a certain amount of relief. The blood " distributed itself " slowly. He attributed the trouble to " wind in the wrong place."

It was in reality a case of mingled hypochondria and anxiety neurosis. The patient was formerly an onanist and then practised coitus interruptus with a widow whom he must not impregnate. He dared not go to a brothel for fear that he might have a " stroke " there and everybody would then know of his vicious life. A speedy recovery was brought about by the use of a condom in his sexual relations.

The relief caused by free discussion as well as the assurance that he was not suffering from " calcification," were probably the most important factors in the cure.

Attacks of *convulsive* yawning can also arise as rudiments of an attack of anxiety on the foundation of an anxiety neurosis. But vertigo, perhaps the positively typical symptom of an anxiety neurosis, appears much more frequently than all other symptoms and can lead to the strangest diagnostic mistakes. In its slightest form it is simply a " staggering sensation," a swiftly passing shock of the static sense. *Freud* describes it (l.c.) as follows : " The vertigo of an anxiety neurosis is neither a revolving giddiness, nor does it, like the *menière* vertigo, cause particular planes and directions to stand out. It belongs to the locomotor and co-ordinate vertigo, like that felt with paralysis of the optic nerves ; it consists of a specific discomfort accompanied by a sensation of a heaving floor and sinking legs and an impossibility to stand upright any more ; the legs are as heavy as lead and tremble, or else double up. *This vertigo never causes a fall.* On the other hand I should like to maintain that an attack of that type of vertigo can also be substituted by an attack of profound faintness. Other conditions akin to faintness in an anxiety neurosis can be dependant on a heart collapse. An attack of vertigo is not infrequently accompanied by the worst kind of anxiety and is often associated with respiratory and cardiac disturbances. Vertigo at high altitudes, vertigo on mountains and near abysses, is also manifested, according to my observations, in an anxiety-neurosis ; and I do not know if it would be justifiable to acknowledge a vertigo a stomacho læso in addition."

Vertigo is a very frequent symptom of an anxiety neurosis and physically expresses the idea : I am not sure of myself, I cannot stand firmly, I shall fall. This fall is the " fall of man," and most patients therefore state that they are drawn towards the *left*[1] (the side of sin).

Vertigo resulting from fish, sausage and meat poisoning is very marked. *Sausage poisoning* especially can show such slight symptoms in the digestive region, that vertigo becomes the most conspicuous symptom and the one that causes the greatest anxiety.

No. 53.—A lady of sixty-seven awoke in bed one night with violent giddiness. She felt as if the whole room were revolving with her. The arteries were rigid, the pulse highly strained, decidedly arhythmic. She repudiated the suggestion of a mistake in her diet. After a detailed enquiry she admitted having eaten a thin slice of sausage the previous evening, of which all the members of the household had partaken without harm. Only after a few days did the symptoms of sausage poisoning make their appearance (fever, gastric disturbances ; no tumour of the spleen ; widal negative !) The severe vertigo lasted for three weeks and only yielded very slowly.

No. 54.—The following case offers a contrast to this observation. Mrs. A. R., a widow of sixty-two, fell ill one day with excessive giddiness. She felt as if the bed were rising and falling and sometimes as if her head were quite low and her feet quite high. The arteries were rigid, considering her age ; the pulse hard, well filled, normal tension, slight arhythmia. She had never before suffered from attacks of vertigo. There was no fault of diet. She had not eaten sausage, fish or tinned food for weeks before the attack. The stool was regular. A purgative and salol with menthol had no effect, neither had iodide of sodium which was given her some days later. After a week the attacks of giddiness stopped of their own accord.

About six months later I was called to the same lady. She complained of a harassing smell in the nostrils which made her quite unhappy. Objectively no bad smell could be found. The nose and the naso-pharynx where,—as a result of the interesting statements made by *Kirstein* concerning disagreeable subjective smells,—purulent spaces were sought, proved to be perfectly

---

[1] Cp. the Chapter, " Rechts und Links im Traume " in my book, " Die Sprache des Traumes." (J. F. Bergmann, 1921. 2nd ed.)

normal. The smell could neither be driven away by internal nor external means. The patient was quite desperate. " Every time my son is here," she cried, " must I get so ill ? " This exclamation put me on to a track. " Was your son there last time, too, when you suffered from giddiness ? " " Of course ! It was quite uncanny. As soon as he arrived I fell ill— and the day after his departure I was perfectly well again."
" Doesn't your son live in Vienna ? "
" No—he lives in Germany throughout the year. He only comes to Vienna occasionally to visit me. You see—he did not get on with his brothers and sisters, they are really step-brothers and sisters."
" So he is the eldest ? "
" Yes, by my first husband, whom I unluckily lost so young."
" Well, but you soon married again ? "
" Yes, but it was not the same. The first marriage was a love-match ; the second a *mariage de convenance*. Both were good men, but the first . . ."
Her face lighted up. We went on talking. I learned that she was sexually anæsthetic in her second marriage, that she always thought of her first husband. The second one had been a " weak " man, always ailing. She suffered much from anxiety conditions. She admitted that she had repeatedly had sexual dreams even in recent years, which quite shocked her and of which she was ashamed. A woman of her age ! She was intensely irritable, was always in a state of anxious suspense and often spent sleepless nights. (Pavor nocturnus.)
The first attack of giddiness with all its symptoms (the rising and falling of the bed) was now quite comprehensible to me. The son stood before her as the living image of the father. The ardent love for her child brought her whole passion, never yet chilled, into being again. The vertigo was a symptom of an anxiety neurosis which often continues from the climacteric years into old age. But what could be the meaning of the bad smell ?
In this case I tried a certain method which I shall mention again later and which is an improvement on the association-method of *Jung*.[1] I asked the patient : " Tell me some words that happen to come into your head. The first word you say must be ' Smell.' Now then : *Smell* —"
She began, " *Smell—stench—repulsive—sickness—nausea—heartburn—loss of appetite—*" these words followed each other in fairly rapid succession. Then she paused. About half a minute later more words followed, at marked intervals : " *Rosa, Danube, river, professor, booking office, sympathy.*" A longer pause, then : " *Son, daughter.*" Then she stopped.
I followed the associations suggested by her words. " Smell" to "loss of appetite " was perfectly clear. It was a fact that she suffered in those days from anorexia and continually struggled with feelings of disgust, as the horrible smell was mingled with all her food. I now came to the pause. According to the investigations of *Jung* this is always a suspicious factor. It was a case of significant resistance to unconscious complexes. " Who is Rosa ? " I asked innocently.
" Rosa ? Don't you know ? The wife of my son. My daughter-in-law."
" Which son is that ? "
" Why—the one who has just come."
" Oh—and what has this ' *Rosa* ' to do with the ' *Danube* ' ? "
" I don't know. That just came by chance into my head. You said that I should name the words that happened to occur to me."
" Yes—but there is no chance in these matters. Does not your daughter-in-law suffer from a woman's disease ? "
" Why do you assume that ? "
" Because ' *Danube* ' is followed by ' *river*.' "
" True.—How curious ! She has suffered for many years from " weissen Fluss " (leucorrhea). Do you know, between ourselves, my poor son is to be pitied ; the odour is simply unbearable. The amount of money that it has already cost him ! All the professors of Vienna have attended her ! "

[1] Diagnostische Assoziationsstudien. Leipzig, 1906, Y. A. Barth.

" Are you still surprised that you always have this bad smell in your nostrils ? You have been tormented by this smell since your daughter-in-law is in Vienna. Cannot that be traced to a repressed idea, that would approximately be expressed thus : ' Here is this repulsive person in Vienna again, with her stinking disease. My poor son, how can you stand that ? ' "

" But, Doctor !—"

" Please let me finish. You now demonstrate before your son how such a smell can embitter one's life. You do not get on well with Rosa in any case. I'll bet : You were jealous."

" Well, not exactly. I only get annoyed because she deprives me of my son's love and talks against me. Perhaps I was slightly jealous at the beginning, but there is no trace of that now."

" Now I understand. Your son does not live in Vienna because you do not get on with his wife. Is that so ? "

" It is."

" Then the other is right, too." . . .

By the following day the revolting smell[1] had completely disappeared. The patient ascribed this cure to a popular remedy recommended by a neighbour.

No. 55.—Mr. L. M., a man of sixty-four, with a youthful appearance, whose beard only contained a few grey hairs, came into my consulting room armed with a large piece of paper. This was a list of remedies and cures that had been prescribed against vertigo and pains in the feet. The list was very imposing and filled four folio sheets. His troubles were as follows : He could hardly walk more than a few steps without beginning to limp on account of the violent pains in his foot. But if he happened to have a fairly good day, he was overcome with vertigo instead.

" Which direction does the vertigo take ? "

" Always the left. And I can stand on one leg and shut my eyes at the same time. Have you ever heard of anything like it ? My own doctor sent me to Prof. O., who told me I suffered from " arterio-sclerosis," as I had an " intermittent limp." But it is not at all intermittent ! I always limp. And I used to love Nature so passionately. Now there is no more joy left for me. If it continues like this I shall commit suicide. The professor also forbade me to have any sexual intercourse whatever. Why should I live· at all ? "

" How long is it since you have had intercourse with your wife ? "

" With my wife ? Good heavens ! Not for twenty years. Although I love her very much. *If she were to die to-day I should at once commit suicide.*"

" So if it was not your wife ? . . . "

" I know of a place where I can go regularly without danger of infection."

As I had found no trace of arterio-sclerosis I consoled the patient and recommended him to go on walking and take no notice of the pains.

I had soon discovered that the pains were " safe-guards " against the walks to his mistress. He felt he was sinning against his wife. He was already an old man and said to himself : It is time you stopped and became a sober man. But he had not the strength to stop and took refuge in the malady wherein he was supported by the professor's advice not to have any sexual intercourse ; this, however, caused violent psychic conflicts, for after every relapse into sin he would reproach himself severely that he had shortened his life, etc.

I recommended him to take up regular intercourse again and had the pleasure, some weeks later, of finding him looking very much better and even more youthful than before. He only came to thank me. Since his consultation with me the pains and giddiness had left him as if by magic .

But after a few months he returned. The attacks of vertigo had become so severe that he could not trust himself to go out alone. I made further investigations and discovered a most remarkable fact. This man lived for

---

[1] Cp. *Erwin Kobrek,* " Ueber subjektive Kakosmie." (Med. Klinik, 1908, Nr. 48.)

twenty years—*twenty years*—with two wives! Neither had any notion of the existence of the other. One was his legal wife with whom he could have no intercourse on account of a woman's disease she had. The other was his mistress with whom he associated under a false name. He respected his wife and loved the other one passionately. But he was a swindler in a double sense! He lived in the continual fear of his mistress or his wife discovering the double game he was playing and had not the strength to break with his mistress. The repressed desire for the death of his wife appeared in caricature as anxiety for her life. He took refuge from this irremediable conflict in his illness. Some days previously he had concluded from a remark made by his mistress that she knew his real name.

I advised him to tell her the whole truth. " Is she a clever woman ? "
" I should think so ! "
" Well then, she probably knew the truth long ago and only lets you believe that she is ignorant of it."
The patient emphatically denied this. But a few days later he came to me, blissfully happy : " You were right. She knew everything and only laughed at me. Now I feel a new man again."
The vertigo had vanished entirely. It had really drawn the poor man in the left hand direction and he was a swindler in the true sense of the word.[1]

In other descriptions of diseases we read of acute manifestations of vertigo with feelings of anxiety and violent perspiration. (In the lavatory during defecation, at the writing desk, on an excursion, on the edge of a precipice, etc.) Sometimes vertigo, which in the following case, besides the toxic basis has also a psychic origin, is followed by a more or less profound fainting fit. This tendency to faint is characteristic of the anxiety neurosis.

No. 56.—The psychogenesis of fainting fits is explained by the following observation : Mrs. M. B., aged thirty-five, of healthy parents, had never been seriously ill, had been married since she was eighteen and had had five normal accouchements. Since the birth of the youngest child, two years previously, she suffered from attacks of anxiety. Suddenly she felt " bad," as she expressed it, and had a violent attack of vertigo. This happened almost every week ; but also in the day-time if she stooped quickly, she felt slightly giddy and her heart troubled her. Any great excitement would be followed by a worse attack, accompanied by loss of consciousness. These attacks began with violent palpitations and lasted from twelve to fifteen minutes. A certain agitation of the heart lasted for hours after the attacks. Besides this the patient suffered from sudden congestions. Her face became crimson and she had a sensation of blood being poured over her. In addition she complained that phlegm stuck in her throat. Now and then she had fainting fits accompanied by a " sweet "[2] sensation.

I had an opportunity of witnessing one of the patient's severe attacks which had occurred after a quarrel with the housekeeper, who had called her eldest son a " *dirty lout !* " It was the characteristic form of an attack

[1] Stekel here makes use of the two words " Schwindel " (Vertigo) and " Schwindler " (Swindler).

[2] The " sweet " fainting fit here betrays itself as a substitute for coitus. Violent attacks of hysteria, which are induced by the same psychic mechanism, can also be introduced by a similar " sweet " aura. I therefore do not regard *Dostojewski's* severe attacks as organically epileptic and in this I disagree with Dr. *Tim-Sigaloff* (Die Krankheit Dostojewski's, München, 1907). Dostojewski's joyful sensations before an attack were so great that he would have given up years of his life for them. . . . It is my opinion that the fine frenzy in which the poet's eye rolls, is that piece of hysteria which we all carry about with us.

of hysteria.   The following day I asked her why she had excited herself so much.

"Well," she answered, "because it was my eldest son who is already in the third class of his school. He is no lout. He is a man already."

I gained the following anamnestic information : She professed to have been an inexperienced girl and had never masturbated. Complete amnesia existed concerning her experiences before puberty. However when she was fifteen years old she had an " attack " after her mother had told a gruesome story about deaths-heads.   When she was sixteen she went into the service of her god-father.   One day he called her into a distant room and wanted to violate her. She screamed loudly and a watchman, who chanced to be coming that way, saved her before it was too late.   From that hour she never had a quiet moment's sleep.   She always hid in the corner of a barn for fear of being caught and overcome.   Finally she wrote to her parents and begged them to take her home, for the god-father's wife also worried her with jealousy.   Soon after this she became acquainted with her husband, whom she married without love, but only in order that she should be provided for.   He was fourteen years older than she and apparently not very highly sexed, for he had already lived with her for over a year without intercourse.   She also stated that she was anæsthetic and added that that year, as her husband had left her in peace, had been the " happiest year of her life."   Intercourse had never afforded her satisfaction, especially latterly.   Altogether, to tell the truth, she was sometimes disgusted by her husband, although he was otherwise a good man.   Especially did she reproach him if he completely undressed himself, saying that it was not the thing to do before the children, but in reality because she wanted to spare herself the sight of him.   When I cross-questioned her she admitted that she had masturbated, but that she had read books since her marriage warning her against it.   She had given up that vice because she did not want to contract an abdominal disease.   It was since then that the " sweet " fainting attacks had occurred.   But she did not love her husband at all, as she had once heard a conversation that she could never forget ; he had said to his friends : " I only married my wife out of spite, in order that I can often see her sister whom I cannot have."   Since then she could not endure him any more.

The malady was caused by the psychic trauma and by suppressed incestuous thoughts concerning her own son.   She therefore became hysterical when her son, who was the embodiment of her sexual ideal, was called a " lout."   She was troubled by the anxiety neurosis because she could find no outlet for sexual excitations in consequence of having given up masturbation.   The congestions were anxiety equivalents.   In her fainting attacks she appeared to re-experience the scene of seduction with the god-father, to a successful termination.

The anæsthesia was a relative one, as is mostly the case with women. In consequence of her dislike of her husband she could feel no libido. I afterwards learned that a friend of her husband had courted her and although she felt profound sexual excitement in his presence, she had always resisted him and had altogether given up associating with him. She could not injure her good husband in " such a way." Her dreams revealed an abundant, an even superabundant sex life.

After a psycho-therapeutic treatment, there was a complete disappearance of the bad attacks. But the " sweet " fainting fits persisted.

No. 57.—Mr. J. L., aged thirty-two, of healthy parents, was in perfect health up to his thirtieth year. Then he began to suffer from vertigo and anxiety attacks. The vertigo mostly occurred in the morning after a long sleep. A tension in the head, as if it would burst, preceded the attack.[1] Then came a sensation of heat ascending from the stomach to the head, followed by *a wonderfully pleasant intoxicating loss of consciousness in which the remembrance of recent events disappeared.* " I am filled with a sense of general well-being. I ask myself : What is now ? What was yesterday ? For a short while I am unable to recognize my surroundings. Remembrance gradually comes back to me. I still feel a pressure on the stomach, am very weak and look quite pale."

Mr. J. L. obviously experienced a certain sexual scene during this attack, which however could not be traced analytically, as he had to go on a journey after the first consultation.

Another picture !

No. 58.—Mr. J. H. complained that for four weeks he had suffered from palpitations and anxiety feelings in the street. At night, on going to bed, he had an anxiety feeling before falling asleep, as if he were about to die, as if the heart were about to stop and the breath to give out, as if he were to fall asleep for ever. His wife shook him violently until he recovered.

His wife described the attack as a slight faint. His sexual life was quite normal. He smoked twenty or thirty cigarettes daily. The attacks ceased six days after he gave up smoking. The anxiety feelings also disappeared.

No. 59.—I should like to close these little pictures with a typical case of fainting as a result of an anxiety neurosis.

Mrs. D. T., aged fifty, the mother of seven children, fainted one day without any apparent cause. The doctor who was summoned found that her pulse was very strong and the colour of her cheeks was remarkably good. After a few seconds she recovered without the slightest feeling of unpleasantness. On the contrary ; it seemed as if a rush of heat were streaming through her body. She then felt a slight sense of anxiety and an irritation in the vagina. After that she fainted every month and sometimes suffered from attacks of sickness, dryness in the mouth and shivering fits. Now and then also vertigo. She then thought : " Now I am going to die. Death is not so terrible after all." Most of the attacks culminated with violent hiccoughs or yawning. She became very anxious, and worried about everything ; whether the business would soon be ruined ; whether the children would die of some disease. At other times she appeared to be indifferent and almost egoistical. A cure at Marienbad had no effect. Carbonic acid baths excited her terribly ; and finally she feared severe chronic heart disease.

---

[1] Symbolic expression of the inability to keep back a repressed thought. It is continually noticeable that long sleeps do not agree with neurotics. The unconscious desires chafe and struggle for too long a time. With this patient, too, the long period of sleep released a condition of twilight in which the repressed complexes tried to force themselves into the conscious mind, which was prevented by an attack of fainting and amnesia.

The anamnesis revealed an important fact : her husband had been completely impotent for two years. She had numberless erotic dreams. She was a very plump, almost youthful looking woman and still menstruated regularly. The fainting fits always occurred a day or two before the period. A speedy cure without any treatment whatsoever followed the menopause (masturbation ?).

A violent struggle takes place in every human being between "forbidden thoughts" and the "ethical censoi." The "moral-ego" does not allow the "instinctive-ego" a chance. Vertigo arises from the fear that the instinctive-ego might overpower the moral-ego. The conscious mind struggle against the demands of the unconscious. Vertigo and faintness arise from the "fear of oneself." In both maladies the unconscious conquers the "moral-ego." With vertigo the conquest threatens, but the conscious mind retains the mastery after a few seconds' struggle. With faintness the mastery slips from powerless hands, the instinctive-ego accomplishes its mission in a dream from which it is sooner or later relieved by the reality.

The view, expressed by *Freud*, that the lack of sexual gratification or frustrated excitations are directly responsible for this symptom of disease, cannot be retained. Anxiety is not primarily of libidinous origin. It arises from a fear of the claims of the inner, primitive man. This fear of oneself clearly explains the mechanism of every "nervous attack." Attacks are crises in the eternal struggle between primitive and civilized man. The neurotic then employs the fear of vertigo and faintness as self-protection against his instinctive-ego.

CHAPTER XI

CLINICAL PICTURE OF ANXIETY NEUROSIS: TREMBLING AND SHIVERING, PARASTHESIAS. HOW DO THE RUDIMENTS OF ANXIETY ORIGINATE?

A N anxiety neurosis can sometimes occur as a result of intercurrent causes. *Freud* instances in this connection the moment of overwork, of exhausting strain, *e.g.*, after vigils, sick-nursing, or convalescence after serious illnesses.

All these exhausting situations are associated with severe psychic conflicts. A case is known to me in which a young woman suffered from a severe anxiety neurosis after nursing her sick husband. Added to the injurious results of abstinence and vigils came the struggle with a tormenting thought that continually gnawed away in the unconscious : " If your husband dies now, you can marry Mr. W., who is more suited to you." How did the workings of this unconscious idea, which only occasionally rose to consciousness, find expression ? As a reaction to this sinful desire, an exaggerated love for the sick man made itself felt and was manifested in a neurotically exalted anxiety. If the temperature rose a few tenths the doctor was " most urgently " telephoned for. A different professor had to appear each day. On no account would she share the nursing with anybody else. She allowed herself no rest, no sleep, no suitable nourishment ; she was, in short, the potential ideal of a self-sacrificing nurse. Our virtues often—one could even presume to say almost always—originate thus, as a reaction to suppressed vices, and the good deed has often missed being a crime by a hair's breadth. It is interesting to note that the patient nearly gave herself away once by a symptomatic action. One night she had given her dear patient a whole teaspoonful of morphia instead of twenty drops. Of course she was desperate and inconsolable. But such symptomatic actions are now quite comprehensible to us since *Freud's* explanations. They correspond to a repressed desire which has expressed itself all the same. Not long after this I had occasion to intervene in a second case of poisoning, which was equally premeditated by the unconscious. A child lying hopelessly ill with phthisis was to have a teaspoonful of a weak morphia solution to calm him at night. For he had been harassed for many weeks and the parents were really waiting impatiently for his death, which would be a relief for all concerned..

A few days before his death the terrified mother discovered that she had given the child turpentine instead of the medicine. This woman, too, manifested all the signs of an anxiety neurosis. But it was again neither the vigils nor the nursing of the child that were the cause of the neurosis, but rather the psychic conflict between the mother love and the egoistic desire : " Oh, may the child-die ! " The following example very clearly shows the influence of psychic conflicts :

No. 60.—Mr. M. S., aged fifty-two, with no hereditary taint, suffered for years from malaria. In the tropics, when he was younger, he had stood it fairly well. Suitable doses of quinine kept him well for a considerable time, but this year he contracted malaria again during a voyage to the tropics and according to his account was unable to recover as quickly as before. At night he suffered from slight attacks of vertigo. He had a sensation as of a veil being drawn before his eyes. Then he was able to rest for a time and felt perfectly well. But when he returned home he found the business had been greatly neglected. He was obliged to work until late at night and was greatly agitated. One morning he had an attack in a tram which scared him very much. *For a moment his hand went to sleep and dropped slackly, as if it were paralysed.*[1] Two days later was the Day of Atonement. As a devout Jew he fasted and to this he attributed a violent attack of vertigo that overcame him that day. He felt that he would fall, and clung to his wife. It was all over in a few seconds. The following day he again had an attack, a sensation of ants crawling all over his right hand. Here and there he felt a violent irritation, as if an electric current were streaming through his whole body. At night, too, he was sometimes awakened by an acute pain. (Pavor nocturnus of adults.) At times he could not sleep for excitement. But he had no direct, obvious feeling of anxiety. His greatest torture was the darkness that veiled his left eye. The most frequent symptom was, however, a slight *feeling of faintness*. That was especially the case in his previous office. He attributed it to dark, ill-ventilated rooms.

An oculist examined his eyes and found them normal. Neither did a thorough internal examination reveal any organic foundation for his disorders. The anamnesis proved, on the other hand, the indubitable existence of sexual disharmonies. For about fourteen years, with the exception of the years of pregnancy—*i.e.*, every fifth year—he had practised coitus interruptus. His anxiety neurosis was only manifested in the slight attacks of faintness which he had attributed to bad air. But even with a normal coitus he felt slightly faint. He only evinced the normal anxiety-components (*Fliess*)[2] of desire. Only with weakened powers of resistance (malaria, fasting, etc.) did the symptoms of the anxiety neurosis assert themselves. Every month he suffered from a recurring coated angina, with violent febrile symptoms. The symptoms of faintness only appeared during the days of convalescence. These signs could be imputed to weakness, but the success of therapy clearly proved the etiology. A complete and rapid cure was effected by the regulation of the sexual life (use of a mensinger pessary).

A few months later there was a slight relapse, in spite of the pessary and normal gratification. Armed with a better knowledge of the facts I was then able to discover his psychic conflict. His wife was very jealous and forced him to dismiss a charming typist because she got on too well with him.

[1] Dead fingers and limbs that have gone to sleep are the symbolic expression of impotence or a wish for the death of some member of the family. Such symbols play a large part in hysteria. I once had a woman under observation who always suffered from cold feet. She then learned to know and love an officer and her feet ceased to be cold. She laughingly admitted : " Yes, I could never feel any *warmth* towards my husband."

[2] *Fliess*, Der Aufbau des Lebens. Vienna, 1906. Deuticke.

She herself learned typewriting in order to compensate him for his loss. It was then that the first attack took place. *They were death wishes against his wife.* (Paralysis of the right hand ! His wife is his right hand in the business !) In his attacks he clung to his wife (over-compensation of criminal wishes by love !) He took refuge from unbearable thoughts in a fainting fit. I have been able to prove the existence of a similar mechanism in pseudo-epilepsy of a hysterical nature.[1]

Another attendant symptom of anxiety neurosis frequently met with (here and there as anxiety equivalent !) is the trembling of an arm or hand ; sometimes the entire body is thus affected. Cases of shivering fits are of not uncommon occurrence, as, for example, in Case 50. Shaking in the legs is another well known symptom of anxiety.

No. 61.—Mr. S. C., a lieutenant, twenty-four years of age, with no hereditary trouble (a sister suffered from hysteria and anxiety neurosis) complained of cardiac pressure. His heart felt as if it were beating too violently. He was also troubled in the night with feelings of anxiety : dread of a stroke, of being attacked by robbers who might stab him. Sometimes, in the street, he felt as if he would fall down ; trembling in the left hand, varying in intensity, was also experienced. (The trouble commenced after the death of his father, to whom he was much attached, and after other very agitating circumstances). He was moreover easily excited and very irritable. Excitement made him tremble, his legs shook, and he was unable to speak. The most trivial causes often induced this state. A soldier failing to salute smartly enough was cited by him as an example of the provocation of such excitement, reducing him to such a pitch of agitation that he was in danger of falling down.

Analysis elicited in the first place the fact that the patient is a man of cold temperament and not highly sexed. He was quartered with his garrison at a solitary fort, where there were no women, and for a whole year had felt no inclination for sexual intercourse. Even formerly when living in a large garrison town he had only had intercourse once every three months, and then very reluctantly and without any pleasurable sensation. He had masturbated early on entering the cadet school, and was obliged to visit a brothel with his companions because he was ashamed not to do as they did.

The women he met there were always repugnant to him. It always took a considerable time and various manipulations to achieve an erection at all.

He had never been in love in his life, and preferred the society of elderly women (!) to that of young girls. He was, in fact, a woman-hater.

Further investigations pointed to a distinct homosexual tendency. He loved his father more than his mother, his brother more than his sister. It was his greatest pleasure in the cadet school to see certain boys undressed. The swimming school was his chief delight. He had formed a pure friendship with one of his comrades which was almost of the nature of a love affair, although they never spoke about " such things."

He could remember no dreams of a homosexual character, but experienced the typical violation dreams, such as unsatisfied women dream. (Burglars entering the window, the man with the dagger, wherein dagger, knife, revolver, sword, bow and lance always represent the dream symbol for the penis).

This is a clear case of anxiety hysteria. The hysteria was engendered by strong repression. He was not conscious of his homosexuality. There was also evidence of incestuous thoughts directed on the eldest sister. The latter was very energetic, had masculine habits and a masculine appearance. Hence his predeliction for elderly women, with whom he evinces, relatively, the strongest potency. This form of erotism is often present with incestuous thoughts directed to the mother. In this case, as was proved by analysis,

[1] Cp. the Chapter : " The Psychic Treatment of Epilepsy."

it was the eldest sister, twenty years his senior, who chiefly responded to his homosexual and masochistic tendencies. It is interesting to note that this sister suffered from the same malady arising from the same cause. Total amnesia in all experiences prior to his cadet school life was accountable for the hysteria. In short, he sought in every man his sister.[1]

This patient was a homosexual unconscious of his homosexuality. He was unable to find adequate satisfaction and therefore fell a victim to anxiety neurosis ! As in so many homosexuals he is fixated to his mother and sister. Homosexuality is his means of escape from Woman, whom he cannot differentiate from his nearest relatives. His life was thus spent between two erotic goals, both of which were unattainable for him.

A series of symptoms owed their origin entirely to sexual abstinence. He had been an habitual onanist, and had abandoned onanism in consequence of information obtained from books. But he was incapable of leading a life of abstinence without suffering for it. Individual symptoms admit of a simple psychologic explanation. He trembled when a man saluted him carelessly. It came out afterwards, in course of examination, that it happened to be the handsomest lad in the company who had thus aroused his erotic feelings, and at the sight of whom his repressed thoughts had been awakened. He was inwardly agitated by an affect from the unconscious. He transferred the affect, however, to a secondary phenomenon. The soldier had failed to salute him with due respect. But what he really desired from the soldier was not respect but love. The trembling of the left hand is a typical anxiety equivalent, which I have observed in a considerable number of patients. It affords us opportunity of examining more closely the origin of anxiety equivalents from the psychologic point of view. This officer was ashamed of his anxiety. He endeavoured to suppress it as such, and the anxiety equivalent arose from the repression of that anxiety. 'Nor is the choice of the left arm a mere coincidence. He was accustomed to masturbate with the left hand (he was left-handed !) This hand was to a certain extent his erogenous zone. The feeling of anxiety is here transferred to organic sources. The heart must be diseased, or the brain affected.. But the mechanism of the origin of anxiety equivalents is connected solely with the violent reaction against the anxiety and the transference of the sensations from the sphere of general sensations produced by *sexual* excitement, to that of one or more erogenic zones. I do not maintain that this is always the case. But it is of very frequent occurrence. The causes of the equivalent formation are obvious : some particular symptom predominates over the entire disease. Which symptom ? Why that particular symptom ?. That is just the question.

Janet also is acquainted with the phenomenon of the anxiety equivalent, and if we substitute his " Psychasthenia " for anxiety neurosis we can form a clear conception, from his descriptions, of the localisation of anxiety and its remarkable metamorphoses. He describes the following case :—

No. 62.—" This woman of thirty-five had a great variety of pains. At the age of seventeen she showed symptoms of respiratory disturbance, resulting from excitement. She suffered from a feeling of suffocation of an unpleasant character, which left her with a violent and alarming pain in the breast, about the middle of the sternum.

" This was followed by pain in the gullet, so that she could hardly swallow her food ; at the age of twenty the pains moved to the stomach. The act of digestion was attended by considerable suffering and ended with the vomiting of lumps of whitish phlegm. *At twenty-three the seat of the pain was the uterus. She experienced the unusual phenomenon of the discharge of an*

[1] I was unable to solve the deeper roots of his homosexuality at that time (Hatred of Women—Sadism).

enormous quantity of fluid from the uterus. These discharges resembled nasal *Hydrorhoe* and must not be confused with metritis. At thirty the pain had extended to the back, and is now established in the face."

The examination of the face proved the condition, as far as sensibility was concerned, to be normal, with no changes in the surface of the skin.

" Where is the seat of the gnawing pain ? " The patient herself supplied the answer : : " I feel it mostly in the breast, because I am suffocating, in my heart because it palpitates, and in my head, because I am losing my reason." The seat of the pain, therefore, was not the face, but the entire body, *the alleged pain in the face is really general anxiety. This is proved by the fact that the pains in the various organs were identical ; when she complained of pains in the uterus or back, the actual phenomenon was always the same anxiety, as now when the pain is localised in the face.* But what part is played *by that organ which is the seat of the pain ?* It adds a nuance to the anxiety " *en y melant ses sensations propres la douleur que ressent la malade c'est de l'angoisse en pensant au dos, au ventre ou bien l'angoisse en pensant a la figure.*" Just as Tic is a motor excitation attached to the conception of a particular member of the body, so are algias merely *systematised* conditions of anxiety, in which the general anxiety is merged with the presentment as some particular organ which *appears* to suffer pain.

No. 63.—Another case illustrative of this form of anxiety equivalent. Mrs. M. S., aged fifty-one, a well-preserved, robust widow, was subject to severe attacks of ague almost every month. Her whole body trembled and she tried to obtain warmth by additional coverlets, by hot-water bottles and hot tea. She experienced no specific feeling of anxiety, but felt extremely ill. The heart seemed to stop beating, and she feared an attack of pneumonia. I was usually called in on these occasions and found the temperature both in the rectum and axil to be normal. After the administration of twenty drops of validol all alarming symptoms quickly vanished. On the following day she was conscious of a " pleasant " feeling of tiredness and lassitude, so that she was obliged to remain in bed. These attacks occurred, curiously enough almost always before Sundays and holidays, so that it was in no way inconvenient for her to lie in bed, whereas otherwise she could ill be spared from her business.

The anxiety neurosis was, in this instance, engendered by long abstinence. The act of coitus produced in her sensations over the entire skin, she was very ticklish, and was obviously dermographic. (The skin as erogenous zone !)

At one time she was laid up with a whole series of such attacks. They occurred on four successive nights and were of a most severe character. This was—naturally enough—on her wedding anniversary, and had originated by contrasting the past with the present. The attacks show, in other respects, a certain tendency to periodicity, in which male and female periods alternate.

There were also passing attacks of anxiety with vertigo, and violent migraine. Excitement produced slight urticaria in the neck.

Cases of *pruritus-parasthesia* are also not infrequently to be observed in anxiety neurosis. They often accompany the anxiety affect, but they may sometimes occur as the rudiments of a serious attack, without any attendant symptom, giving the anxious patient cause for a variety of hypochondriacal uneasiness. Parasthesia can sometimes be so troublesome as to give rise to insomnia.

Pruritus vulvæ is very frequently met with ; it then induces scratching, which may be regarded as a disguised form of masturbation. The pruritus ceases with a slightly pleasurable feeling which has a tranquilizing effect on the woman's previously excited nerves, and she finds that she is then able to go to sleep. *Sudduth,* also, lays stress on the soothing effect of onanism. The case of *Scheuer* is worthy of note. (On a case of masturbation, caused by Pruritus genitalium. Münchener med. Wochenschr., 1909, Nr. 25.) In this instance the pruritus occurred after the masturbation. Such an inversion of the symptoms is not unusual in hysteria. In the same way the strangest sensations are experienced in the skin, generally a form of sexual excitement in disguise. The following case is in this respect very instructive :—

No. 64.—Mr. V. S., an officer of twenty-eight, with no hereditary ailments, complained of a troublesome irritation and " crawling " feeling in the face. He was not troubled with it in the day-time. But when lying in bed the boring, burning, twitching, and tickling in the face used to begin, so that he was prevented from sleeping. All remedies hitherto resorted to were without effect. Neither general treatment (bromide, opium, cold water cure), nor local applications of menthol, cocaine ointment, alcohol and ether applications, gave any relief. On the first night the remedies gave relief, and then, being unable to sleep, he ran up and down the room ; towards morning he obtained a few hours' uneasy sleep, troubled with anxiety dreams. He found an article on parasthesia in an Encyclopædia. The diagnosis was written on his chart at the Nerve Clinic he was attending for treatment. The information he obtained from the Encyclopædia was to the effect that parasthesia may be a prodromic symptom of paralysis. The skin becomes withered and shrunk. The muscles atrophy. This information greatly alarmed him. Every few minutes he looked in the glass to ascertain whether there were any evidences of the results of " parasthesia." When on duty he was obliged to control himself, but at home, or in a restaurant he stared into the mirror for half-an-hour at a time. Eventually he discovered minute indentations, which he had not hitherto observed. He even made use of a magnifying glass in order to examine them more closely.

He showed me these " distinct " little indentations in his face. When I replied that I could see nothing but a normal skin, he was very indignant and said he would not have things suggested away ; he was still in his right mind.

His mania was of an almost paranoiac character (hypochondriacal delusions, paralogia). He had been accustomed at one time to masturbate frequently, but suffered afterwards from psychic impotence. An attempt to accomplish the sex act with a *puella publica* was unsuccessful owing to a feeling of intense repugnance. He visited the girl later, in anxious expectation of the result. Hypnotic treatment by *Krafft-Ebing* was utterly unsuccessful. The inhibition was so strong that it would not admit of any suggestion. He suffered greatly, however, from abstinence. The perusal of instructive literature on the subject of onanism was the source of the gravest self-reproach to him, and, believing that he had injured his health, he gave up masturbating. During the first month of abstinence he fell ill with agoraphobia, from which he recovered in a few months, only to fall a victim to other forms of anxiety of an indefinite nature.

He was also subject to occasional anxiety attacks with a slight feeling of giddiness. All these symptoms then disappeared to give place to parasthesias.

The cure was effected by a fortunate chance. He was always subject to violent erections in the early morning, a symptom which enables us easily to distinguish the psychic from the organic impotence. One morning his housemaid, an elderly, not very attractive individual, entered the room to fetch his clothes which lay on a chair near the bed. Half awake, he stretched out his arms to her. He had been greatly attracted by her for some time past, and had been distinctly encouraged by her, but he had not ventured to make any advances for fear of making a fool of himself. But when in the dim light of the room he touched her lightly, she bent over him and kissed him on the forehead above the eyes, *just as his mother had been used to do* and just on the spot where he had suffered so much from the parasthesias. This prelude led to coitus, which he performed (still as in a dream !) perfectly normally, and with astonishing potency. The next morning he felt happier than he had ever felt in his life. On the following night he performed the sex act ten times in succession, without experiencing a trace of exhaustion or tiredness the next day. He then came to me, radiant with joy to report his recovery. The cure proved to be permanent ; he changed from an agoraphobic into a so-called " gay dog." He became a Don Juan, married, but always had other attachments besides his wife.

This case is, in several respects, interesting and instructive· It provides a clear demonstration of the generation of the rudiments of anxiety. Parasthesia occurred in an erogenous zone. *His mother had been accustomed to kiss him daily on his forehead and closed eyelids.* This innocent act of tenderness awakened, however, in the child feelings of an erotic nature, which made of that particular part of the skin an " erogenous zone." This zone was later on the seat of the parasthesias. It was there that he saw, symbolically, that for which his senses longed—it was all over " dimples " (indentations). He stared into the mirror because it was there that he conjured up (unconsciously, of course) memories of bygone happy days. Sexual feelings were mingled with this anxiety, as it is also always linked with the libido.

Fliess says : " There is always a touch of anxiety in the surging, tumultuous pleasure of the normal sex act, in the form of a slight feeling of oppression, an acceleration of the heart's action and a light outbreak of perspiration from the pores. This condition becomes enhanced in the great attack of anxiety with all its attendant mental and bodily suffering. This enhancement takes place when the full discharge of sexual feeling is inhibited, and a portion of it is stored up." Anxiety, according to his conviction, is due to the *sexual element* in our libido. It is to this heterosexuality that he attributes the various conditions of anxiety (senium, childhood, etc.). He has also observed that an anxiety attack is frequently preceded by dilation of the left pupil. The left side of the body is, according to *Fliess*, always the hetero-sexual side. We will avail ourselves of this opportunity to insert a few observations. We would ask ourselves how these anxiety conditions and anxiety rudiments came into being ? *Freud* sees the mechanism of anxiety neurosis in the deflection of the somatic sexual excitement from the psychic sphere, thereby causing an abnormal application of anxiety. There is a fragment of anxiety floating about which attaches itself to those ideas which are capable of assimilating it.

Now, what is *Freud's* conception of this transformation of the libido into anxiety ? How can a somatic excitation change into an affect ? I must confess that I regard *Freud's* libido theory as a beautiful myth, which I was only able to believe until my professional experience convinced me of its untenability. Let us return to the example of the patient who sees dents in his face, spends the whole day in observing them and is now afraid that everybody will notice them. We cannot say that the libido has established itself in the erogenous zone of his face. What are we to understand by these mysterious psychic charges and metamorphoses? Clarity and facts are essential to the medical profession. We have, unfortunately, a superfluity of theories.

The patient is merely afraid that his evil thoughts may be revealed to the world. He has a longing to be kissed on the face—and this desire—as I did not learn till afterwards—was associated with his housekeeper, who was the wife of his paternal friend, and therefore a mother-imago. His bad conscience tells him that his friend might guess this thought. The transference to the housemaid is a fact of extraordinarily frequent occurrence. Any person living in the same house may become the object of a transference of this kind whereby the circumstance of " living together " supports the idea that the person in question is desirable. It is a matter of " substitution," a very common phenomenon in the world of neurotics. Once the cure had been effected through the medium of the house-maid, the auto-suggestion of impotence was undermined and replaced by a number of the beloved objects (Don Juanism) the object previously lacking.

I had at that time, however, failed to recognise the homosexual component of the malady. He imagined, as a woman, that there were " holes " in him which had to be filled in, and expressed this in his fear that his face was all over " holes." These " holes " represented one single " hole "—that of the anus.

I did not then understand his homosexual tendency, his transference to my own person, which once manifested itself in a violent discharge of affect. He was eternally wandering about, he needed some form of activity to satisfy him. Nor did I realise at that time that the constant longing of the patient to be hypnotised was in reality a desire for homosexual experience in hypnotism (according to the theory evolved by me " pleasure without guilt ") and that his incapacity to be hypnotised arose from his dread of experiencing what he desired.

We are approaching a unanimous understanding of anxiety phenomena. I said : " Fear is always attached to some object, Anxiety has no object." This is correct only up to a certain point. The object of anxiety is a desire of the unconscious or a suppressed wish. Anxiety is not a transformation of the libido, it is the libido itself, for every sexual wish is the expression of a desire, every wish is a desire, the fulfilment of which produces satisfaction (satiety). The wish is hunger, the libido, the expression of sexual hunger. When this hunger is of an asocial character, when it is a matter of sexual impulses rejected by the conscience, these desires manifest themselves as anxiety.

Whenever two wishes, a moral one (dictated by the conscience) and one dictated by the instincts, are fighting for supremacy, the repressed wish is compelled to express itself as anxiety. This anxiety is the fear of God's punishment, of social consequences, of the fall into the depths of criminality. The patient was afraid of being hypnotised because he feared to become a homosexual. He desired hypnotism because his homosexual impulse demanded satisfaction. He had only fallen in love with the wife of his paternal friend because he really loved the friend himself and the wife was merely the common vessel out of which both might drink.[1]

Anxiety rudiments are always engendered when the unfulfilled desire tries to reveal itself in some form or other to the world. They are symbolic transformations of a fact, which has to be concealed from consciousness. A lover will find expression in the organic language of the heart; disgust of a paraphilia manifests itself as stomachic neurosis; a burning sensation in the anus and dread of rectal carcinoma are masks for homosexual impulses, and the desire to be examined by a doctor.

They are purely psychological mechanisms, which have nothing to do with the libido, as such.

Anxiety need, however, show no connection with the libido. It may be fear of one's own criminal thoughts, it may be dread of death, as has been demonstrated by the trembling neurotics in the war. But *Freud* has developed his "Libido Theory" powerfully and evolved an entire system, such as his "Vorlesungen zur Einführung in die Psycho-Analyse" (Third Part. Allgemeine Neurosenlehre. Leipzig and Vienna. Hugo Heller, 1917) prove.

A connected presentation of his libido theory from his own pen was hitherto lacking. We now have it in his "Vorlesungen zur Einführung in die Psychoanalyse." Freud's libido is no mystery as is the libido of Jung, but just the good old eternal sexual instinct, pure and simple. According to his conception this libido is always striving for fixation on an object of the external world. If this means of relief is denied to it, if, in other words, the individual fails to find the sexual pleasure he was striving for with others, the libido has to be dammed up. It takes up the old, childish positions (thus giving rise, according to Freud, to the transference neuroses, anxieties and conversions, "hysterias" and "compulsion neuroses") or it results in love of their own ego, in narcissistic neuroses (dementia præcox, paranoia, melancholia). Hysteria, therefore, may be said to be generated by the reversion of the libido to childish positions; infantile experiences (traumas), would then acquire, by the new psychic charge, fresh significance. As, however, these experiences are kept back from the conscious mind, that is to say are unconscious, the libido stream is diverted into the unconscious. The task of psychanalysis would be to release the fixation on childhood and the unconscious,

[1] Compare Vol. II, the important Chapter, "Masken der Homosexualität."

and to render possible for the libido a new fixation on the present, or an intellectual sublimation. This would be a rough outline of the foundation of the *Freudian* Neurosis = and Libido Theory. Now how does this work out in fact? Are all neuroses merely disturbances of the sexual instinct? The Great War has provided a clear and irrefutable answer to this question. There have never been so many male hysterics as in these days. Careful analysis of these cases shows, however, that it is a question of conflict between the instinct of self-preservation and the sense of duty. Hysterics give the idea of illness as a refuge which enables them to conceal the real motifs (anxiety, distaste for work, blighted ambition, etc.) in the unconscious, so that they are capable of believing in their own illnesses and of pretending to long to be restored to health—a condition which deceives the doctor and their own conscience. The libido plays no part in these cases, or at least only that of a pleasure premium which life promises to the survivor. In no way does the sexual pleasure regress to infantile forms; except when the illness as such is an expression of infantilism.

I would submit the following example, which we may regard as coming under the head of hysteria. All definitions are nebulous, however, unless they can be substantiated by living examples. That is the great error in the above-mentioned work of *Freud*. It is a philosophy of psychanalysis and not an introduction. It is instructive for the initiated, but misleading for the uninitiated and students. Now to our example :—

No 65.—A lady sought my advice in the matter of a peculiar malady. She was less sensitive on the right half of her body than on the left half; she believed also that she had less power on the right side than on the left. On pressing my hand on the right and left sides I could perceive no difference. The lady then informed me that there was no actual weakness,—that the condition was "imaginary." She merely *felt* that the left side was stronger than the right. It also seemed to draw her, towards the left. The trouble had commenced three years previously, there had been some temporary improvement after treatment at a Sanatorium which she had undergone on the advice of an eminent professor, but it was now worse than ever. If she could not be cured, life was not worth living. She was wrestling with suicidal impulses. She eventually confessed that she was very happily married and was the mother of three children. The lady suspected some serious spinal trouble. After a thorough examination, which proved the condition not to be neurological, I said to her: "No. It is a question of hysterical disorder."
She. "What is the meaning of hysteria? What kind of disorder is it?"
"A malady in which psychic conflicts manifest themselves as physical disorders."
"What conflicts am I suffering from?"
I have learned, in the course of many years, to translate the organic language of the soul. Now and then I am tempted to reconstruct the life's romance from the symptoms of a patient. In this case the task was a simple one :
"Three years ago you made the acquaintance of a man with whom you fell in love. But you remained faithful to your husband. You respect your husband and could not deceive him. But even now you have not forgotten your lover. You still love the other man. But your children and

your husband prevent you from following the dictates of your heart. Life without your lover does not seem worth living to you, and suicide would be a welcome means of escape, putting an end to all conflict. Moreover, you are religious, a fact which makes the conflict all the harder."

The woman paled and looked at me with wide eyes as if I were a wizard : " Every word of what you've said is true. How could you have guessed it ? "

" I read it in your symptoms. The right hand side represents your husband and your duty : the left hand side stands for love and your lover. You have no feeling on your right side, but you are drawn towards the left. Shall I translate the disorders from the physical into the psychical yet more fully ? "

" No, I understand. . . . I have thought for a long time that my malady must be connected with my love. But the professor did not ask me about my experiences. How did you recognise that I was religious ? "

" Because it is only moral, pious people whose health suffers from such conflicts. If you were more easy-going and less inclined to inhibitions, you would not have come to a doctor. Hysteria is, in point of fact, the conflict between morality and impulse " . . .

But enough of examples ! Where is the objective physician to find, in this instance, the reversion of the libido to the infantile sphere ? No ! He finds merely conflict and an attempt at the manifestation of such conflict through physical channels. The malady enabled the woman to complain openly of her trouble, even to her husband, without betraying herself. In the same way, a soldier suffering from "trembling neurosis" admits his fear of death without this being regarded as the humiliating confession of a coward. And we now realize that hysteria is the life-long lie of civilization, is that play-acting through which those who cannot cope with life turn their tragedies into comedies.

It is a question of typical conversion-hysteria. The idea, " I love the other man better than my husband. I have more feeling for the wrong (left) side than for my lawful possessor, but I am continually being drawn towards my lover," was converted into the above-mentioned physical sensory disorder. But was this sensory disorder an infantile position ? It was only a " clever *façon de parler*," the typical organic language of the soul. The root of the trouble is the " psychic conflict," the sole cause of neuroses, as I have maintained in my little article " Die Ursachen der Nervosität " (" The Causes of Nervousness ") (Published by *Paul Knepler*, Wien, 1907). But *Freud* differentiates between Actual Neuroses (Neurasthenia, Hypochondria and Anxiety Neurosis) which can only be traced to some injurious form of sexual life, and the Transference Neuroses, with their psychic super-structure. I have not been able to discover these Actual Neuroses of *Freud's* in practice. Wherever I found a neurosis, I found also the psychic conflict, which very often had its origin in the sex life, but also its equivalents in other instincts (ambition, instinct of self-preservation, avarice, etc.). The preceding case is itself an example of actual neurosis, which owes its existence to an actual conflict between love and duty. But *Freud* insists that : " The libido is shut off and must try to flow off in some direction, where in obedience to the pleasure-principle it can find a discharge for its energy."

The symptoms are supposed to originate in a kind of sexual activity and a compromise-formation. Now, does this theory accord with our case ? The compromise is only effected between that which one may and that which one may not say. The left side is not, in reality, charged with stronger erotic feeling than the right. The gain from illness is merely the possibility of an incomprehensible confession.

Freud emphasizes, more and more distinctly, the significance of the " ego-impulse in contradistinction to the sex-impulse." I must confess that I do not understand this distinction. In my view the sex-impulse is the same as the ego-impulse ; the distinction is artificial, theoretical, and not corresponding to actual life. That *Freud* traces all anxiety to the act of birth is no novelty ; but the conversion of my formula : " All anxiety is fear of oneself " to the phrase : " All anxiety is the fear of one's own libido," is new.[1]

Under *Freud's* hands everything is converted into a libido theory. What is sleep ? A condition in which all psychic charges of objects, the libidinous as well as the egoistic, are relinquished and withdrawn into the ego again ! . . . This is supposed, by *Freud*, to have thrown a new light on the recuperative powers of sleep and on the nature of fatigue. But his hypothesis is false. In dreams, objects psychically charged with affect are presented with extraordinary strength ; we dream of some beloved person, we desire her, we awake with our hearts throbbing, and think of her. Why should we have relinquished the blissful isolation of intra-uterine life nightly conjured up for us by our sleep, as postulated by *Freud*, in favour of an actual love emotion ?

No, the libido alone does not offer sufficient explanation of the anxiety equivalent. In the majority of cases they show a distinct connection with the sex life, but not in all. We can only admit the following facts from the *Freudian* Libido Theory, in the majority of cases :

Every sexual excitation with repressed libido is converted into anxiety. Where the *libido*, as such, does not reach consciousness, where it is disguised, where it is experienced as painful and dismissed from consciousness, it manifests itself as anxiety. The neurotic whose sexual goal is barricaded by æsthetic inhibitions, who loves his mother, his sister, the wife of his friend, or inclines towards the perverse or homosexual without experiencing this inclination as a sexual impulse, experiences it as anxiety.

The anxiety of the inexperienced at the first encounter with the sex problem, the anxiety of the old men who are ashamed of still feeling sexual excitation, the anxiety of children, are instances of the fact that the sex impulse of the unconscious mind is expressed by anxiety. *Anxiety is the fear of one's own libido. All anxiety is fear of the criminal ego.*

[1] Mostly discussed in the first edition of this Book.

The task of psycho-therapy is to unmask the anxiety affect as a sexual excitement and inhibited criminality, and to restore the libido from the unconscious to the conscious mind. The " free-floating anxiety " of Freud is an anxiety which represents a suppressed wish. This piece of " free-floating anxiety " is at the disposal of other objects and presents itself in consciousness with false associations. Anxiety equivalents which run their course apparently without anxiety affect, are again a translation of sexual excitement. It is a question of excitation of the erogenous zones ; the libido has come, to a certain extent, into " consciousness " in a disguised form, the contribution of the unconscious diminishes or is scarcely perceived, or is taken for a symptom of organic disease.

An anxiety equivalent is, therefore, generated :

(1) When the libido is suppressed and separated from its rightful sexual goal.

(2) When the liberated unconscious component of the libido, anxiety, occupies another position. This position may be an erogenous zone or a locus minoris resistentiæ (an organ weakened by illness).

(3) Through conversion.

(4) When a painful thought wants to find expression through the " organic speech of the soul."

There takes place, in this manner, a displacement of affect or of the sexual conception originally experienced as painful, to some other conception more indifferent to consciousness. It is actually the same mechanism, as in the compulsory-ideas which are for the most part falsely associated, transferred erotic desires and reproaches for lustful ego-strivings or criminal wishes.

Sexual excitement in dreams manifests itself so frequently as anxiety just because the unconscious component of the libido in the realms of the unconscious is more easily expressed in dreams as anxiety. Because all repressed sexual and criminal desires, because all libido becomes anxiety in the unconscious through the censor of the conscience.

Also the " traumatic neuroses," the fright-hysterias become comprehensible to us. Fright succeeds in freeing, for a moment, all repressed libido. Tourists describe the sensation of falling down a terrible chasm as a voluptuous feeling, those who have been hanged are found to die with a pollution, and " psychic trauma " and fright work in a similar manner through the deliverance of the anxiety accumulated in the unconscious. We can thus understand the individual disposition to traumatic neurosis.

CHAPTER XII

CLINICAL PICTURE OF ANXIETY NEUROSIS: VASO-MOTOR PHENOMENA. PERIODIC EMACIATION AND CONVULSIONS. INFLUENCE OF THE MENSES ON ANXIETY ATTACKS AND EQUIVALENTS OF ANXIETY.

HECKER also mentions parasthesias as anxiety equivalents. Among others he describes " coldness and numbness of the limbs." I myself know a woman of thirty-five, suffering from anxiety neurosis, who has been treated unsuccessfully for years for chilling of both forearms. Her husband is completely impotent. I believe that the enigmatic disease which goes by the name of " Acroparasthesia " may have intimate connection with anxiety neurosis.

Flatau (Angstneurosen und vasomotorische Storüngen. Med. Klin. 1913) observed two groups of disease in which associations between anxiety and vaso-motor disturbances were in evidence. (1) Women with Urticaria and swelling of the joints. (2) Pathological blushing and a feeling of impediment in speech.

The pathological blushing will be dealt with separately under the Phobias. But anxiety neurotics are also otherwise disposed to vaso-motor phenomena. They nearly all evince distinct symptoms of dermographism, they easily change colour, sometimes turning pale and sometimes dark red. This vaso-motor lability is the cause of countless parasthesias.

Extremely instructive examples of parasthesia in anxiety neuroses are provided by *Hartenberg*. (Le nevrose d'angoisse. Paris, 1902, Felix Alcan).

The following is one of his observations :—

Nr. 66.—Mrs. M. married at eighteen. After the marriage she soon began to grow thin. One child died of meningitis. One night after Christmas she awoke with palpitation of the heart, impaired breathing, and bathed in cold sweat. She felt terribly frightened and cried : " I feel as if I am going to die ! " The crisis ended with *a copious evacuation*.

The morning after the crisis she felt a kind of indefinable shame, a perpetual anxiety which never left her.

Six weeks later the same attack was repeated, and a third after some months. The fear of dying during one of these crises was never absent from her. She was seized with such anxiety while in the street that she was obliged to hire a cab, only for the sake of getting home. She lost weight perceptibly. Treatment by suggestion effected an almost complete cure.

Two years later she experienced a severe psychic shock. (Her drunken husband threatened her with a revolver.) She became again very run down until complete peace was again restored to her by the death of the brutal husband. In another eight years she fell ill once more. This time with violent and prolonged fits of yawning, alternating with attacks of vomiting. She sometimes experienced cold shivers of unusual intensity. On another occasion trembling of the muscles, cramp and general sickness. *Eventually her hands and feet seemed to " die off,"* she was not able to feel the needle with which she worked. She rapidly lost flesh.

This case contains the whole repertoire of anxiety neurosis. Hartenberg draws special attention to the symptoms not mentioned by *Freud.* Attacks of *numbness in fingers and toes, yawning fits, periodic emaciation.*

The circumstance that the woman was anæsthetic at the commencement of her marriage, that she practised normal intercourse and that she occasionally lived in total abstinence, appears to Hartenberg contrary to a sexual ætiology. But this very anæsthesia is a sign that she was never satisfied by her husband or that she did not love him.

Hartenberg's account of this case clearly proves anxiety neurosis to be a " disease of the conscience." The anæsthesia at the commencement of the marriage shows that this woman did not love her husband.[1] Women of this kind look upon their child as a burden and desire its death. They suffer from " Maternity neurosis "—a complaint which we will deal with later on. They wish to see the child dead, who is a burden and a hindrance to them, and who symbolizes the indissolubility of marriage. Such death wishes manifest themselves symbolically as " mortified limbs." The patients pretend that the limb is dead. The craving for satisfaction expresses itself as anxiety and anxiety diarrhœa which attaches itself to a dream occurring in the early hours of the morning, after all inhibitions have been overcome. Hence the indefinable shame felt by this patient after such an attack of diarrhœa. But the death wishes against the husband were also a source of severe conflict to this woman.

It was not until his death that she was released from all conflicts, until opportunity arose for another conflict with its attendant " bad conscience."

It is useless to attempt to explain the dying-off of the limbs by the libido theory. The explanation can only be a psychological one.

I would draw particular attention to the very interesting phenomenon of " periodic emaciation " to which Hartenberg, the French scientist, first gave prominence. As a matter of fact it is never a primary symptom. It occurs only as the result of stubborn anorexia, which, in its turn, owes its origin to secret disgust. Loss of appetite and aversion are, nevertheless, sometimes denied, so that the conspicuously rapid emaciation can scarcely be accounted for. If we then seek for further symptoms of anxiety neurosis, especially for irritability, want of breath, palpitation, syncopic

---

[1] For further details of this see Vol. III, " Die Geschlechtskälte der Frau."

conditions, anxious anticipation and other forms of anxiety, we shall soon discover that the rapid loss of flesh is merely an acute incipient anxiety neurosis, which we must regard as the expression of a guilty conscience.

No. 67.—A corpulent, lively woman of forty began to lose weight with conspicuous rapidity and complained of troublesome night-sweats. Careful examination by her family doctor gave no grounds for attributing this emaciation to a somatic cause. Condition of urine found to be normal. She was referred to me for my opinion. I learned that she had been very nervous for two months. She would not go into a dark room, and looked under the beds before she went to sleep. In the street she experienced curiously uneasy sensations, as if black men were coming after her to rob her and carry her off. She practised coitus interruptus with her husband, with whom she was absolutely anæsthetic. It had done comparatively little harm to her. She had formed an attachment for some months with an old friend of her youth. The latter was unable to use a contraceptive, and she lived in continual fear of impregnation. During coitus which is preceded by great sexual excitement she is possessed by but a single thought : " If only nothing happens." She experiences no pleasure because her anxiety will not admit of any other sensation. A deflection, therefore, from the somatic to the psychic sphere. She gave up the liaison and regained in a few months her former balance and perfect health.

The severe psychic conflict between love and duty or a guilty conscience had obviously played a significant part in the generation of the neurosis.

One of the characteristics of anxiety neuroses is the fact that anxiety equivalents can substitute each other. If we follow such a succession of anxiety attacks we shall have little difficulty in establishing a certain periodic sequence in some cases, as has been clearly demonstrated by *Fliess*. The very fact that various parasthesias occur on periodic days proves them to be anxiety equivalents. I was first convinced of this in the case of a lady suffering from anxiety neurosis, whose great attacks occurred at long intervals. There were, however, days in these intervals on which she complained of trembling of the hands and a numbness in the thumbs. On other occasions she was attacked by violent sneezing fits, which disappeared on the following day without a trace. It seemed as if this numbness in the thumbs might be open to symbolic interpretation, as having originated through conversion. The thumb (which in folk-lore figures as "thumblet") is a symbol for the penis. And, in point of fact, the lady in question was ill-adapted for widowhood ; her "thumb" had atrophied too soon ! In another case the patient's finger with which she had been accustomed to masturbate, atrophied.

I have already made several allusions to this symbol as frequently representing a death wish.

Hartenberg (l.c.) describes a similar case resulting from sexual abstinence. I quote it here because it is illustrative of a rare symptom of anxiety neurosis : perineal cramp. This symptom, together with nervous tenesmus, urge to urinate, irritation in the vagina, pain in the testicle, irritation in the urethra, and the coccygodyce belong to those rudiments of anxiety neurosis which are rare and very difficult to detect. I only met with one case of perineal cramp before the composition of the first of these books, but I had no understanding of these things at that time, and regarded it as nervous over-excitement. Since then I have had occasion to observe six cases, of which I will introduce one here. But let us now take Hartenberg's case:—

No. 68.—Mrs. L., aged thirty-seven, complained of a condition of morbid excitement and incessant restlessness. She was tortured by groundless anxiety, arising at every opportunity, on the receipt of a letter, whenever she heard a shout in the street, when she thought her purse was lost (of course symbolic. Purse = omit; pocket = vagina). She suffered from frequent palpitation, stomachic and intestinal cramp. As she had lived for two years in complete sexual abstinence, she was troubled by excessive libido, and very painful perineal cramp. She was a singer. For some time past she had developed a phobia and was always ill for some days before appearing in public. At the moment when she began to sing she felt a contraction in the throat and in the breathing muscles which prevented her from doing justice to her powers. [1]

The patient showed no signs of hysteria, neurasthenia or organic disease.

In the course of treatment the conditions of her life underwent a change. She was no longer abstinent (" elle reprit ses habitudes sexuelles "), and six weeks afterwards had completely recovered. The morbid anxiety and anxiety conditions disappeared.

Perineal cramp often ends with a fairly intense feeling of pleasure. A colleague of mine thus describes his attacks of perineal cramp : " I often suffered as a child from diarrhœa. I had a bad attack of this malady when I was six years old, complicated by severe tenesmus. This tenesmus remained with me and occurs from time to time without any special cause. I feel a strong impulse to defecate, but am unable to do so. A violent contraction in the rectum causes such pain that I could cry out. *This pain gradually resolves itself into a pleasurable sensation, which ends in an actual orgasm. Sometimes the cramp occurs only in the perineal region, which, when it reaches a crisis is combined with a mild feeling of pleasure.*" [2]

This case is interesting because it also introduces very characteristic disorders of the bladder. My colleague suffered among other things from such violent polyuria that he was obliged to urinate every ten minutes. This symptom is very common and is indicative of great sexual excitement and the transference of anxiety to the genital tract. In this case there was also intense pain in the urethra which increased during urination and then, too, resolved itself into a feeling of pleasure.

Disturbances in the bladder in the form of cramp in this organ,

---

[1] We frequently find this connection between sexual disturbances and impediments in speech and singing. We shall later on meet with a very interesting case in the analysis of Phobias. It is a question of transference from *lower* to *higher*. (*Freud*).

[2] These perineal cramps are associated with unconscious homosexual phantasies. In all these patients, the anus and nates, as well as the perineum are the favourite erogenous zones.

are also well-known to urologists. Gonorrhœa particularly may greatly complicate anxiety neurosis and delay its cure. Sometimes gonorrhœa brings to light some latent anxiety neurosis. These patients often suffer from dreadful cramp in the bladder and at the same time produce a perfectly clear second urine. (Two-glasses test!) One can only confirm *Gyon's* statement that " Gonorrhœa is ' *the touchstone of a weak brain.*' "

The prostate also is the seat of neurotic phenomena which indicate the existence of anxiety neurosis. The prostate feels to the patient like a stone or foreign body. The sensitiveness of the organ increases during walking and may reach such a pitch that the patients are unable to sit down. (Acathisia). These attacks drive them to distraction.[1] The cramp may pass from the bladder to the anus and then to the prostate or *vice versa.* It is generally due to re-pressed homosexual tendencies. This would account for Preyer's case of a man getting cramp of the prostate while watching copulating dogs.

The organs of the urethra are especially subject to anxiety neurosis. The first symptom of anxiety neurosis is often a frequent desire to urinate which is sometimes so imperative that the patient is liable to wet himself, as he can never reach the lavatory in time. These patients develop a phobia : they are afraid that this weak-ness may attack them in public, and therefore shun society, never going to a theatre, because the very thought of urination produces the desire to urinate and they eventually suffer from dread of anxiety. Many patients are troubled with fear that they cannot urinate, that they may become incapable of urinating and func-tional paralysis of the detrusor vesicæ is the result.

We meet with cramps of all kinds in anxiety neurosis. I myself once observed a case of Pseudo-Cholelithiasis, and cases of so-called " *false appendicitis* " are legion. Fear of appendicitis may induce a very similar condition.

No. 69.—Mrs. S. H. came up from the country in order to undergo an opera-tion. She was suffering from " Abdominal cramp," the cause of which was attributed by all the doctors to an attack of appendicitis. Professor X., of Vienna, had recommended complete rest in bed for two weeks. The patient lived in Hungary and would have to return home at once otherwise the suppurating appendix would burst and she would become seriously ill. So home she went !

The journey involved *two hours'* shaking in a ricketty country vehicle, for the purpose of remaining so quiet for two weeks that, according to the sur-geon's orders, she was not even to turn round from right to left (!). The pain, notwithstanding, increased in intensity, and the patient decided to have the operation.

I was called to the hotel to see her the day beforehand. The lady wanted my opinion, as she was very nervous and was afraid of the anæsthetic.

On examination there was found to be *great sensitiveness in the Mac Burney region. But this pressure sensitiveness was confined only to the skin. When the skin was pinched the patient cried out, but intensive and deeper pressure if imperceptibly increased occasioned no pain.* She also evinced a *gradually*

---

[1] Cp. the case of acathisia in Vol. IV, *p.* 466.

remarkably increased peristalsis. She frequently dreamed of men cutting open her stomach with a big knife. She was an unsatisfied woman whose husband was completely *impotent.* The pains were an anxiety equivalent and of a purely neuropathic nature. The appendicitis was non-existent.

I prescribed a normal diet for the woman, who had been living for weeks on bread and milk. Trembling with anxiety she eat a cutlet in my presence. It was only when I pointed out to her, logically, that she was in Vienna, that the surgeon was at hand, that she was running no risk and would be operated on in any case, that she was induced to eat. After a few days she had overcome her anxiety and enjoyed everything she ate. In two weeks she left Vienna. Some years later I saw her with a strong, bonny little boy in her arms.

In the category of rare cases of anxiety rudiments are also included convulsive contractions of the gullet (with or without singultus) and cramp of the œsophagus.

No. 71.—Hecker (l.c.) described a case of this description. "M. S., a medical student of twenty-two, with no hereditary affection, suffered from his tenth year from fits of depression with violent attacks of anxiety in which he tore his hair and sma'shed things. Since the commencement of his malady he suffered from a peculiar obstruction in swallowing, which only occurred when he partook of solid food. He had the greatest difficulty in swallowing *meat* and *bread-crumbs,* but, curiously enough, he was able to manage the *crust* of bread."

This case is of obviously hysteric structure. Especially the circumstance that the patient could not swallow " meat," lends itself to symbolic interpretation. He was likewise unable to eat the crumb of bread, while he found the crust easier to swallow. *Freud*[1] has made an excellent analysis of a similar case.

No. 72.—" A woman who was living apart from her husband, was accustomed, when eating, to leave the best part, *i.e.,* she would only eat the skin of roast meat. This abstinence was explained by the date of its origin. It happened on the day when she gave up sexual relations with her husband, *i.e.,* renounced the best part."

I have met with several cases of anxiety neurosis which gave the picture of an œsophagus neurosis.

No. 73.—Mr. L. L., merchant, thirty years old, noticed that for some time past, his food had " stuck in his throat." He experienced at the same time a violent feeling of anxiety and was obliged to drink a glass of water in order to get the food down. Sometimes he brought the food up, after which he felt considerably relieved. He had lost 10 kg. in two years.

The surgeons suspected malignant neoplasm. But the complaint remained stationary for two years, and the probe passes the œsophagus without difficulty.

The diagnosis of œsophagus diverticle was also considered. But a careful œsophogoscopy revealed the condition to be quite normal.

The patient was eventually given bougie treatment daily, which afforded him some relief, so that he gained some kilos in weight.

The trouble could be traced to a homosexual fellatio phantasy.

[1] Zwangs handlung und Religionsübung (Zeitschrift für Religions-Psychologie, Bd. I, H. 1.).

CHAPTER XIII

CLINICAL PICTURE OF ANXIETY NEUROSIS: MUSCULAR CRAMPS, TICS, AND PAINS

MUSCULAR cramp frequently accompanies anxiety attacks. The patients complain of various disorders : the hands become stiff, a leg contracts convulsively, there is cramp in the calves ; cramp, and cramp-like conditions in the muscles underlying the sympathetic—intestines, stomach, bladder, heart. These cramp-like conditions are easily comprehensible to the physiologist. It is merely a question of the degree of stimulus. The cell reacts to stimulus first with excitement, but when the stimulus limit is over-stepped, it reacts with paralysis. Excitement and paralysis are both manifestations of reaction to external and internal stimuli. Fear and slight degrees of anxiety are expressed by excitement ; great anxiety-affects, fright and horror, by paralysis of the muscles. A timid person screams, but a frightened one loses his voice. The various muscular cramps are indications of anxious excitement, *e.g.*, the action of the sympathetic muscles may be excited, and that of the voluntary muscles inhibited. The transference from the psychic to the somatic sphere takes place most rapidly in a beaten track. People who are susceptible to cramp in the calves are likely to experience it during an attack of anxiety.

But this is not applicable in all cases. One sometimes succeeds in discovering a psychological explanation for the development of a particular cramp in a muscle-group. The following case is also of some interest in another respect :

No. 78.—Mrs. M. V., aged twenty-nine, mother of four children, no hereditary taint, was subject to conditions of nervous anxiety. The outstanding symptom was excessive irritability, under which her children, husband and servants suffered a great deal. She also complained of palpitations, emaciation, and constipation. I elicited the information that she practised coitus interruptus with her husband, and prescribed an occlusive pessary, whereupon there was a rapid improvement in the conditions. The woman became quieter, gained in weight, and the bowels worked spontaneously without laxative remedies.

After about two years I was called to the patient at night. I found her deathly pale, bathed in perspiration, and sitting up in bed moaning. She had awakened out of an anxiety dream with violent palpitations and severe pain in the shoulder. She felt *just as if she were going to die.* A cold sweat broke out all over her body, and she had fallen out of bed almost insensible. But the unbearable pain had brought her to herself again. *Her right arm was entirely numb, as if it were dead.* She could not move it.   She was seized with excruciating *cramp in the muscles* radiating from the neck.

She also held her head in the familiar distorted position peculiar to contraction of the strenocleidomastoideus.   The part behind the mastoid process was so sensitive that the slightest touch produced a fresh access of cramp.   After half an hour the cramp subsided (hot compresses) the excited heart calmed down, and the patient's cheeks regained their fresh colour.

I found no difficulty in arriving at the explanation of this remarkable case. But I was obliged to acknowledge, to my shame, that it was not the occlusive pessary prescribed by me which had brought about the temporary improvement in the patient's condition, but the co-operation of a third factor, which I had left entirely out of account.   Among her husband's friends there was a tall, handsome officer, who used to make ardent love to her.   She resisted all his temptations, although, or because, in her intercourse with her feebly potent husband she was generally completely anæsthetic.   (It was only by picturing the officer in her mind that she was of late able to attain any feeling.) It was at this period that her anxiety neurosis broke out.   She fought shy of adultery for the one reason that she was afraid of bearing children.   She had had enough with four children.   She would moreover have considered it a grave sin to introduce a " strange " child among her own.   (She was religious and went to church daily, but never to confession !)   But when she obtained the pessary her resistance broke down.   She yielded to her lover and found complete satisfaction and the complete restoration of her health.   But the love of a Don Juan, accustomed to the adulation of women, soon wore off.   Their meetings became rarer until with the exception of necessary visits to her husband—he severed all connection with her.

There was then a recurrence of the nervous conditions.   She took a dislike to everything ; her children, her husband, her pleasures, her beautiful clothes. The anxiety feelings, her irritability and constipation recommenced.

She had long ago given up conjugal intercourse with her husband under the pretext that he must take care of himself.   (He was a weakly and ailing man.)   On the evening before the attack, he had " come in to her again " after a long interval.   In order to provoke libido she had imagined herself with her faithless lover and became intensely excited.   But her husband's ejaculatio præcox prevented the normal discharge of the increased libido and left her unsatisfied and unhappy.   She sobbed herself quietly to sleep.

The association with the muscular cramp was as follows : As long as she resisted him, the officer used to kiss her on all the uncovered portions of her body.   Especially on her neck behind the ear.   He called this spot his " favourite," and maintained that she had the prettiest neck he had ever seen.   During the first coitus he had bitten her so hard in the neck that she had cried out with pain.

Thus the cramp was accounted for.   After the abortive coitus she dreamed of a second one with her lover.   The anxiety attack was the complete substitute for a coitus.   And the pains were the same as those she had once experienced, except that they were more intense and lasted longer.   The muscular cramp corresponded to a sympathetic excitation of the nerve in question.

But this is not the end of this remarkable story.   The pains increased to such an extent during the morning that I was again sent for.   The husband, in his desperation, had instinctively turned to the officer (who was an intimate friend of his) for help.   When the latter saw the woman in the throes of such cramp he promised to come again in the afternoon.   I was obliged to go again in the evening to administer a morphia injection.   Her lover was sitting by her bed, holding her hand, and consoling her.

The next morning I found her completely recovered.   She had not slept, although the injection had made her very sleepy.

" You will laugh when I tell you why I couldn't sleep.   My nose tickled so all night."

Now irritation in the nose is a well-known phenomenon in intoxication. In this case, however, the symptom was over-determined. In Vienna it is supposed to be an infallible sign of an impending quarrel. I therefore asked her : " Have you decided to give somebody a piece of your mind to-day ? " " I should think I have ! " she replied automatically.

We see how life complicates the cases. If we had attempted in this instance to strike a balance with an unknown factor, we would never have arrived at the truth. Type cases are only to be found in text-books. Each new case provides a fresh problem.

Another marked symptom of anxiety neurosis which also played a part in the above-mentioned case is worthy of special note : the dying off of the right arm. I have occasionally observed this symptom in women whose husbands were ill or dead ; similarly the feeling of *a dead right hand* (numbness of a finger is more frequently met with[1]: *e.g.*, see case 66). It seems to be a question of conversion in which the idea that the right hand (the bread winner !) will die off plays the principal rôle. Cases of weakness of the left arm are also met with, but they have not the same psychic origin. (Cp. also chapter VI., similar phenomena in Arteriosclerosis). The following case is a striking example of weakness in the right arm alternating with muscular cramp :

No. 79.—A very corpulent lady of forty-five, who had to nurse a sick man, awoke one night with a violent anxiety attack. Her right hand seemed paralysed. She thought she had been seized with a stroke. The doctor who was called in said she must have been lying on her arm. Since that occasion she suffered from frequent numbness and painful *muscular cramp* in the arm, which also occurred during the day, together with slight feeling of giddiness and palpitation. After the death of her husband she came to me for treatment. Typical anxiety neurosis with severe heart attacks ending in fainting. Her condition grew worse when she consulted another doctor who diagnosed fatty degeneration of the heart in an advanced stage and prescribed· a cure in Marienbad. She then attributed all her anxiety feelings to her heart. A common saying with her was : " I shan't live long," or " I shall die soon." Frequent sighing was likewise attributed to the fatty degeneration.

A hydropathic cure, validol, an apparatus for cooling the heart and re-assuring psychotherapy had brought about a general improvement in the condition. In her fiftieth year the menopause took place without any particular trouble. On the contrary, from thence forward the heart attacks subsided and were succeeded by a complete restoration of health. The weight remained the same. It was impossible to make a thorough investigation of the size of the heart on account of the enormous mammilla. The heart beats were perfectly pure and loud.

I asked her subsequently about the first attack when her hand had died off. It happened—she said—during the night after the family physician had so alarmed her. He had informed her that her husband was suffering from calcination of the arteries and had advised her to refrain from conjugal relations on account of· the danger of excitement. Some years previously the husband's potency had considerably diminished. The " dying off of the right hand " was a prophetic symptom. Three years later the husband died of a heart seizure in the night and she was left entirely alone, and badly provided for, with a business beyond her capacities. The alleged symptoms of fatty degeneration were merely symptoms of an ordinary anxiety neurosis

[1] A well-known phallic symbol.

consequent on frustrated excitement and abstinence. She was a voluptuous, sensual woman who looked much younger than her husband and was very attractive to men. She must have harboured unconscious death wishes, for her period of mourning was unusually protracted, and in every respect exaggerated. She wanted to dedicate her whole life thenceforward to good works, wore only black clothes and never went to a theatre. She then came into an inheritance and left the whole fortune to the church. I learned subsequently that she had had a lover during her husband's life-time; but afterwards would have no more to do with him. She lived a life of remorse.

Allusion may here be made to a variety of phenomena which should be of great interest to the psycho-therapist. I refer to the various cramps which embody a particular representation. When, for example, a woman makes a negative sign with her head, we will endeavour to discover what is concealed behind this movement. We learn that these cramps were first experienced during an anxiety attack when the patient cried : " I shall die—I shall never get over it." We then infer that the cramps represent the remembrance of an act of infidelity in which she said " yes "—to her subsequent regret. She denies the traumatic occurrence and is now continually saying " no." It is as if she were trying to protect herself against a fresh temptation by saying " no " in advance. It is a frequent symptom of " *subsequent correction*."

These phenomena really come under the category of " Tics." As Brissaud has ably demonstrated, the Tics represent a " systematic " movement, they are substitutes for an act. This distinguishes them from the cramps, which are isolated muscular contractions. (Janet).

These Tics play an important part in anxiety neuroses and phobias. But they are of comparatively less frequent occurrence in this country (Austria) than in France. Janet records a variety of interesting facts concerning the most remarkable Tics. There is, for example, the person who is perpetually saying " Yes," and another who says " No " ; a woman with a torticollis which disappears when she presses the little finger of her left hand on her chin ; distortions of the feet and legs, muscular cramp of the spinal column which has the deceptive appearance of skoliosis ; men who tear their hair, women who simulate coxalgia. In all these cases, unfortunately, the psychologic explanation, such as I was able to supply in the case of the woman who always said " No," is lacking.

The cramp (or the Tics) may affect the eyes. The patients are incessantly blinking, as if they were trying to dislodge some foreign body. Some movements are positively comical. Charcot says rightly : " The Tic is a caricature of an act." (Janet : Les Psychonévroses.) Others pull at their noses, or pluck at their clothing, etc.

I once observed a patient who, during an anxiety attack, would stretch out his arm in front of him as if he were shooting. This man was possessed with the idea that he would shoot the man who had seduced his wife. These cramps always subserve some unconscious idea. If a patient suffers from cramp in the œsophagus it is obvious that she doesn't want to eat because she is tired of life. Many of these cramps are *resistance movements* and *protective measures*. A very instructive example is afforded us in vaginitis. What a number of hypotheses have been formulated in explanation of this phenomenon! It was eventually agreed to regard vaginitis as a symptom of hysteria. Vaginitis is less known as a symptom of anxiety neurosis. It often occurs in young married women whose husbands are inexperienced, relatively impotent, or maladroit. The women become irritable, tearful, apprehensive and complain of palpitations, vertigo, fainting attacks, migraine, etc. It is well known that anxiety neurosis is very liable to break out in young married women if they are still anæsthetic, *i.e.*, if the sexual aversion is not yet overcome. This is the most important underlying cause of Dyspareunie.

Kisch (l.c.) makes a sharp distinction between *vaginitis, sexual anæsthesia*, which he always regards as a pathologic symptom, *i.e.*, as the result of spinal complaints or diabetes, etc., and Dyspareunia, formerly known as anaphrodisia. I cannot see any particular difference. With the exception of organic disorder, it is always a question of *conversion* symptoms.

Wherever sexual aversion has the upper hand we shall always find sexual anæsthesia, especially in hysterics, but also in anxiety neurotics. *Vaginitis* may likewise be due to unconscious psychic causes. A woman who has been mortified by the unskilful attempts of her husband will deny him intercourse with her. *Vaginitis is sometimes only a symptom of fear of coitus.*[1] This fear can only be overcome through love for the husband. A lady of my acquaintance exhibited vaginitis in her relations with her husband, but experienced no difficulties with a friend of her youth. She had married her husband from cold calculation and without love, but she loved her old friend passionately. She once told me that she would like to bear her lover a child. That was the psychic root of her vaginitis. We observe that, in reality, it has the same psychic motivation as nervous vomiting, as abdominal cramp, as prejudices against flesh-foods, etc. Difficult cases of vaginitis require psychanalytic treatment.[2]

Besides muscular cramps, muscular pains play a certain part in anxiety neuroses. *Freud*, in his work on anxiety neurosis, points out that many so-called rheumatic pains are only symptoms

---

[1] These remarks on vaginitis in the first edition were confirmed in Professor Walthood's work on " Die psychische Aetiologie und die Psychotherapie des Vaginismus " (Münchener mediz. Wochenschr. 1909, No. 39). Walthood, who did not know my book, came to the same conclusion—*i.e.*, that vaginitis is the result of a phobia.

[2] Dealt with fully in Vol. III.

of disguised anxiety neurosis. The same might be said—and with even greater justification—of the " gouty " pains now so fashionable, gouty neuralgia, etc. Such uric pains are often miraculously cured by medicinal baths. But that is only because the women are removed from the injurious effects of coitus interruptus and form new connections here and there in the health resorts ; and because the men satisfy their desires in a normal way out of wedlock. These enigmatical " rheumatic or gouty " pains arise, as in the case of the parasthesias, through a form of conversion, *i.e.*, by the transformation of psychic phenomena into somatic.

No. 80.—I knew a lady who suffered for seven years from an unpleasant muscular pain and muscular cramp in her right upper thigh. Massage, electricity and painting with iodine were ineffectual. The lady had been under my treatment for anxiety neurosis for some years. Apart from the outstanding symptom of excessive anxiety she was troubled with palpitations and slight attacks of vertigo. She suffered from time to time from insomnia of a particularly obstinate character which greatly pulled her down. One day I made an attempt to approach the enigmatical pain psychanalytically. To my surprise it proved to be a case of conversion. The patient was unsatisfied in her marital relations. Not that the husband was impotent. On the contrary ! He was very highly sexed—but she remained anæsthetic with him. (This phenomenon is frequently to be observed in women who have been forced to marry men whom they neither love nor desire). Once, during a summer holiday, a friend of her husband's had made love to her and sought to win her favour. When they were resting on the grass during an excursion, he threw himself upon her and wanted intercourse with her. She screamed as loudly as she could, for though she was prepared for a harmless " flirtation," or possibly a kiss, she would not go to extremities. She screamed therefore and achieved her purpose. The man (whom she loved) released her. But some months later the anxiety neurosis made its appearance and she began to complain of pains in her upper thigh. It was on that spot that she had felt the powerful hand of her tempter. The pain was the result of conversion. She had had a burning sensation there for days, which had produced great sexual excitement in her. The pain also induced her—after she had *suppressed* the remembrance of the painful episode—to speak to her husband about the unpleasant matter which had so disturbed her. She had hitherto had no secrets from her husband. She had suppressed the affair with the friend because she had not been guiltless, because she had tolerated the first advances, and even a few kisses without resistance. But the episode caused her such tribulation that she told him all, though only in a symbolic disguised form. The pain therefore reminded her of the experience, without bringing its painful side to consciousness. The analysis successfully disposed of the pains. Many rheumatic pains might be thus accounted for by conversion, and cured by elucidation.

No. 81.—A similar and yet more interesting case. A lady of thirty-six had been suffering for fourteen years from dorsal pains of such an unbearable character that she was obliged to stay in bed for weeks at a stretch. A celebrated gynæcologist diagnosed the case as one of " adhesions " and suggested laparotomy. She came to consult me. I questioned her, after I could detect no somatic affection, as to the psychogenesis of the pain. A significant fact then came to light. She was unhappy with her husband, a neurotic, who had married her not for love but for convenience, and was now, for some unknown motive, making her suffer for it. She had experienced the violent pain for the first time on the wedding night. On that occasion her husband (who had caused her intense pain during the defloration) had cried out : " *You have deceived me ! You are no longer a virgin !* " She had almost forgotten this painful episode. She never spoke of it. But the pain in her back was the fixation of the unpleasant scene. Her illness was the husband's punishment, for the cures she had undergone had been a great expense to him. After the discovery of the psychogenic cause (*in seven days !*) the pain entirely vanished. But there was a relapse following a violent scene with her husband. The pain was, however, not so intense, and subsided after two days, never to return.

The so-called " cardiac pains " which young people suffer from, are, in the majority of cases psychic pains, which have become projected on to the heart as the seat of all emotions. In older people who suffer from arteriosclerosis, a differential diagnosis is, as I have already shown, much more difficult to arrive at.

But the statements : " My heart hurts me "—" something is weighing on my heart," " something is pressing on my heart," lead one to suspect " unhappy love," and one should never omit—as I demonstrated in the chapter on cardiac affections—to seek for psychic causes.

But muscular cramp, which we know as occupation neurosis, may have a similar source of origin : anxiety neurosis due to psychic motives. *Janet* terms these conditions *Tics*.

No. 82.—I remember a patient who, though highly sexed, abstained from intercourse from fear of infection. He exhibited the typical symptoms of anxiety neurosis (vertigo, palpitation, oppression in the head, dyspepsia, tendency to be easily fatigued, rachialgia, insomnia). He also suffered from writer's cramp, which at first occurred only on certain occasions and then with increasing frequency, thus hindering him in his profession. He had up till then given up his entire earnings to support his father (whom, for various reasons he hated) and the whole family. The father should be compelled to work. The anxiety proceeding from the anxiety neurosis was then transferred to the writer's cramp. If he had to answer an advertisement he was haunted all day with the thought that he might be seized with cramp and thus hindered. There was no escape from this vicious circle. He was soon incapable of remembering the details of certain commissions. Formerly he had been able to keep mental notes of everything. But he might still have dictated the orders at home to his mother, of whom he was very fond. But his misfortunes were increased by rapid loss of memory. He could not remember a single number or a single price. He gave entirely wrong figures so that he was obliged to cancel large orders. He was utterly unfitted for any position and went and sat with his father by the fire. His sisters then supported the household in which were these two men, both incapable of working. At the same time he protested that he would be so glad to work, and wanted to be well again ; if only he could be free of this confounded fear of writer's cramp ! An attempt at analytical treatment failed, for the patient ceased his visits after a few sittings. The inner resistance to the cure was greater than the will to health.[1]

I do not wish to generalise. But it is my belief that certain conditions of cramp necessitate still more careful analytical investigation. Another form of occupation neurosis shows in a like manner

[1] *Janet* makes a very pertinent observation in describing a case of writer's cramp, which reveals something of the *unconscious* motives of the cramp : in this patient, who earned her living by copying, the writer's cramp was preceded by another symptom, which in my opinion was of great significance, and occurs more frequently in writer's cramp than one would suppose. She experienced an intense deep-rooted antipathy (dégoût) for her occupation, she had hardly the spirit to work at her copying, and would have preferred to do any other work (n'importe quoi !).

the power of unconscious resistance. I refer to the remarkable *laryngeal cramp* to which singers are liable who do not love their profession. I knew a very intelligent young man who studied for the stage against his rich father's wishes. He received a very moderate salary and was scarcely able to make both ends meet. Suddenly his powerful, beautiful voice began to lose its strength, and after a few clear notes he was unable to produce a single proper note from his throat. I pointed out to him, in the course of analysis, that he was feeling remorse and would rather return home to his father than continue to suffer privation abroad. He denied the imputation vehemently. A few years later I met him again. He had in the meanwhile become a doctor, was reconciled with his father, and wished to devote himself to psychanalysis.

A young singer of good family, still attending the Conservatoire, came to consult me for the same reason. This lady was likewise unfitted for her profession. For she had a narrow-minded "bourgois" morality and was afraid of the erotic dangers of stage life. I counselled her to give up singing and take up another profession. She took my advice, and, after being happily married, regained her voice in a few months.

It is these occupation neuroses in particular which throw such a strong light on the "will-to-illness." We must not allow ourselves to be led astray by the complaints and lamentations of the patients who are perpetually protesting that they would be overjoyed if they could only play or speak again. A pianist was seized with cramp after playing the piano for an hour, complained of "excruciating pain," and was unable to continue her practising, escaped by her illness, the necessity of appearing in public, and of supporting herself. A violinist managed to escape in like manner from the promptings of his ambition, and thus induced his parents to support him. In all these cases there lies concealed behind the cramp a resistance to the profession, and fear of appearing in public.

Among the war neuroses which came under my observation were various forms of muscular cramp which were positively ludicrous. With them illness was always the means whereby they escaped military service and the trenches. I could never detect any sexual component of these cramps. It was simply a psychic conflict, between the instinct of self-preservation against and compulsory military service. This self-deception was as common among officers as in the rank and file.

CHAPTER XIV

CLINICAL PICTURE OF ANXIETY NEUROSIS: SLEEPLESSNESS

GREAT excitement of the central nervous system reveals itself, in severe forms of anxiety neurosis, by psychic irritability, and quick changes of mood, so that the clinical form it takes is sometimes that of mania, and sometimes slightly resembles melancholia. The patients are strung to such an intense pitch of excitement that they will sometimes attempt to commit suicide—fortunately with no serious intent. *The tendency to fly in a passion*, the conversion of anxiety into anger, is a characteristic psychological factor in the life of the anxiety neurotic.[1] They are a type of people dominated by their affects, and every neurosis is a disturbance of their affectivity. A life of high emotional pressure brings them more easily into conflict than normal people. An underlying element of hate generates death wishes and becomes the source of endless self-reproaches and a tormenting sense of guilt. It is then that the affects become inhibited. Anxiety neurotics may give the impression of melancholia because of their seemingly complete indifference, their inability to enjoy life. But this mood is never sustained for long. And it is just this rapid change of mood which is such a typical feature of anxiety neurosis. Other cerebral and spinal symptoms are likewise in evidence : migraine (even as a typical anxiety equivalent with excessive vomiting), yawning fits, insomnia, marked increase of all reflexes, and hallucinations (especially in childhood and in combination with hysteria) are no unusual phenomena.

It sometimes happens that a serious psychosis develops on a foundation of anxiety neurosis. But these cases are of rare

[1] The connection between *anxiety* and *rage* is more close than we think. There are anxiety attacks which end up with a violent outburst of rage. Every anxiety neurotic is easily aroused to fury and is afraid of his own temper. It is difficult to believe that behind blushes and shyness are hidden overwhelmingly strong criminal instincts. Anxiety is, then, fear of the active criminality within. Rage is the direct outburst of the criminal component—destructive hate. Some people when angry will beat the table or break something : they must ,anihilate something *symbolically*. There is no proof of my statement :—"every anxiety is the fear of one self," better then these connections between anxiety and rage. Active criminality becomes passive anxiety. It may also happen the other way round. *Cowardice* is transformed by the motor system into many a beautiful example of heroic *courage*.

occurrence, and anxiety neurosis in particular is distinguishable from all other neuroses by the ease with which it can be cured. When the injurious causes·are removed, the repressions made conscious and disposed of, the conflicts mitigated, an improvement of the distressing conditions rapidly takes place. The apprehensiveness of the patients often takes the form of a conviction that they are suffering from spinal disease; their memories are affected; they feel threatened with a serious mental disorder. These fears cannot be dispelled by reassurances from the doctor as they are compulsion phenomena for which psychic investigation and analytical treatment are absolutely essential. The pangs of conscience, the disposition to doubt, the typical moral over-scrupulousness, and mania for brooding, all arise out of the tendency towards rumination and anxious expectation. These anxiety conditions lead, among other things, to *insomnia*. Nor must we leave out of consideration the most important cause of insomnia—*insufficient sexual gratification*. Concealed behind all these problems, that appear insoluble to the patient, there often lurks the one important problem—that of sex.

Uniformly (as over-valued idea) or in rapid succession (almost like a flight of ideas) thoughts course through the mind at night, when the anxiety neurotic is withdrawn from the distractions of the day. The general anxiety is increased by the terrors of the night. All the accumulated anxiety clamours for release; the night is, in a measure, reserved for prohibited and especially sexual thoughts. It is at night that the "secret criminal" makes his appearance.

Insomnia is one of the most unpleasant symptoms of anxiety neurosis. If it occurs as the result of an anxiety affect it is easy to diagnose. The patients are seized with a feeling of anxiety before falling asleep, which they generally attribute to some organic cause. They are afraid of something horrible happening, that they will be seized with a stroke; that they are on the verge of a severe illness; that their heart will cease to beat. "This must be the end." "This is how one feels when about to die." The anxiety thoughts chase one another in riotous confusion, or else only *one* thought—sometimes an isolated meaningless word—roves monotonously through the field of consciousness.

The study of these isolated words, which are only apparently meaningless, is very interesting. There was one neurotic who incessantly repeated the word "*Mortateller! Mortateller!*" This is the name of a sausage, but signified in this instance murder (*Mort¹-a* [ein !] *-Teller* [plate]) and refers to his poison phantasies. A lady who felt impelled to hum a melody for hours at a stretch and could not sleep, sang me this melody. I at once recognised the familiar song: "I am a widow, a little widow," etc. Concealed behind this harmless melody were death wishes against her husband.

¹ Murder.

It more frequently happens that those suffering from anxiety neurosis fall asleep and are then awakened by an anxiety dream. The familiar sensation of falling from a height and the sudden fall in which the whole body makes a convulsive movement are sensations generally occurring in the first stages of sleep, and are very frequent symptoms of anxiety neurotics. *The anxiety neurosis only subsides when the ætiologic factors have been changed.* The anxiety neurotic falls asleep again when his libido has been satisfied, or if his pangs of conscience are set at rest. If such is not the case sleep can hardly ever be induced. Bromide is the most effective soporific, as it reduces the libido and the cerebral excitement.

His sleep is generally restless, full of wild, confused dreams out of which he awakes with a throbbing heart and bathed in perspiration, after which it is a long time before he can fall asleep again. The dreams that trouble him are often of a typical erotic nature. Women dream of men who pierce them through the breast, of great savage men who pursue them, of gigantic steers that follow them, of neighing stallions, etc. Men dream that they are in a position of great danger, that they fail to pass an examination, that they are standing as prisoners at the Bar. Here and there incest dreams or perverse impulses (homosexual dreams)· frighten the moral ego and compel consciousness to reassume its control. But the dreams betray still more. The neurotic dreams of murder, of corpses, of criminals. When once we have mastered the language of dreams and gained insight into them, we are amazed to find what a severe contest the anxiety neurotic is engaged in against his criminal impulses. I repeat :

All anxiety is fear of one-self !

The criminal thoughts come forth at night and demand realisation. They want to be more than mere phantoms. It is then that the neurotic becomes afraid of himself. He sees before him the yawning abyss of his soul. Perhaps he cannot sleep because he fears the evil thoughts in his dreams. *Janet* reports a case of this description in which the patient, after a few minutes' tranquil sleep awakes with fearful anxiety feelings and passes the whole night in sheer endless misery. Similar cases have proved to me that such patients are afraid of their own phantasies. The analysis of these dreams betray these phantasies to us.

We shall have an opportunity, in discussing the complicated phobias, of analysing a number of these anxiety dreams, but we must not lose sight of the fact that an anxiety dream may precede a severe infectious illness.

As a medical student I once had a violent anxiety dream. I cried out in my sleep for the first time in my life. I was then in the early stages of a severe attack of typhoid.

These dreams should be regarded as a refined perception of the brain liberated from the function of conscious thinking. There is no foundation for the assumption that these dreams are prophetic.

My son (aged nine) awoke one night from a violent anxiety dream. A dragon had pursued him and "wanted to bite him." He could not sleep that night for anxiety. Two days later he was seized with a severe inflammation of the throat.

An unexpected anxiety dream, followed, possibly, by sleeplessness, should always suggest to the practitioner the incubation stage of an infectious disease.

Feverish dreams, of course, betray the same complexes as normal anxiety dreams. An analysis of the various fever phantasies would form a very profitable task for the analyst.

It is perfectly marvellous how quickly the insomnia of some neurotics vanishes when their excitement is allayed by sexual gratification. There is always a certain amount of anxiety dissipated by the sex act, which, if it accumulates makes people ill. This is especially to be observed in women whose husbands are away. As long as the husband is not there they sleep badly. They attribute the insomnia to the fact that they cannot sleep alone, and have a relative to sleep with them because they are "afraid of burglars." The psychology of this anxiety is transparent! (Cf. Case No. 85.) When the (potent !) husband returns they sleep excellently. *Nota bene* only when sexual relations are normal and the anxiety neurosis is due only to abstinence. Otherwise (in cases of ejaculatio præcox and coitus interruptus) the cessation of the injurious stimulus without gratification, which only rouses the libido and provokes fresh anxiety, often brings about the desired rest and healthy sleep. I had a case of this description :

No. 83.—Mrs. H. C., aged thirty-two, had been suffering for four years from severe anxiety attacks. She suddenly turned pale, her heart beat violently, and she was seized with such giddiness that she had to lie down. "I feel as if some force stronger than I were pulling me backwards," she said. In this condition she often cried : "This must be the death struggle." "The death struggle must be like this !" or "One of these days I shall lie like this and go to sleep." Of late years she had had a feeling, before the attack, as if her feet were swelling. *This was no hallucination ; the soles of her feet were often swollen.* I saw them myself in this condition.[1] At the same time all the blood would rise to her head and deprive her of breath. She had no hereditary taint, and, apart from an ulcus ventriculi and secondary severe anæmia, had never been ill. She had three children. Since the birth of the last child (five years) coitus interruptus had been practised. She was of an extremely jealous disposition, and, like all jealous women, insatiable. She also exhibited a strong homosexual component. (Deepest root of jealousy !) She declared that she was absolutely anæsthetic. "She had no taste for such things." But I had the real facts of the case from the lips of her husband, who had once consulted me about an attack of gonorrhœa, and asked me if it could be the result of excessive irritation. On that night—each time on his wife's desire, and after corresponding manipulations—he had been obliged to perform the conjugal act ten times in succession. She was now very irritable and made his home a hell. The husband, who used always to be at home, then took

[1] *Freud* told me of a man suffering from agoraphobia (anxiety hysteria), who, after crossing a road exhibited extensive œdema in both legs. If his family physician accompanied him he could walk for three hours without a trace of œdema occurring. Of course, then he felt no anxiety.

to travelling about, and often left her for six weeks alone. On his return he only slept with her twice a week. She was always accusing him of infidelity. " You give yourself out elsewhere, and in consequence have nothing left for me ! "

The potency of this man was so great that, in spite of the coitus interruptus with her he was able to produce two orgasms. In his absence she was entirely sleepless but without anxiety. As soon as the husband returned and fulfilled his marital duties she slept peacefully and dreamlessly. After long intervals, *i.e.*, during the menses—she also suffered from insomnia, or only fell into a restless sleep towards morning.

There was an interesting explanation for the premonitory swelling of the soles of the feet, which occurred with her also as an anxiety equivalent. Her husband was accustomed to tickle her—she was extremely ticklish— with his big toe on the soles of her feet when he desired to stimulate her erotically. That was his way of inviting her to the "love-dance." This symptom was also the prelude to the anxiety attack. The periphery nerves were so highly sensitive to excitement that a temporary transudation was caused. (Angioneurotic œdema !)

I have frequently observed œdema in cases of anxiety neurosis partly as a correlative symptom and partly as equivalent.

No. 84.—Mr. A. K., a twenty-two year old medical student, whose father had died of progressive paralysis, had been suffering for four months from insomnia. He had been troubled for a year with *vague feelings of anxiety.* He also complained of trembling in the hands, of general weakness, and especially, of lack of energy. He was incapable of concentrating his thoughts for any length of time on a particular subject, and, in consequence, could not continue his studies. His attention was always wandering. *Melodies* would run in his head which he felt impelled to whistle, phantastic pictures appeared before his mental vision in rapid succession. A mad confusion of pictures, ideas, reminiscences and wishes distracted his attention. All these phantasies were always accompanied by some particular melody.

Before going to sleep he experienced severe orthopnœa. He would fall into an uneasy sleep from which he would awaken after a few hours with palpitation, shortness of breath and anxiety feelings. Then it was all up with his sleep.

" What melody prevented you from studying to-day ? "

He whistled a Viennese song, the text of which he could not remember. I knew it very well. The words run : " Wiener Frauen, hold und schön— ach wie herrlich anzusehen." He had heard the song repeatedly and forgotten the words.

All other melodies proved in like manner to be connected with the erotic complex.

The young man was exceptionally highly sexed. He had masturbated daily for years and later on performed coitus twice a week.

He learned from lectures and pamphlets of the dangers of sexual intercourse and resolved to remain chaste until his marriage. A few weeks after the abstinence, which he found extremely trying, the first symptoms of anxiety neurosis made their appearance, and increased to such an extent that he was unable to work. The fact that his housekeeper, a young and lively widow, seemed to be amorously inclined towards him, made his self-enforced abstinence all the harder. The melody which disturbed his studies had reference to the housekeeper. Finally, youth and impulse got the better of all chaste resolutions. After a few days he was quite well again and slept soundly and regularly for ten hours.

The sexual abstinence movement has two sides to it. Some men avoid infection only to become neurotics. For them it is a choice between the two evils of neurosis and infection.

Let us turn to another picture !

No. 85.—Mrs. N. Z., aged thirty-two, mother of two children, dress-maker, suffering from troublesome nervous symptoms. She had experienced severe mental shocks. She had been obliged to separate from her husband, a man of great sexual potency, because he, being a regular Don Juan, spent enormous sums of money on other women and involved her in considerable debts. After the separation she became gloomy, pensive, very irritable and wept at every opportune and inopportune occasion. Her life was so lonely ; she hadn't a soul to turn to—no sympathetic friend. Those were her usual complaints. She began gradually to suffer from insomnia. Bromide, veronal, trional brought only moderate relief. A change of circumstances occasioned by a journey to the North Sea resulted in a notable though temporary improvement. The patient returned home almost well, fresh, and in good spirits. Then she had to undergo a small operation (peringorrhaphy). This was followed by absolute sleeplessness. She betrayed her character in the nature of her dreams. For example, she recounted a dream in which she was to be bound naked to a tree by several men, a reproduction of the situation during the operation, with which her sexual phantasy was much occupied. On another occasion she was unable to sleep despite the veronal (0.60). She was so terribly anxious. Why ? Because the landlady (she was living in a boarding-house) and the house-maid were not at home on that night and so many men were living in the house. She was at that time the only woman there. How easily might one of these young men make a mistake in the doors, and come into her room ! I pointed out to her that there was a very good means of preventing such an occurrence—by locking the door. Her excuse for not doing so was that she might be taken ill in the night and no one could get in to attend to her. This fear of the young men resolves itself, therefore, into a concealed, suppressed desire. When I represented it to her as such, her first question was, whether she might " have intercourse " again. I told her that she could. From that day onwards she was completely cured. She had made the acquaintance of a man during her visit to the North Sea, who became her lover. Her anxiety neurosis and insomnia were simply the result of *abstinence*.

Insomnia very frequently occurs after an operation. This insomnia was regarded, for a time, as the result of fear, anxiety, and the toxic effect of chloroform. From my analyses I can draw but one conclusion : *The anæsthetic and the operation are a severe trauma for the sexual phantasy of the patient.* Imagine what it must be for a modest woman to lie naked before a lot of men and allow herself to be operated on. It is such a complete break with everything that has hitherto been so bashfully preserved, that the phantasy must be greatly excited. Dreams after an operation prove that the operation is the point of issue for violation and prostitution phantasies, which all come under the category of " Pleasure without guilt."

No. 86.—Miss K. B., aged thirty-six, spinster, shop-keeper ; some hereditary taint (mother with religious mania). This woman suffered for seven years from insomnia, which afflicted her especially when she was about to undertake anything. Even a visit to the theatre was liable to excite her to such a degree that she could not sleep. She would walk about with the fixed idea that she could not sleep. During the menstrual period the patient's sleep was uneasy and restless, even when there had been no mental excitement. When she went to bed, one thought after another raced through her brain. (Flight of ideas). She put questions to herself, and answered them.

The patient never complained of anxiety, although she experienced disagreeable feelings. Sometimes she felt tired of life, and found her work distasteful. In fact her grievance was that her work was so futile; even an imbecile could do it.

The patient had an erotic experience at a very early age. When she was seven years old she overheard the performance of coitus between her father and mother, and thought to herself : " That is what grown-up people speak of." She had a dim remembrance of crying out on that occasion. She menstruated at fourteen years, and used to feel erotically excited when reading novels. She masturbated by means of the thighs. Further, as a child, she used to experience voluptuous sensations when she saw another child being beaten or when she read about tortures in books. This used to excite her tremendously. When she was nineteen she met a man of her own age whose slightest touch greatly agitated her. But he never let things come to a climax as he " did not wish to break the flower," as he expressed it. " Although I pretended to be asleep with him and would have given him all, he did not touch me."

The parents of this young man got to know of the affair and forbade his friendship for Miss B. K. The latter was so mortified at her lover's submitting to his parents' judgment, that she gave herself to a friend whom she did not love in the least. She did this out of revenge, but during the whole intercourse was entirely anæsthetic. A year later the man died ; and she then continued to masturbate until her twenty-seventh year. Then followed another liaison which she found tolerably satisfying. When this affair was broken off (she had made a terrible mistake in her choice) she came across certain books, all warning her against the practice of onanism, and describing the frightful consequences thereof. She resolved to give up masturbating, in which she was only partially successful.

This was a case of typical anxiety neurosis resulting from sexual abstinence. Whereas masturbation was comparatively harmless for her, she was unable to endure abstinence.

This is one of the most frequent causes of insomnia. In innumerable cases that have come under my observation, I have repeatedly found that the patients were onanists struggling to break themselves of the habit. After an act of masturbation they were able to sleep peacefully. I know people for whom masturbation is the only effective soporific. The most obstinate cases of insomnia occur when the habit of masturbation is abandoned. In its place there is often an increase of nocturnal emissions. But all emissions are merely onanistic acts with the elimination of consciousness. (Pleasure without guilt—the old familiar Leitmotiv of all neurotics !)

No. 87.—Mrs. L. P.—no hereditary taint—married—no children—an abortion eighteen years previously. After bronchitis she suffered for three weeks from *insomnia*, shortness of breath, a stabbing pain (within the mammilla) and oppression over the heart. She used to awake with a start after falling asleep, and with an outbreak of perspiration in the hands and feet, loss of appetite for a week, constipation, congestion of blood in the face, nervous twitchings in the night and depression. She was always thinking of illness and death. Unhappy marriage—husband quick-tempered, brutal, ejaculatio præcox—no orgasm. Masturbation in the first years of marriage—abandoned eighteen months ago. She was very sensitive (her parents had been very happily married !). Neglected herself, became apathetic and " lost interest " in everything. Murderous thoughts against the husband.

During the three weeks when she lay in bed, the desire to masturbate which she so dreaded, was reawakened. She then learned from a doctor of the harmlessness of onanism practised in moderation and after two weeks she was perfectly well again and was able to enjoy peaceful sleep. This patient also was unable to exist without masturbation. In place of pleasure anxiety appeared as its equivalent.

This form of anxiety equivalent is alluded to by *Hecker* (l.c.). In this instance the insomnia was the result of a condition of sexual excitement. Lack of satisfaction, as in libido with no outlet is one of the principal causes of sleeplessness. In this case the anxious anticipation of the sex act, the one thing that she really longed for, was transferred to the small affairs of life. Without knowledge of the mechanism of this process of displacement almost all phobias and compulsion phenomena would remain a mystery to us. Freud has demonstrated, however, how the affect is deflected from the repressed idea on to a less painful one, which, for the sake of simplification I have called " displacement," an expression coined by *Freud* and applied by him in the Interpretation of Dreams in a similar sense.

How important a knowledge of a " displacement " is for therapy is demonstrated in the following case of the insomnia of an anxiety neurotic :

No. 88.—Mr. C. W., aged sixty-eight, hereditary taint on the maternal side—had been suffering for eight months from sleeplessness. At first he experienced an intense feeling of anxiety in the evenings, accompanied by palpitations ; he felt as if he were going to be seriously ill or that some great misfortune threatened him. After thoroughly examining him and finding no organic defect I enquired whether there was not some definite trouble or grievance that prevented him from sleeping. He denied this and said that he was merely extremely excited. He found noises particularly irritating.

" What kind of noises ? "

" Well," he replied, " its rather strange ; I don't mind the rattling of vehicles. Even when one noise predominates over others in the street it does not trouble me. *But what I cannot stand is the banging of doors.* It irritates me to such an extent that I can't go to sleep."

" Well, that is easily remedied. You need only request people not to bang the doors."

" But it doesn't occur in my flat, but in the one below, which is occupied by two fast young men who come home late at night, make a noise, and bang the doors without any consideration for others. That excites me and keeps me awake."

" You say, ' fast young men.' In what way are they fast ' ? "

" I only know that they come home late. Besides one hears things about them in the house. But that has nothing to do with the case."

" You are mistaken—everything has to do with or may have to do with the case. What is said of these ' fast young men ' ? "

" Oh, that they've both got an affair with the housemaid."

" Ah—now I understand your excitement. You imagine the young men going in to the house-maid."

" I don't imagine. I *know*. I know for certain that first one goes in. Then I hear the door shut again. . . ."

There was then a motive for the sleeplessness. The old gentleman was in the highest degree sexually excited when he heard these sounds. But there seemed to me to be a disparity between the intensity of the affect and the facts revealed. I investigated further, with discretion.

" Have you never suffered from insomnia before ? "

" Oh, yes—as a little boy I was once three months without sleep."

" Did you sleep in your parents' room ? "

" Yes, always—until my tenth year."

" Did you overhear things that were not intended for you to hear ? "

" Yes, I did. I used to wait anxiously for my parents to ' have a tussle.' I didn't know anything about such things."

" Did you let your parents know that you were awake ? "

" No. I said nothing about it at that time. I don't know why. I then became very run down and they noticed that I was not sleeping."

" And did you never suffer from insomnia in later years ? "

" Yes, six years ago. It was when I was greatly concerned about my son. He was a clerk in a large firm. It was very difficult to obtain this position for him. And the expense he was to me before this was achieved ! At last he was independent, and then he brought this shame upon me, eloping with the wife of his chief, a woman fifteen years older than himself. He is now living with her in America."

After a pause, he continued :

" Unfortunately, he also tampered with the funds. In order to preserve the honour of my name and to save him from legal proceedings, I was obliged to replace the greater part of the sum involved. Oh, the trouble I have gone through with that boy ! "

" So you don't sleep because you are thinking of your son. Now, has not the door-banging some connection with this son ? "

" Of course. Once—he was then barely eighteen, and just such a gay young spark as the two boys in the lower flat—I heard a door slam. I got up quietly and saw that my son's bed was empty. I suspected something was wrong, went into the kitchen and found my son in the maid's bed. Well, you know, doctor, I was no saint myself when I was a boy, but I never did anything of that sort in my own house. Moreover, the girl, whom we turned out of the house, had a child by another man. And who had to pay for its keep ? I, of course—on my son's behalf."

It would take too long to go into a detailed analysis of this case. The cause of the insomnia was complicated. All his life he had been a very highly sexed man. The ill-sustained abstinence of the last ten years had made an anxiety neurotic of him. The slamming of doors awakened repressed ideas in him : the scene in his childhood at home, the memory of the thoughtless behaviour of his son. A yearning for his child arose in him—the child who had been such a bitter disappointment to him and who had brought shame upon his name.

But the most important point was that he was *still struggling against temptations*. His secret thoughts ran on house-maids.[1] (His son had inherited this tendency.) He had always had a special predeliction for maid-servants, even for those in his own home. There used to be violent scenes and his wife died—so they said— of a broken heart in consequence of the sorrow he caused her. And even still, as an old man, he was a prey to temptations. The slammed door reminded him of his own house-maid. He was afraid that the dissolute young men might come and visit his cook. He was, in fact, jealous.

The analytic method was in this case triumphantly successful. When I had solved the problem of " the slamming doors " for him, he was soon pacified and able to sleep the whole night through undisturbed.

[1] " The predeliction for maid-servants " is attributable to fixed infantile experiences. Men of this description have received vivid erotic impressions in their youth from the servant-class.

No. 89.—A commercial scholar of twenty-four, suffering from uneasiness debility, pains in the head and back, constipation and loss of appetite. He was incapable of following the lectures in school, or of studying. He felt as if an iron band were encircling his head and was " dreadfully " despondent. His parents thought he had been over-exerting himself—too much study—he was too ambitious. They asked me to prescribe a few weeks on the Semmering for him. After a lengthy investigation I could discover no physical root to the trouble. He had had regular sexual intercourse until a few weeks previously. *But he was now so depressed that he could not think of such things.* The motivation appeared to be somewhat unsubstantial. I asked if he had been " crossed in love." This he laughingly denied. He went to the Semmering and came back after a few weeks perfectly well and ready for work.

How great was my astonishment, when, a month later, I had occasion to treat his brother, a law student, for an identical complaint. I at once thought of identification. Such cases are very frequent. From various motives ! Mostly envy of the sympathy lavished on the sick brother, etc. In this instance I thought : " Aha ! this boy wants to be sent to the Semmering, too, for a few weeks."

I suggested therefore to my patient that he should go for a few weeks to the Semmering, which had done his brother so much good.

To my surprise, he replied :

" I absolutely refuse to leave the house. I am about to stand for my examination and have no time to pay court to the pretty ladies on the Semmering."

" You think that your brother—"

" I don't think—I know. He kept up the affair in Vienna."

" Does your mother know about it ? I know she is very strict."

" Mother doesn't bother about things that go on outside the house. But on the other hand, *in* the house jealousy is an absolute disease with her. Would you believe it, she takes the house-maid out with her when she goes out ? She is afraid I might make love to her."

" Have you never given her any grounds for her suspicion ? "

" Grounds ? Mother doesn't need any grounds. You have no idea how she pestered my brother with her jealousy of our extremely pretty house-maid. The poor boy had no peace, night or day. He was genuinely in love with the girl ! She (my mother) used to come into our room, sometimes, and into the girl's room to keep her eye on us. Especially in the night."

" Are things better now ? "

" Yes, now I am left in peace. *I have given my mother the word of honour of an officer* (he was a lieutenant in the reserve) *that I will have nothing to do with Mali. No, only that I will not enter her room.*"

" Now I understand your trouble. You regret having given your word. *You are unable to sleep because you are worried by the thought : I might be going in to Mali now. It was only when you were forbidden to touch her that you began to find her desirable.* For it is forbidden fruits which taste the sweetest."

" You are right. I used not to give the girl a thought, and laughed at my brother. But now my mother has forced my thoughts to turn in her direction. But the mere fact of telling you about all this will prevent my sleeping. What do you advise me to do ? "

" To go away. I will tell your mother that you are unable to study in your present quarters and that you must rent a small room elsewhere."

" What are you dreaming of ! My jealous Mama would never consent to that. *No ! I will not leave the house.*"

Of course I knew that the boy didn't want to be separated from Mali, and I prescribed a little Pantopon for the insomnia. The trouble lasted a while longer and then subsided rather rapidly.

I had the opportunity of speaking with him alone. " How do you stand with the girl ? "

He gave a forced laugh. " Well, its rather strange. You know that I promised Mother not to go into the servants' room, but I've found a way out. Mali comes into my room two or three times a week. Mother does not suspect anything because I make myself very unpleasant to the girl and protest that she ought to be dismissed for her slovenliness. That is why Mother keeps her ! "

" And what about your health ? "

" It is excellent. I sleep like a top and eat like a bear."

Thus we see into what severe conflict a poor youth may be brought by an oath. An oath of this description is really a mild form of blackmail. It is interesting, too, to note the jesuitical trick he uses to pacify his conscience and preserve his honour as an officer intact ! This case is important for the understanding of insomnia. It was not merely a matter of unsatisfied libido with the two brothers, for the law student had sexual intercourse outside the house. But his desires were centred on one person in particular. In such a case the libido may be non-existent where anyone else is concerned and sexual intercourse with others, even when phantasy conjures up a " Mali," never affords complete satisfaction. The simplest formula for insomnia is therefore : *Ungratified wishes and psychic conflicts (anxiety for the future, fear of legal procedures, or of moral and social disaster), prevent the neurotic from sleeping.*[1]

[1] This subject is fully dealt with in my essay, " Der Wille zum Schlaf." (Altes und Neues über Schlaf und Schlaflosigkeit.) Publ. by J. F. Bergmann, Munich.

CHAPTER XV

ANXIETY NEUROSIS IN CHILDREN

SO far we have only discussed anxiety neurosis in adults. Anxiety neurosis in children is not so well known, and very little investigated. In children it usually expresses itself in a sudden fear of darkness and of being alone, though they have never before experienced this anxiety. In other words—a little child is instinctively frightened of darkness. In his book, " Drei Abhandlungen der Sexualtheorie," *p.* 65, *Freud* emphasizes the fact that this feeling is at the root of all anxiety feelings.

" Fear in children is originally only the feeling of missing the person of whom they are fond, they therefore fear strangers. They fear darkness because they cannot see the person they are fond of, but are calmed if that person holds their hand in the dark." This applies to all children, to strong and nervous alike.

Suddenly, without any special reason, a certain irritability and a kind of exaggerated anxiousness appears in children, who although used to being happy in the dark, suddenly refuse to remain alone or to enter any room which is dark. They begin to feel shame and to ask many questions : " Daddy, why are the trees green ? " " Mother, why do people not have four legs ? " and so it goes on and on without ceasing. Behind those endless questions is one which begins to occupy the mind of the child, they have come in touch with the sexual problem. They feel a sexual excitation from the Unconscious which appears in consciousness as anxiety. That fear corresponds to an unsatisfied " libido." And one question which occupies their mind could be expressed as follows : " Where do children come from ? " Some other signs of cerebral irritation appear : glittering of the eyes, slight convulsive (choreatic) tics, grimaces, an extraordinary restlessness which had never been noticed in them before, absent-mindedness and lack of attention during lessons in the case of children already attending school. Religious problems also begin to come forward, such as : Whether God sees everything ? Whether everything is real and not a dream ? Such children become sleepless and begin to suffer from " Pavor nocturnus," or " Somnambulism." Sleeplessness is the first and the only distinctly outstanding symptom of infantile anxiety neurosis. J. Zappert in his study of " Disturbances of Children's Sleep," mentions that even suckling babies have the quick convulsive movements of which we have spoken already as noticeable in adults, and which to my knowledge can be traced to alarming dreams (in adults—tumbling down, falling, wild animals, abysses ; in older children—dragons, black men, ghosts, bogies, devils, etc.). The infantile form of anxiety expresses itself often in fits of screaming in the night. *T. Zappert* sees in these manifestations a sign of neuropathic constitution. " Pavor," he says, " represents only one form of the psychogenical illnesses of childhood of which the most acute is Hysteria. However, like enuresis,[1] these sudden fits of pavor nocturnus at long intervals can be regarded as the first symptoms of epilepsy."

Thus he describes a little girl of eight who at intervals of weeks or months used to call out several nights in succession : " Not so quick," directly after there had been a flickering in front of her eyes (aura ?). During the day she occasionally had fainting fits, described by *Zappert* as " petit mal."

According to my experience, the prognosis should not be such a bad one ; in such cases one could easily trace a sexual etiology. They are mostly cases of anxiety neurosis, and often even of decided, phobia. This could be proved by a closer observation of the cases. Such observation results in a very rational therapy and prophylaxy of " pavor nocturnus " and of sleeplessness in children.

Bendix ("Lehrbuch der Kinderheilkunde," Urban and Schwarzenberg, 1907) recommends in his excellent handbook a number of proved remedies for pavor, so much dreaded by parents. (1) A spacious bedroom ; (2) A hard bed that is not too warm ; (3) A moderate supper some time before going to bed ; (4) Attention to regularity of stools and passing water before going to bed ; (5) Avoiding exciting shows ; (6) Treatment of anæmia ; (7) Bromide.

All these measures are surely only of secondary importance. Any system of therapeutics that deals with the causes of disease must seek the hidden roots of this somewhat common malady. Once more I emphasize that " *pavor nocturnus* " *is the infantile form of anxiety neurosis, and appears when children come into touch in some way with the sexual problem, or feel the prick of conscience because of some criminal phantasies.* An analysis of anxiety dreams, a close examination of hallucinations always show the same cause : sexual excitement through parents, tutors, irresponsible servants, playmates, or by accident. The terrifying stories of the "black man " can also play a certain part. But what part ? Just as with adults—because they act as a means of release, or because they are a ready object for already available anxiety. The same is true for the exaggerated consequences of a sudden fright (by a cat or a dog, a noise, a stranger, etc.). In any case, sexual excitement had already paved the way for the development of neurosis. (False connection of an available affect). The

---

[1] This enuresis, which reappears after a period during which the child was quite clean, represents typical symptoms of infantile anxiety neurosis. It represents in a certain way an equivalent of the sexual act.

only cause that comes into consideration besides the sexual is the criminal. We will return to that question later on. Anyhow, we have arrived at the following formula : The causes of " Pavor nocturnus " are the first repressions from consciousness of unbearable ideas and the struggle against criminal tendencies.

I know that most children's doctors are of a different opinion, and that they maintain that " Pavor nocturnus " is caused by constipation, cold in the head, overloading of the stomach, adenoids, opticushyparesthesia and carbonic acid intoxication. But the experienced *Henoch* (" Vorlesungen über Kinderkrankheiten," Berlin 1893), whom I consider one of the finest and most reliable observers among children's doctors, says very aptly : " In most cases of ' Pavor nocturnus ' I could not trace any disturbance of the digestive organs, neither could I discover any unhealthy condition of the respiratory and circulatory organs, and in particular I was unable to find adenoids in my cases."

Furthermore : " A hereditary tendency is often undeniable —children of nervous parents are especially liable to the illness."[1] Thus *Henoch* hits the nail on the head, It is an undeniable fact, and *Zappert* emphasizes it also, that : *young patients who suffer from " Pavor nocturnus " are often the children of nervous parents.* But the connection is generally quite different from what the partisans of the theory of " hereditary taint " believe it to be. A close examination of the home surroundings in which the nervous children have grown up, proves that there exists a typical way in which these poor children are made nervous by nervous parents. It is mostly due to a father suffering from anxiety neurosis, hysteria or compulsion neurosis, deficient potency, or to an unhappy marriage in which the parents do not suit each other. In such a marriage the wife feels discontented, and she generally succumbs to anxiety neurosis. Her unsatisfied longing for caresses expresses itself in great irritability towards her husband and an exaggerated love for the child, who serves to satisfy all her need for tenderness. The way such mothers behave with the child is simply disgusting. It is constantly being kissed all over its body, even bitten or licked. I have even seen a mother kiss the child on the anal region. It is inevitable that the child of such a mother becomes unhappy. A very acute observer, a children's doctor in Breslau, Mr. *Czerny*, in a little book worth reading—" Der Arzt als Erzieher des Kindes," Vienna, Deuticke—1907, describes the dangerous consequences of blind mother love during the first years of life, and maintains that in many cases separation of the child from the mother is the best treatment for sick children. It is the duty of children's doctors duly to impress on mothers the injurious consequences of *exaggerated* tenderness. (We only deal with these exaggerated cases here.)

---

[1] Also Mosso, " La Paura," Milans, 1901, says : " Vi sono predisposti i figli di genitori molto eccitabili o affetti da malattie nervose."

Much has been said lately about infantile sexual trauma since *Freud* pointed out the pathogenic significance of these facts in his " Studien über Hysterie." Such evidently harmful injuries must certainly be taken into consideration. We will shortly deal with them more fully. But there is such a thing as chronic trauma, too! The so-called " tenderness " of mothers can under certain circumstances exercise just as harmful an influence. By perpetual caresses, kissing, licking, fondling, petting, etc., the erotic instincts of the child are prematurely awakened, that is to say, of any child who, as *Freud* so well expresses it, is inclined to be " polymorph perverse." Equally harmful is the bad habit of constantly taking children into bed with one, and even letting them sleep in the same bed with adults. Of course, most doctors know nothing about the harmful consequences of such proceedings. But we psycho-therapists, who get to know the whole and intimate life history of men, who are concerned with their infantile impressions and their effect, we know the devastating influence of such passionate unnatural caresses on the psyche of the child. We are grieved to see that so many neurotics are suffering from a severe psychical conflict of incest phantasy, and that the compulsion neurosis and conversion hysteria in individual cases are to be traced to this sort of infantile experience.

I was always able to find the cause of anxiety in a suppressed *sexual excitement* or in criminal phantasies. According to the opinion of *Freud*, anxiety neurosis often begins when young girls come in touch for the first time with sexual problems. An obscure erotic emotion expresses itself in children in a feeling of anxiety. Therefore, children could sometimes easily be cured of those fits of anxiety if they were taken away from the bedroom of their parents and put to sleep in separate rooms. Children often overhear incidents of married life when the parents think that they are fast asleep and can hear nothing. Unfortunately one still imagines a child as an asexual being. In my essay, " Koitus im Kindesalter " (Wiener med. Blätter, 1894, No. 1) I have many years ago strongly emphasized that among other conditions required, children must never sleep in their parents' bedroom. To-day, after thirty years' experience I can maintain the necessity of this with still more emphasis. Harmful influences come not only through parents. Other persons of the opposite sex can under certain circumstances exert on the child a sexual influence, of which he is not aware, but which is strong enough to release an anxiety affect from the Unconscious. One cannot be too cautious in dealing with children. This also applies to children of the same sex. *A sexual impression on a boy from his father or from a tutor*, as I found out from my investigations, *can be of great importance in building up a permanent homosexuality.* An important suggestion for a tutor is not to let himself go " sans façon" before children. Sleeplessness and " Pavor nocturnus " have the same etiology and can also be observed together.

No. 90.—Thus I knew a boy who remained for a long time sleepless at night. He could never fall asleep before 1 a.m. All the remedies prescribed for him by famous children's doctors remained useless. If he were forced to sleep one night by a narcotic, the next night he returned to the same state. During the night the boy would awake with a " Pavor nocturnus." He would sit up in his bed and vehemently cry out, repeating without variation one word : " *Snake, snake, snake!* " Anyone who is acquainted with the symbols of the sexual life by dream analyses, who can read the symbolic language of fairy-tales, will know that " snake " is one of the words most often used as a sexual symbol. Even the Bible tradition of Eve becoming seduced through the serpent indicates that this conception has dwelt in the mind of the people for thousands of years. This boy slept in the same room as his young and very pretty governess whom he worshipped. His mother took him by surprise as he was passionately kissing the governess's arm. Four days afterwards, when the governess was replaced by a tutor, the fits of sleeplessness completely disappeared.

The boy simply used to wait until his governess undressed herself, and thus created for himself erotic feelings of pleasure which came out in dreams transformed into feelings of anxiety.

Other children see during the attack, *fire, especially burning stoves, glowing balls, large knives, toads, red-hot glowing caves, bulls, " black men," wild animals, devils, thieves, robbers and assassins, corpses, blood, wounds and single parts of the body.* Some talk confused words. If one would take the trouble constantly to investigate in this direction, one would come across some surprising things. *Alfred Adler* told me of a child who made a noise during the fit : " *piss, piss, piss,*" which onomatopoetically expressed passing water. That child had certainly watched adults passing water, which apparently strongly impressed him. Further, the calling out of " fish " (tail ?) and " Not so quick ! " (Reproduction ?) seems to me also suspicious as regards sexual etiology. It is very likely to be reproduction in the exclamation : " Ah, now it comes ! " (*Hesse*). An overheard coitus may cause the exclamation : " Oh, I am dying ! " —" Faster, still faster ! " One of my colleagues heard a child calling out : " *He will crush me !   Too much !   I cannot stand this !* " I knew a child of six who exclaimed : " *There are little pigs in my bed and they are digging in my mattress !* " The analysis proved that the child had overheard some obscene doings of the servants. He wanted to tell his mother of his observations but the latter declined to listen to him, giving as a reason that " a good child should not speak about such piggish things." Hitschmann tells of a child who, during fits, saw letters on the walls changing in size from *large* to *small* and *vice versa*. (A symbolic representation of erection !) Another child who suffered from anxiety attacks used to call out : " *No, no, I have not touched the pipi.*" Another always saw *mice* at the time of the attacks. The analysis showed that this was due to seeing his mother naked doing her toilet and that her vulva (the mouse, " la souris ") made a great impression on him. A child of four used to call out, " *A monkey is not a Chinese !* " The Tertium comparationis of monkey and Chinese was the long tail. He touched the penis of his father while sleeping

together. Other phantasies reveal death-wishes, and criminal
ideas. Thus one of my colleagues tells me that he used to suffer
from anxiety hysteria and to feel very hostile against his father :
" I always saw hearses in my dreams." He used to call out during
' Pavor nocturnus ' :—' A hearse comes galloping into the room !
Mama ! Mama ! ' I became quiet at once when my mother took
me into her bed, and was delighted."
  I am now attending a doctor who in his childhood suffered for
years from " Pavor nocturnus." He has still the habit of starting
out of his sleep, also of talking confusedly and screaming. He often
awakens from anxiety dreams. This patient used often to watch
the coitus of his parents. The influence that this trauma had on
his psyche can be seen from a quotation of a scene from his childhood, which I repeat literally in the analysis of this colleague.
  It also throws an interesting light on the children's wish to become
" grown-up."

No. 91.—" I experienced the emotional complex of megalomania for the
first time when I was eight, and indeed with an intensity such as I have
never felt again.
  I had a slight cold or stomach trouble at that time and had to stay in bed
for several days. One night I had a high temperature and became delirious.
I remember that I had an impression of my body being enormous and heavy.
Arms and legs were like towers, each finger appeared to me like a rock. My
breathing and the slightest movements seemed to have almost the power
of an earthquake and I felt my body as an enormous weight on my bed.
Added to this I seemed to hear a perpetual and very unpleasant whizzing and
roaring. Apparently it was the result of my over-heated blood. Every
slightest noise that came from outside, whether a distant noise in the streets
or the ticking of the clock was of a particularly unbearable character,
which was very characteristic, but difficult to describe in words. I might
perhaps compare it with the nervous sighing of someone whose patience was
tried to the utmost and who could not express this indignation in words.
I felt a very unpleasant strain in my fingers and toes. These are the
phenomena, which in their combined effect in the day-time, or at night, in
bed, or in the street, produced a more or less strong attack of megalomania.
  " During that first attack I had also some characteristic fever dreams.
Sometimes I imagined myself lying at the foot of a mountain, from which
rolled down large yellow tree-trunks, which threatened to fall on my breast
and crush me.
  " Another time I dreamed of my father, who completed some violent deed
which made me feel an immense respect for him. Then I saw him shaking
large sacks of nuts and heard the same whizzing in my ears as I had heard
before from the rolling of the trunks.
  " As my nurse told me the morning after, I kept calling out during this
dream, ' Shake my nuts ! Help me to shake my sack of nuts ! ' and
between those sentences : ' Ah, father ! He can do it ! He can ! '
Then I remembered exactly these exclamations.
  " This violent action of my father, that seemed confused in my mind,
sometimes like the rolling of trunks, another time like the shaking of a large
sack, stirred up in me a mixed impression of astonishment and horror and at
the same time a desire to be able to imitate him. The origin of this ' megalomania ' is to be found in the reminiscences of the early childhood, when
parents must appear giants to a child. Parents are the first love objects
of a child, hence the wish to be as big as they are, to imitate them in every
way, briefly—identification with father or mother. The real feeling of the

tremendous bigness, and the weight of one's own body is to be taken as a symptom of hysteria, as the realisation of a wish that has become unconscious, because repressed as a hallucination of the tactile and bodily sensations and even of hearing. Then the peculiar roaring is probably due to the rushing of blood felt by the strongly excited child in his ears, when he watched a coitus of his parents, or to the noise that the parents made during the coitus.

" The feeling of being a heavy weight is identification with the father who crushes the mother, and the fear of being crushed is identification with the mother, the pressure in the extremities is the result of the pressure of the excited blood of the child, during the original experience.

" The trunks of the trees appearing in the dream are symbols of the penis of the father as well as of his whole body and the body of the mother. The yellow colour corresponds to the colour of the skin. The nut sacks of unbleached canvas are, according to the principle of multiplication, symbols of the body, eventually also of the scrotum. The shaking of the sacks means the movements during coitus. My exclamations can be explained as astonishment at my father and as a wish to imitate him."

Listening to the parents' coitus can lead to strange manifestations of anxiety. In one of the cases observed by me, the child believed that it was an earthquake which he had heard mentioned before. The attacks of " Pavor nocturnus " generally frighten the parents in such a way that they overlook certain of its peculiarities. Even doctors are so bewildered at the sight of the screaming, frightened child that they fail to discover the psychical roots of the fits.

The procedure is practically always the same. The child jumps up in bed, very often uncovers itself, screams in many cases and seems to be absolutely unconscious. It behaves like a somnambulist. Children act at this time from unconscious sexual motives in a most clever way. They betray a part of their sexual life in a hidden way. They undress themselves and thus indulge in their exhibitionistic inclinations, which are known to be very strongly marked in all children and are repressed only by education. And what is the most important of all, they entice the beloved nurse (whether mother, father or governess) to their bed while they themselves are in a very exposed night costume. If they are left alone and no one troubles about them, the attack stops astonishingly quickly. If they are thus purposeless and the little hysterical imp does not gain anything by it.

One of my patients told me that as a child of five he used to scream terribly at night. He wanted to be in bed with his nurse. He remembers very distinctly that touching her pubic hair gave him great pleasure. That patient is unable to perform coitus unless the woman puts his penis in the vagina with her hand. The cause of this frequent relative impotence is in this case to be sought in certain tricks of the nurse[1] who tried to introduce his penis. The

---

[1] The second cause is the emphasizing of the passive factor. The neurotic has checked his aggressive activity and seeks external aggression. He wants to be passive in order to lessen his guilt. He has this excuse in his heart : " But I am not guilty, *she* has done it." The same applies to women whose ideal is violation—the most ideal form of " Pleasure without sin."

first infantile impressions are decisive for the individual form of sexual life !

These principles account also for ordinary sleeplessness (without " Pavor "). Children mostly do not want to go to sleep because they want to watch the undressing of the adults. Thus they pretend to be asleep and wait for hours to watch the various scenes of married life. In many cases the "not wanting to sleep " of children has this motive. One child demands that a light should be left on, otherwise it cannot sleep ; it wants to see the undressing. Another child demands violently that the governess should snuff the candle : it wants to see the governess in her night-gown. A third child cannot go to sleep because of the fear of " black men " : it wants to go into the bed of the person it loves. One can hardly believe how much astuteness children develop in order to be taken into the beds of adults. When a grown-up person suffers from fear of thunderstorms, the phobia is often due to this infantile experience. During a thunderstorm a child is generally taken into the adults' bed, and the father, or mother, or some other beloved person takes it in his arms and fondles it. When this child grows up the erotic and delightful excitement that he used to feel expresses itself, because of repression, as displeasure and as *fear of thunder*.[1] Neurotics often tell us such infantile experiences when questions are put to them. Thus I learned from a barrister who suffered from compulsion neurosis, that during a heavy thunder-storm the cook took him into her bed and this made such a strong erotic impression on him that he still dreams of that event after eighteen years.

We are thus mistaken when we consider that only crude sexual excitements are important. Even such insignificant occurrences can influence the whole life.

Freud told me of an hysterical woman who at the beginning of a psych-analytic treatment followed with interest different shadows on the walls. It turned out that this hallucination was due to an important experience in her childhood. This explanation came out during the treatment a few months later. This patient had as a child a governess, whose bed was separated from hers only by a folding screen. Every evening the girl wanted to watch the process of undressing which was hidden from her. This was possible only by the shadows which clearly showed every single phase of the performance. Even after many years in a convent she managed to continue this watching with the help of shadows.

One can see that children have many reasons for " not wanting to sleep." I will mention only a few : the wish to see (these are called " voyeurs ") ; the wish to listen ; the wish to be taken into an adult's bed ; the wish to have the person they love near by. There are also unconscious sadistic reasons to be considered (to annoy the person they love).

One can hardly understand how doctors so constantly overlook the sexuality of the child. Moll, who wrote a long book about this,

---

[1] Another root is the "fear of the punishment of God."

G

"Das Sexualleben des Kindes" (Berlin, 1909, H. Walther) meets the complicated circumstances of the child's sexuality with but little understanding, while Strohmayer "Vorlesungen über die Psychopathologie des Kindesalters, für Mediziner und Pädogogen" (Tübingen, H. Laupp, 1910) takes advantage of the knowledge which he owes to psychanalysts and them against excessive sexual excitements: "In this direction much harm is often done thoughtlessly. People who show exaggerated fondness, do not know that by caressing and constant kissing of the child, by patting and fondling it, especially when it is done mostly on erogenous zones (ear, mouth, throat, neck, or even anus) they are stirring up in the child erotic instincts which lead to masturbation. Few teachers and very few doctors know that such awakened frustrated sexual excitement can take the form of anxiety, sleeplessness or ' Pavor nocturnus ' in the child. If they realised, surely many parents would be more careful in guarding the mysteries of their marriage bed and of not exposing their whole body or part of it in front of their children. It is surely remarkable that some cases of ' Pavor nocturnus ' can be cured at once when the child is removed from the bedroom of its parents or is taken away from a pretty and tender-hearted governess, and that so many cases of children's hysteria with convulsions and delirious fits, show during the attack, erotic imitations or directly imitate the coitus. It is due to Stekel that attention was drawn to this subject."

The perverse predisposition in the child is unfortunately also often forgotten. And it is positively certain, that children from three to five years can have distinctly marked masochistic or sadistic sexual feelings. A single whipping on the bare nates, or the sight of any pedagogic cruelty, also the biting of children, which is sometimes done as a joke, can serve as a well defined step in the development of sexual perversity.

No. 93.—A boy of thirteen gets ill, following an appendicitis operation, with eczema of the penis. The eczema was extraordinarily stubborn and would not yield to treatment. During the day the boy behaved very quietly. His mother sat beside his bed, read to him aloud or tried to distract him in some other ways. At night when everybody had settled for rest and his mother had gone to her room, he used to sleep for about half-an-hour or lie still in bed with open eyes. Then he would begin an extraordinary childish miserable sing-song which drew his mother immediately to his bed. " Why are you crying, Max ? " enquired the mother. " It itches so that I cannot stand it ! I must scratch myself ! " " Scratch ! " was a terrifying word to the mother. She was afraid of the eczema getting worse. Therefore she began to make him fomentations with Liquor Bourowii, etc. The boy had got what he wanted. His mother sat beside him. He exposed himself in front of her (exhibitionismus) and she occupied herself with his organ for hours. Of course the eczema did not improve.

At the same time, the boy had a very evident anxiety neurosis. He was very irritable and frightened, in a state of permanent anxious expectation. Not a word could be spoken in his hearing that had the slightest connection with anything to frighten him. Besides this, he suffered from a stubborn constipation, which made his mother occupy herself with his vegetative functions continually.

A few objective characteristics of sexual excitement could also be observed. The whole time during the changing of the dressing, his penis made strange movements which resembled a half-erection. It changed its original horizontal position for a few seconds to a new horizontal one taking a vertical position in between, and then jerked back again to the original position. The scrotum was in constant movement. The so-called cremaster reflex convulsive movement continued almost without interruption. From time to time pains appeared in the thigh and formication. In the last week he complained of a convulsive tick in his thigh. Briefly, one could see that the nerves of the genitals and of the neighbouring region were in a state of the greatest excitement. The boy was under the treatment of a very efficient specialist. I drew the attention of the latter to these phenomena. I told him nothing new. The boy had already been in a sanatorium under his care for many months. At that time the illness had been cured only after the boy's mother had been sent away and his hands had been tied up during the night.

This time I also proposed to his mother that she should keep away from the boy during the night and entrust the nursing to an old nurse or, if possible, to a male nurse. The effect of my proposal was surprising. The same woman who a few days before had assured me with tears that she would never in her life forget that I had saved her child's life (by advising a laparotomy on him against the wish of the operator ; the boy had already an abscess in the Douglas !) the same woman became my silent but bitter enemy and after a few days when an intercurrent illness arose, she reproached me with having brought it on by my casual treatment. She would not part with her child ! The boy also instinctively felt in me an enemy, who wanted to disturb him in his erotic amusements. When the boy, owing to his constant sleeplessness, got very much worse, of course I was the scape-goat who was the cause of it. Such are the dangers of trying pedagogical methods with a mother who possesses a hypertrophical tenderness. That a mother does not want, in such circumstances, to renounce the pleasure and responsibility which nursing the child gives to her is, of course, natural.[1]

Another child of five could not go to sleep unless it was allowed to play with his mother's breasts. He would call out : " Busti ! " (Bosom) until his wish was fulfilled. When I had noticed this and prohibited it, the boy became my bitter enemy and would never afterwards allow me to examine him. Every time that I wanted to touch his body, he burst out in fits of anger. A similar case where the mother had been ill and the child perfectly well, will be mentioned later when we deal with hypochondria.

Vomiting is another symptom of children's anxiety neurosis, besides " Pavor nocturnus," general anxiousness, strongly marked irritability, eczema, enuresis, attacks of diarrhœa, slight fainting fits, This vomiting generally happens in the morning, when the child has to go to school. It often does not appear on Sundays or holidays

[1] I could produce a great number of observations on the sexual etiology of eczema. Very often the eczema is only a pretence in order to be able to scratch on the erogenous zones and is artificially created by scratching. The skin of the people who go about all their lives with some sort of habitual eczema, is an erogenous zone. In any case, eczema shows a distinct relation with sexual proceedings, as *Oscar Scheuer* shows in his well-known book, " Hautkrankeiten sexuellen Ursprunges " (Urban und Schwarzenberg, 1911) see especially page 77. Eczema and menstruation. There are cases of eczema which become exacerbated at every menstruation. *Scheuer* naturally sees in every case only the influence of the internal secretion and completely disregards the psycho-sexual component of these diseases.

when the child can sleep longer, and is therefore often taken as a characteristic sign of school nervousness. These children are afraid of the school, sometimes of the teacher. They sit there with a brooding feeling of anxiety that if they are examined, they probably would not be able to answer. They often suffer from " nervous diarrhœa " and they cannot contain themselves even in school. They also often are enuretics and remain such when they get older without a trace of epilepsy. We already know the causes of nervous vomiting of adults. Vomiting is especially characteristic in neurosis, when the repressed erotic idea is combined with a feeling of disgust. We must make sure whether the same cause does not apply to children. The teacher also notices that these children have the unpleasant habit of wanting to go every moment to the lavatory. Certainly the fear of school plays a certain part in these cases also. Especially as the child has been threatened for months with such words as : " Wait until you go to school, the teacher will know how to deal with you."

But other children hear the same threats without any effect whatever.

No. 94.—P. S., a boy of six, suffers terribly from vomiting since he began going to school ; the attacks happen always in the mornings after he has had his breakfast. This very nervous child suffers also from sleeplessness, *e.g.*, he cannot fall asleep easily and the temporary measures that I have suggested to help the boy have been declined as unnecessary. He stays in the bedroom of his parents, the light burns as long as the little tyrant wants it. Apart from this, his mother has to come several times to his bed to cover him up. He gets cold so quickly and begins to cough if he is not covered properly. He coughs, strangely to say, only during the night, when he feels the cold, never in the day. He locks himself in the lavatory for hours. I make the suggestion that it is a case of some sexual excitement, but the parents decline this distrustfully. " He is such an innocent, unsuspicious little angel ! "

In a few weeks' time I am called again. The father tells me he caught the boy masturbating his brother, two years his junior. Such was the disposition of the boy, for whose innocence his parents were prepared to take any oath.

Strict watching of the child by an intelligent elderly relative of the family produced a brilliant result. Vomiting and sleeplessness stopped in a few days, the migraneheadaches appeared but seldom. The child was cured astonishingly quickly.

In some children a " school phobia " or " teacher phobia " develops. Certain teachers become the object of neurotic anxiety. Children are seized with anxiety when the teacher looks at them, their whole body shakes and they can never give a proper answer. These are mostly cases of erotic settings. The children are in love with the teacher (male or female) and they often convert this love into hatred, as they believe they do not get enough attention. They suspect slights, imagine that the teacher has a dislike for them, in short, they have an emotional setting towards him.

Very often, changing the school is the only measure that saves the children from such teacherphobia. In a few cases I obtained

a quick cure by using analytic-pedagogic methods. All teachers
ought to know all about these phenomena of child sexuality. They
could act very beneficially towards children.[1] One ought to beware
of wanting to heal these little masturbators by means of fear. Fear
of the consequences of masturbation is often more dangerous than
the masturbation itself. (See the next observation, J. V.) Strohmayer (Vorlesungen über die Psychopathologie des Kindesalters
usw) says rightly : " I warn you against over-loading the young
conscience with the so-called consequences of the ' sins of youth.'
Otherwise the *fear of the consequences of masturbation is worse than
the vice itself.*"

Many exclamations in " Pavor nocturnus " are connected with
warnings against masturbation. For instance : " No, I shall never
do it again ! " or " Nanie, Nanie, go away ! " Here " Nanie "
supplements *onanism*, just as in the case that my colleague *Reitler*
tells me of, where " Onan, the great spirit " meant *onanism*.

One patient told me he suffered also from vomiting when he
was a schoolboy of six. He had already then been a masturbator
and decided to be good when he began school, so that he should
not have any secrets from his parents. He fancied himself so bad
and wicked that he vomited out of sheer disgust.

The moral influence at the time of beginning to attend school
is noticeable in many children. One small patient who as a child
used to play games resembling coitus with a boy two years her
senior (see Case No. 1 of my study : " Koitus im Kindesalter " !)
suddenly refused to play them any longer, giving as a reason that she
was now a big girl, was going to school and such things were not
suitable for a schoolgirl.

Children's doctors know far too little about such matters. They
overlook them. I can give many more similar examples observed
during my experiences.

No. 95.—J. V., a boy of ten, is under my treatment with tuberculosis in
the vertebræ. By order of the orthopædist he lay in a plaster bed, which
he bore quite well. His mother was pleased with his sound, quiet sleep. Afterwards, he was put in a plaster bodice, which in the first few days he also bore
quite well. Already in the first week the boy began to scream violently in the
night. His parents tried to comfort him, asking him where he has pain, etc.
He looked absent-mindedly in a corner and screamed out inarticulate sounds,
then made warding-off movements with his hand, fell into a violent fit of
crying and slept again.

The same performance is repeated every night. Every possible organic
cause had been considered, the plaster bodice loosened, the nose examined,
worms had been suspected and sought for. On closer examination I find
that the boy had been masturbating violently. A few days before, his father
had caught him in the act and shouted at him : " *If you do it again, I will
cut the thing off with a knife !* " And in order to add more strength to his
threat, he took a large penknife from his pocket, so that the frightened boy
began to scream. The child reproduced in his sleep this horrible scene.

[1] Deep insight into development of the child's soul and the first erotic
sensations and school experiences can be found in " Das Tagebuch eines
halbwüchsigen Mädchens " (Wiener psychoanalytischer Verlag, 1920).

The abstention suddenly forced on him produced an anxiety neurosis as it would in an adult. Pacifying of that intelligent boy was quickly acquired by frankly talking over the subject. He also was removed from his parents' bedroom.

Children should always have their own bedrooms when possible. The nurse should occupy a neighbouring room. I consider these measures very important. Especially the "sleeplessness" of children, which is always based on sexual excitement, is thus very easily cured. The quick success of these measures confirms this view. •Experienced children's doctors have known this long ago. Only they think that the cause of the sleeplessness is the frequent looking-in of the mother, and also her nervousness and anxiety, which might be true in some cases. In some cases one must also think of erotic stimuli which come from the nurse, such as either masturbatory manipulations or the unintentional arousal of sexuality by stroking, kissing, or undressing herself in front of the child.

The mother who takes the child into her bed because he happened to have an anxiety dream acts most unwisely. In such cases the child easily gets anxiety dreams in order to be taken into mother's bed. The following observation confirms this:

No. 96.—V. T., a little girl of seven, suffers from frequent anxiety dreams and Urtikaria (Urtikaria is a sexual skin disease *par excellence*.) It reminds one of Urticaria from which Goethe's sister, Cornelia, suffered before every ball when she had to wear a low dress. It is true that there is also a toxic Urticaria originating in the intestines. But who knows, however, if the sexual Urticaria is not also created by toxin?) After a scream of fear the father generally took the child into his bed, after which she soon became pacified. This was repeated every night for months. At the same time the girl demanded all sorts of things, such as she must have several chairs in front of the bed, the electric light must be turned on, the dog must lie on her feet, etc. When the girl was put into a separate room with a governess who was ordered never to take the girl into her bed, the result was that the anxiety dreams completely disappeared in a few days. The Urticaria gradually disappeared. In that case we see that the so-called exudative diathesis comes from constitutional predisposition of the skin and over-excitability created by peripheral irritation of the same. I wonder if all that irritating of the skin like patting, tickling, kissing and fondling could not make the skin into an erogenous zone?

Change of bedroom and of nurse often produces astonishing results. The effect of this simple measure is wonderful and it is so much better than veronal, which is much misused and strongly recommended for children against sleeplessness.

It cannot be too often repeated that in most cases it is only the exaggerated tenderness of the guardians that draws out the first sexual feelings from the child. An unreasonable punishment can also lead to serious perversities (Sadism and masochism). All extremes are harmful. Cruelty of the parents acts in the same way as exaggerated tenderness, because of the too early awakened erotic sensations. The obscure sexual feelings express themselves in fear or rage. Crude sexual excitements can come from a nurse.

Our experiences in psychanalysis prove that this is often done in a most criminal way. I will relate later on of a boy of six with whom the servant of his father used to try fellatio. Such cases are certainly extremes, as is that of the boy of five who had been introduced to me with gonnoirhœa which he had acquired from his sister of thirteen! Such are in reality those children supposed to be without sexuality! And when suddenly in some scandalous law-suit some of the deeds of corrupted children become revealed —one is shocked! One need only have one's eyes open, then it will not be possible to overlook these things!

No. 98.—Carelessness and lack of understanding of parents are sometimes without limit. The case of which I am going to tell now I may call "A picture of German family life." The story is about a boy of nine who is a little anæmic but well otherwise, born from healthy parents ; he had suffered for months from migraine headaches, fainting fits and "Pavor nocturnus." Already a year ago his mother had consulted me about the evening anxiety attacks of that otherwise very intelligent boy. He starts crying in the evening when he is left alone in his room, has creepy visions (white ghosts in white garments!) and is not pacified until he is taken into his mother's bed. A close examination proved that the boy had been masturbating. I ordered watching the boy very closely, strongly prohibited taking him into his mother's bed and drew the attention of his intelligent parents to their being very careful in their talking and their doings in the presence of such a precocious boy. I also gave a little lecture to the boy as punishment. Without frightening him I explained that I knew of his naughtiness and that he should stop doing *those things as they are not suitable for children*. I also told him he was on no account to go into his mother's bed. The boy soon became pacified and the anxiety attacks disappeared. The continuation of this case is interesting and reveals the almost incredible want of judgment in parents as educators. One day I am called to see the boy who is "seriously ill." I find the boy very pale with a suffering expression on his face, sitting and reading a cow-boy story. His mother tells me he is suffering every day from migraine headaches. In the evening he begins to scream, saying : "Ah, I don't feel well! I am fainting, I am dying! Oh, my head, my poor head!" after which his mother takes him into her bed and the boy becomes gradually quiet.

It seems that something is wrong with his head. The boy used to bring home from school the highest marks, now he seems hardly to be able to pass. He often gives to the teacher quite wrong answers. For instance, the other day he said five and two were twenty (the boy is in the fourth form in the school). He also has not been making any progress in piano playing. "And how does the matter stand with his erotic excitements ? " I asked the mother.

"Oh, you wouldn't believe how naughty is the little wretch.[1] On the first floor lives a baroness—we call her this because she is mistress of a baron —she is a very smart and voluptuous woman and she constantly takes the child on her lap. She goes about in the house *en deshabille*, of course. Do you know what my son said yesterday to our cook ? He does not dare to say this to me, the dirty little thing! ' The baroness is a very smart woman, she has a much prettier bosom than mother.' "

"And you allow the boy to go up there every day ? "

"What am I to do ? He has his own ways. Last week we went to the Coloseum to see ' Polkadream.' (It is a very coarse, obscene and unmistakable parody). Of course the boy came with us because my husband wished it. A girl sang a song about a ' wide bed.' When we came home

[1] Viennese dialect expression, which has an appreciable erotic emphasis, cf., "naughty."

· the boy says : ' I know what people want a wide bed for, even if she did not say it.' "

" How does the boy behave when he comes into your bed ? "

" He takes me in his arms, kisses me, and says : ' Now I have no more fear whatever. Sometimes he becomes so boisterous that I must stop him." Explanations are needless. The mother has been warned by me. The family that I am talking of was by no means of a vulgar, common type. In spite of that the mother would not see the connection, because she evidently attributed the fiery embraces of her son to filial love and also did not want to renounce her feeling of pleasure connected with it. In this case I decided to cure fear by making fear. I spoke very severely to the boy and told him that I knew why he went through his performances in the evenings and during the night ; but that he will not succeed in getting what he wants any more. On the contrary he will have to go in a separate room, where he will sleep all alone. I made him understand that I knew of all his behaviour. He even did not try to deny it.

Already the following night, the usual fainting fits disappeared. He always sleeps now perfectly calmly in a separate bedroom. Indeed the best treatment in such a case is to take the boy away from his surroundings, away from his mother. The latter measure seems to me especially important because there are younger brothers and sisters in the house, among them a little girl of five, and they are all in danger of getting too early enlightened on sexual matters, and possibly of being induced to some sexual act.

When we have to deal with children suffering from sleeplessness or anxiety neurosis, we must always think of a possible precocious erotic excitement. Those excitements can be created either by an exaggerated tenderness or by harshness or else by an incomprehensible carelessness of the parents. In other cases one cannot go very wrong in suspecting sexual trauma. It is incredible how often such scenes emerge from one's past memory and how seldom they get to be known by doctors and parents. Sexual attacks play a great part in the children's life.

Children tell but seldom of these attacks, an instinctive shyness keeps them from doing it. It is true that in some cases stories of infantile sexual traumas told by neurotics turn out to be imaginary ones. Anyhow, infantile sexual traumas are much more common than one thought them to be until now. They are also often found in the anamnesis of people with a sound nervous system. Not all children react to such traumas with a neurosis. Like everyone belonging to the school of Freud, I used to over-value the " Sexual " Trauma," and to believe in the traumatic hypothesis of child hysteria. The experiences in my practice have taught me that many forms of neurosis exist which develop without a psychical trauma. Very often the trauma maintains its special meaning only through the neurotic setting of the patient. In spite of that it would be silly and one-sided to overlook the facts that many people are " tied " to their traumas and cannot get away from them. I am thinking of a few striking cases. One very neurotic little girl whose father used to give her his penis to hold and had tried without success a defloration in the seventh year of her life ; a mother who used to play with the penis of her little boy until he was nine and also used to let him tickle her vulva. Seductions can occur through older sisters or brothers, nurses or servants, teachers or even ministers, and can play a considerable part in the dynamics of neurosis.

Anyhow, it would be wise to treat with caution such statements of children about possible acts, and always to make sure first if *desire* alone has not been the cause of sexual phantasies. Thus many quite innocent persons have been sometimes suspected. In such cases the exact knowledge of the infantile form of anxiety neurosis, which is often only an introduction to anxiety hysteria, can serve as a sure point of departure. Fits of " Pavor nocturnus." sleeplessness, fainting fits, bed-wetting, nervous diarrhœas, vomiting, noticeable shyness, urticaria, too vivid imagination, inclination to hallucinations—make those statements very suspicious, of course only when these symptoms have existed *before* the trauma.

In case anxiety neurosis or anxiety hysteria start *after* trauma, those statements of children have a great probability, even though they cannot be proved as certain. The phantasy of a trauma can under circumstances produce neurosis too. These things are so very important because they show us the only way for the time being which can lead us to the prophylaxis of neurosis. " *The example of parents is the object lesson to children* " is a very apposite saying. Czerny (l.c.) had strongly advised in some cases taking the children away from the unfortunate influence of their parents :—" In many cases when it is believed that the illness is hereditary it is often a case of transferring the illness through education."

This applies especially to " only " children[1] as those seldom avoid the great damage done by exaggerated tenderness.

In this way Neo-malthusianism becomes an important factor in the etiology of neuroses. The more children there are in the family the more natural become the relations between parents and children. *Czerny* is quite right in saying : " The constant intercourse with adults is just as dangerous for a child as to be alone." The greatest danger, greater even than severity—and I believe I have proved this—is the exaggerated love of parents or guardians.

We must not, however, be deceived into thinking that children are born asexual and are only made sexual by traumas. This does not correspond with our experiences, which have considerably increased in recent years. According to an apposite and very often quoted expression of Freud, the child is " *polymorph perverse.*" Traumas strengthen this erotic predisposition and fixate paraphilia in those disposed to it. But not in all cases. We must admit that children can endure traumas without suffering any noticeable harm from them. The fact that in one case it comes to a neurosis and that in another the child remains healthy depends both on the

[1] Compare the valuable work of *J. K. Friedjung*, " Die Pathologie des einzigen Kindes " (Wiener med. Wochenschr, No. 6, 1911) and *Neter*, " Das einzige Kind und seine Erziehung " (Verlag Otto Imelin, München, 1910).

" nervous " or " psychic predisposition," and also on the inhibitions which the child receives from his surroundings. That is why children of common parents bear traumas without damage, while children living in a highly cultivated milieu often become strongly neurotic. Religious and ethical inhibitions pave the way for the psychic conflict.

A child represents a stage of primitive man with all the primitive instincts. It feels originally absolutely selfish and hostile towards its surroundings. It wishes death to every person who gets in the way. Children do not look upon death with the same fear as do the adults. A little boy of four used to say : " When Daddy dies I will sleep in his bed ! " A little girl of five said, when her mother was travelling : " Mother must not come back any more. I will cook for father and sleep in mother's bed." These ideas of getting rid of a person often have a sexual foundation. The child's jealousy of parents and also of brothers and sisters is enormous. Jealousy is a feeling of envy which is created when one fancies that another person is loved more than oneself. Children always imagine that other brothers and sisters are loved more than they are themselves and often wish the death of their rivals. In consequence of their bad conscience children are afraid of the punishment of God, Who sees everything and knows everything, and Who will punish them severely for their evil wishes.

The appearance of anxiety in childhood is always a sign that the conscience of a child is awakened.

The anxiety itself is not directly of libido origin. The process of the development of anxiety is the same in children as it is in adults. It only appears more clearly if one takes the trouble to investigate the cases psychologically.

The anxiety of the child is connected with sexuality (it is a fear of the unknown, intangible, incomprehensible). But it also shows an intimate connection with criminality and especially with the subject of *death*. Dead people play a great part in the anxiety dreams of children, and in " Pavor nocturnus." A child begins to think of death very early. This is proved in the strange case of child hysteria which has been disclosed by *Otto Klaus* in the "Wiener Klin. Wochenschrift, 1919 (Ein Kasuistischer Beitrag zur kindlicher Hysterie)."

On July 16th, 1919, at 8 p.m., I was fetched by a peasant from the village A., to see his little boy, who *apparently had a stroke*. An anamnesis gave me the following : Yesterday afternoon the child returned home from picking berries. A few hours before this his mother gave *birth to a baby*. Peperl (the boy's name) had just heard of the event. When he arrived home he was happy and merry, but half-an-hour afterwards he lay down in the middle of the room, let his head fall and his extremities relax, his eyes were closed most of the time, but now and again he rolled them. According to the father's statement the child gets convulsions in a form of tic and moves his limbs as if in a cramp. By further questioning I learn that two years ago there was also a baby born on the same day and another elder child had died the same day, from what cause he could not remember. It also happened that last year his mother gave birth to a baby and on the same day a child of two was laid down on the floor, and died a few days afterwards of meningitis. Now the father thought that this time the same thing would happen again. A baby was born and his boy Peperl became ill the same day and would probably die too. On my question whether the boy knew of all this the father answered affirmatively, because they all had prayed for weeks that the boy should remain healthy.

On my arrival at the house I find nine women busy and lamenting over the boy who lies there in apathy, hardly alive, with closed eyes. From time to time he opens the lids, rolls his eye-balls, makes unco-ordinate movements with his limbs (which have been described as " cramps " by the persons who witnessed it) does not react at all on talking to him and had neither eaten anything, nor talked nor even cried for the last thirty-six hours. When his sister took him up and put him on his feet he drew his legs in and fell down. An objective examination gave an absolutely negative result. During all the time of examination the symptoms of the illness did not change—the child did not utter a sound, nor reacted on pinching his head ; his head wobbled helplessly on his shoulders. After an examination without result I realised that I could succeed only by sudden energetic action and if I did not—any treatment from my part would be useless.

To begin with I asked everyone to retire from the room. When left alone with the child I took him under his arms and shook him slightly, after which he opened his eyes. At this moment I saw him drawing his mouth in a grimace for crying. I put him right on the floor and shouted at him : " Stand up ! " The child gets up and hurries to his father with a cry, " Daddy ! " Half-an-hour's crying releases the tension which had lasted thirty-six hours. One hour later the child asked for coffee and bread, for the first time. How successful was my treatment and how sudden was the change can be seen from the words of his father : " Doctor, you have driven the devil out of the child ! " The night was spent by the child in quiet sleep. On my visiting him the next day I saw that the child was completely cured. A résumé of the story follows :—By chance in one family on the same day of two following years one child had been born and another one either had died or had fallen dangerously ill. When the confinement was expected the coming event was discussed long beforehand and Peperl, a child of three, was treated most carefully and prayed for. The latter listened to the chatter of the relatives. On the day of the birth he literally is taken ill, while his illness takes the form that he imagined his little brother had when he died, which he gathered from the talking of his parents. A suggestive treatment gave a complete cure.

This wonderful case only proves what an important part anxiety plays in the life of children. One cannot be too careful in front of children because they hear everything and assimilate it in their own way. Bad conscience develops extraordinarily early in the child. One could almost think of hereditary conscience when one notices how early the first stirrings of conscience show themselves in the child under the form of " *fear of the punishment of God.*" This anxiety is of the greatest importance in the psychic life of the child. The talion law corresponds to the naïve primitive thinking of the child. If he wishes something wicked, or even death, to a little sister or brother of his, and that one dies, then some signs of anxiety neurosis or compulsion neurosis can soon be noticed.

The significance of death in childhood has been so far overlooked by psychanalysis, which always has observed the sexual moment one-sidedly. When children are taken ill with " Pavor nocturnus " or " anxiety neurosis," one ought to investigate whether there have not been cases of death, either in the family or in the neighbourhood, and one will often come across cases of " Death trauma."

No. 102.—A barrister, aged thirty-three, who suffered from fear of wasps, told me that he had heard in his childhood of a neighbour who had died from the poisoned sting of a wasp.   He himself had wished that wasps should liberate him of a tiresome rival of his—a younger brother.
One of his brothers died of scarlet fever.   But for a long while after, he thought that it had been the result of a wasp-sting.   After the death of this brother he developed screaming fits in the night, during which he fought madly with wasps, trying to keep them off, and he always insisted on having a cloth and a fly-flap in bed with him.   For a while this fear of wasps spread, and became a fear of all insects.

From all these observations it follows that children should be carefully protected from strong impressions.   The bad habit of telling children gruesome myths or tales may also lead to anxiety attacks.   I do not hold with *Czerny's* point of view that fear should be used as a means of education.   Children should never be educated through fear or by means of fear.   A child can only be guided rightly by love.   The secret of bringing up children properly, lies in discovering that proportion of love which, while avoiding neurotic excitement, will yet give the child the tenderness which it cannot do without, and which makes its life more beautiful.

A lack of tenderness makes children as neurotic as a surfeit of love.[1]   Quarrels between parents are just as harmful to the child's psyche.[2]   If a child develops an anxiety neurosis, there is no doubt that some educational mistake has been made in its upbringing. There is no doubt that some children are born with a neuropathic taint, while others seem to be stronger right from the beginning. The highly-strung child appears nervous, moody, obstinate, exaggeratedly sensitive, easily moved, easily angered, contradictory, pugnacious, easily learns to speak and soon becomes talkative.
I cannot close this exposition without drawing attention to the fact that a sudden appearance of anxiety conditions in childhood always requires psychological investigation.   Child suicides become more and more numerous.   Many a suicide could be prevented if the parents and doctors would look upon the appearance of anxiety conditions and upon the changed condition of the child (inattention, absent-mindedness at school, pig-headedness, churlish behaviour, depression) as results of a severe psychic conflict.   I have stated in the discussions on suicide[3] that : " No one kills himself who would not have killed another ! "   The child also, punishes itself by suicide for its criminal phantasies.   Suicide in childhood often shows some connection with giving up masturbation.   The child cannot bring the severe conflict between impulse

---

[1] Sadger : " Ungeliebte Kinder " (Fortschritt der Med., Vol. 34, 1916-1917).

[2] Lazar : " Streit der Eltern." Leitschrift f. Kinderheilkunade, 1914.

[3] Disskussionen der Wiener psycho-analytischen Gesellschaft, " Uber den Selbstmord un Kindesalter." (Publishers, J. F. Bergmann, Wiesbaden.)

and morality to an issue, and so flees from life. Often suicide is intended to be a deep (eternal) punishment to the educators for their supposed lack of love.

In many cases it is jealousy which leads the child into insoluble conflicts. Parents and psychologists do not realise the full strength of a child's jealousy. Jealousy is perhaps the basic phenomenon around which the other symptoms group themselves. This jealousy is chiefly displayed against brothers and sisters, other relations, or sometimes also against the parents. The assumption of the Freudian school that the son is always jealous of the father (Œdipus complex), and the daughter of the mother (Electra complex) is not true. The child is markedly bisexual and jealous *of both* parents. It vacillates in its love between its father and mother and would like to keep each parent for itself.

Much educational skill is required to recognise this jealousy and to make it harmless.

Especially is this the case in unhappy marriages, for the child takes sides very early and soon evolves for itself an entirely false conception of the relationship of man and woman, and builds its neurotic constructions to protect its ultra-sensitive, ambitious, power yearning personality. (Adler.)

Experience shows us that happy marriages rarely produce highly strung (nervy) children. Therefore one ought not to limit oneself merely to saying that the child is "nervy," but one should endeavour to locate the psychic causes of the "nervousness."

It will then be found that in children the reaction caused by humiliation, neglect, unfair punishment, can take the shape of an anxiety attack resulting from suppressed rage, similar to the psychic conflict caused by a sexual trauma.

In no other field can the doctor work with such good results. In the nursery the doctor must be educator as well as doctor, if he takes his calling seriously.

The treatment of childish anxiety conditions is not difficult if one understands the psychology of the child. It is a grateful task because it is the only form of prophylactic therapeutics. This treatment can, and must only, be an analytic-pedagogic treatment.

SECOND PART

THE PHOBIAS

CHAPTER XVI

A FEW SIMPLE EXAMPLES OF PHOBIAS

WE have studied the effects of anxiety on the various organs and covered thereby practically the whole field of the neuroses, which were termed "Neurasthenia" by the old school. Freud tried to separate anxiety neurosis from this neurasthenia. In his opinion both diseases are "actual neuroses," *i.e.*, they arise from an injurious form of sexual life.

But when I brought the first analyses of anxiety neuroses to *Freud*, repeatedly proving the complaint to be "parapathia," a disturbance of the affective life, he felt that his concept was losing ground and suggested as a compromise, that the anxiety neurosis engendered by somatic injury should be affiliated with a second neurosis, anxiety hysteria, which presents the familiar mechanism of hysteria.

The name "anxiety hysteria" was suggested to me by *Freud*. The difference between *anxiety hysteria* and *anxiety neurosis* is still sharply emphasized and adhered to by *Freud*. According to him, it is a *qualitative* one.[1] But in my view it is a *quantitative* one. Since according to my theory there is no room for the concept of actual neuroses it would have been more logical to describe only Anxiety hysteria, and to let the Anxiety neurosis become merged in that. All anxiety would be thus reduced to *one* Neurosis only, which, if you will, might be termed Hysteria. Personally, I have not adopted this course and prefer to preserve the distinction from didactic reasons.

[1] Also *Jones* ("Die Beziehung zwischen Angstneurose und Angsthysterie." Int. z.f. ärztl. Psychoanalyse. Vol. I, *p.* 11) comes to the conclusion : "The fundamental causes of all forms of anxiety conditions consist of a lack of psychic satisfaction of the libido, the anxiety arises from an innate instinct of fear, and the exaggeration of their manifestations is the defensive answer to repressed sexual desires. *In all cases psychic factors play an important part*, in some, in fact, the only part. Physical factors often work in conjunction with them, but they are never sufficient in themselves to induce a condition of anxiety ; moreover these factors include an important psychic side.· The psychic factors are certainly more prominent in anxiety-neurosis than in anxiety-hysteria (phobia, etc.). Anxiety neurosis must only be considered as a single symptom of anxiety-hysteria, which is the wider concept.

The arguments put forward in the second edition (1912), have, as the result of many years of research, been amplified. They are no longer tenable in the form in which they have been presented up to the present. In the first place we have seen many cases of anxiety neurosis in which a distinct conversion was to be observed ; in the second, there is no such thing as somatic conversion of the libido into anxiety, as conceived by *Freud*.

There is only one psychic conflict between various psychic currents, which are manifested as parapathia, *i.e.*, disturbance of affect. *Janet's* view that hysteria is the result of a dissociation of the personality, is the right one. The psychic conflict leads to a dissociation of consciousness, because the ego decides on one of the wishes (generally on the moral ego), while the other wishes remain unconscious (pre-conscious). But it may also happen, as I have demonstrated in other volumes of this work, that the ego decides for a moral life, and that the moral ego expresses itself as conscience in the unconscious.

In all parapathias disturbances of the affective life are to be observed *i.e.*, a fight between two affects. It is never a question of two thoughts in conflict, but of two emotions. (The religious feeling strives against the sex-impulse, which manifests itself as love, and *vice versa*).

Phobia is a compromise in this conflict. It signifies a truce, enforced with the help of anxiety.

It is now my task to illustrate these facts by means of analyses. Let us begin with a case which will clearly demonstrate the difficulties of diagnosis, and enable us to understand the power of psychotherapeutic treatment.

No. 103.—A rather stout man of thirty-four, of healthy parentage, with slight struma, was troubled with violent attacks of palpitation, accompanied by very tormenting feelings of anxiety. Even in his student days he had had himself examined by a specialist in heart diseases, who had diagnosed " a clear case of hereditary tachycardia." The last attack was associated with violent " angina lacunaris." The patient was moreover an inveterate smoker. The Professor who was treating him pronounced him to be suffering from myocarditis infectiosa following angina in a fatty degenerate nicotine-poisoned heart, and prescribed a fat-reducing cure in Franzensbad after a few weeks' rest. The patient followed this advice, left his office in the lurch—he was a Solicitor—and went to Franzensbad. After the first week there he was visited by a frightful attack of anxiety. He awoke in the night with a scream, awakened his wife, and alarmed the whole house. He felt as if his last hour had come. Several doctors and a professor stood round the patient's bed in perplexity, while the latter issued his last instructions. The attack gradually subsided, and the patient returned to Vienna. There he at once went to bed again, and declared he could not walk another step. He was quite convinced that he would die if he went a step further. During every attack he held his wife tightly by the hand, and would not let her stir from his side. Another Professor diagnosed vagus-neurosis, and prescribed large doses of bromide, which gave the patient temporary relief. But he suffered for a considerable time from insomnia, and eventually could not exist without bromide.

Three years later I took him in hand. With the exception of the slight degree of tachycardia already mentioned, I could discover, *in corde objectiv*, nothing of a pathological nature, diagnosed " anxiety-hysteria," and suggested psychotherapeutic treatment. The patient consented, and, after a short time, was completely cured.

Despite certain unpleasant symptoms resulting from abstinence, he gave up the bromide which he had been taking daily, on the advice of the professors, for three years. (*About six kilogrammes* of bromide altogether !) Analysis disclosed a number of remarkable factors which all played a considerable part in the generation of anxiety hysteria. Before the outbreak of his illness he had practised coitus interruptus for six years, and in such a manner that ejaculation was postponed in order to effect his wife's full satisfaction. But this did not exhaust the etiology of this case. During the great attack in Franzensbad he had the sensation of standing for trial in a Court of Law. The attack was, in fact, connected with this dream. *Sanctis*[1] would have called this a case of dream neurosis—for he actually speaks of dream psychoses (reversing cause and effect). Our patient dreamed he was being tried before a judge and jury. Despite the fact that he had informed the doctors in Franzensbad of this dream, it was regarded as a *result* of his heart affection, and the psychic root of his anxiety was not sought for. The psychanalysis of this case afforded us a full explanation. That the trouble was centred in the heart can be explained, in *Adler's* sense, by the fact that it was an inferior organ. The patient had suffered since his student days from tachycardia ; a brother was similarly afflicted with heart neurosis and tachycardia. Coitus interruptus was the original cause of the anxiety neurosis.

A new and important psychic factor was added in the shape of a painful occurrence which initiated the illness. The lawyer had behaved badly to one of the lady clients of his office. This became known to strangers who threatened to inform the magistrate and bring him to Court. His whole position was threatened. He felt as if he had fallen into the hands of blackmailers. The scene in Court of which he had dreamed was merely the anticipation of his waking fears. His anxiety was fear of a social death. He could not remain in Franzensbad because he was afraid that in the meantime action might be taken against him in Vienna, without his being able to retaliate in time. He could not leave his house because, from various indications, he imagined—certainly without foundation—that his neighbours knew something of the affair. Because, in fact, he was ashamed of himself.

Each of his neurotic symptoms was, therefore, of " conscious " origin. But the power of his repression was so great that he was continually transferring them to his organic malady. He said nothing about these unpleasant circumstances to his doctors, simply because they did not ask him about them.

But the analysis revealed still more. He once had a dream in which he saw himself *lying beside himself*, ·bloated, cyanotic, with the death rattle, at his last gasp. He awoke out of this dream with palpitations and anxiety. The interpretation was easy. Who was that part of him, his " second self," that he saw lying beside him ? Just his wife, whom he grasped tightly during the anxiety attack, to whom, in fact, he absolutely clung. In the dream he saw her as a cyanotic dying woman in her last hour. This dream denotes a powerful unconscious desire. His wife had been dangerously ill several times with an ulcus ventriculi. The wish[2]—if she would only die—was on several occasions nearly fulfilled. He had married his ugly wife when she was a poor girl, out of love. He was intensely interested in painting ; was more artist than amateur, and she stood in the way of his artistic endeavours. She was an obstacle to his love affairs. It was for this reason that he toyed unconsciously with the thought, " supposing she were dead." The reaction

[1] *S. de Sanctis*, " Die Traüme." *Karl Marhold*, Halle, a.d. S.

[2] This wish plays a great part in anxiety-neuroses and anxiety-hysteria. An excellent description of this psychic condition is afforded us by *Sudermann* in his Novel " Die Geschwister."

thereto was manifested by *exaggerated tenderness*. He clung to her with the cry : " Do not leave me ! " because he desired the contrary. Criminal impulses may possibly have played their part also. I did not investigate on those lines, but I thought I detected a criminal poison-complex from his neurotic dread of nicotine poisoning. The dream of the rattling body seems to point in that direction also.

This is a phenomenon which is found in every case of anxiety hysteria. We have only to investigate, and a death-thought will always make itself manifest. It generally concerns the death of the other partner, but sometimes also that of the children or of relatives. The anxiety neurotic mercilessly disposes of all obstacles in his dreams. He plays with death. His anxiety is the suppressed wish and conforms with the secret play of psychic powers which desire the annihilation of an otherwise beloved individual. It is, in short, the " guilty conscience."

Investigation of the deeper layers brought to light the fact that the patient, and his brother as well, suffered from remarkable attacks of suffocation, which only occurred during the night. He awoke with shortness of breath and whooping a few times. This seemed horrible but was soon over. These attacks of laryngospasmus familiaris were a simulation of a sound which he had heard his father make at home during intercourse. Hence their occurrence in the night, during sleep, and hence their occurrence in his brother, who had shared the same youthful impressions. It was therefore an hereditary trouble due to environment, which obviously played a much greater part than the much maligned hereditary trouble originating in the germ-cell.

We see from this example how many factors contribute to the generation of anxiety hysteria—for this was obviously such a case. The coitus interruptus, which was the cause of the feeling of dissatisfaction, the well-founded dread of a painful law-suit, the severe psychic conflict between ethical inhibitions and criminal death wishes, the burden of a sexually exciting impression of his youth.

There are certain types of anxiety hysteria which are only revealed to the doctor through dream pictures. I could give at least a dozen examples of this description. Let us take one of my list at random.

No. 104.—A woman who suffered from the phobia that she could not go out alone. She could not even remain alone in a room. She was an elderly lady, and had already two big sons over twenty. She sat for years in her room, and could hardly be persuaded to go out in the evening, the explanation she gave being that " she would be taken ill in the street," she would get another " attack." She had had several attacks in the street and in her room, which the doctors declared to be due to her nerves. She used to stand and tremble, turn pale, and complained of palpitation. She felt as if she were dying. Her condition temporarily improved at a health resort, and she was able to take long walks and on one occasion even went to a concert at which she managed to stand for two hours in a dense crowd (!) After this passing improvement, her condition grew worse. A psychotherapeutic attempt to treat the patient met with strong opposition. She related an insignificant anamnesis of no importance, obviously concealing the chief part. She had practised coitus interruptus for fourteen years, and had become, of late years, totally anæsthetic. This is a condition very frequently found in women who habitually practise coitus interruptus. They protect themselves against the injurious effects of frustrated excitation by complete anæsthesia, which will not admit of any excitement. It is just these people who can deceive the nerve specialist who seeks to investigate their sexual life,

by protesting : " I am absolutely cold and unfeeling, it is a matter of complete indifference to me whether my husband cohabits with me or not."
We are in this way enabled to detect a whole series of anxiety neuroses, whereas a superficial analysis might lead to the inference that there is no connection between sexuality and anxiety. In reality, however, the anæsthesia is only relative, that is,·it is confined to one object, the one who performs the act of coitus, and to this particular form of the vita sexualis. If we do not allow ourselves to be deterred by opposition and proceed carefully with our investigations, or if the patient brings us one of her dreams, which she will do unsuspectingly the first time, it transpires that the phantasy life of these patients is occupied essentially with sexual things and to an altogether hypertrophic extent, and that *behind the apparent anaesthesia, unrestrained sexual phantasies flourish in profusion, and especially those concerning incest and perversions.* Needless to say these inmost secrets are not very easy to confess. But if we succeed in lifting the veil, and releasing the repressions, we are enabled to effect a distinct improvement in the condition.

In the present case the patient emphatically emphasized her sexual indifference. The motives for the anxiety states were not discoverable until she brought me her first dream. It ran as follows :

" I see my son lying on a sofa without a head ; I am quite horrified. · He says, ' Fear nothing, the doctor will give him another head.' " She awoke with a frightened scream.

The dream was connected with the events of the previous day. Mother and son had had a violent dispute. He had said excitedly : " You can't set another head on my shoulders." She decided to complain to me about her son. We see how this wish was completely fulfilled in the dream. The son gets me to set a new head on his shoulders (for I am the doctor of the dream). Since he said it himself, it is a proof that he accepted this service. But this by no means solves the riddle of the dream. If this dream fulfils her wish, why did she awake with a cry of fear ? Anxiety is a repressed wish, generally of a sexual character. Where is the repression in this dream ? I asked her why she cried out. She then recalled the fact that the head lying on the ground had begun to scream. It was not till then that she felt afraid. This brings to her mind her son's circumcision ; the child screamed dreadfully on that occasion also. The operator was very unskilful and had nearly cut away a portion of the *head* (glans penis). Now let us not lose sight of the fact that the *head* (through transference from below to above) is a symbol of the *tail*. The dream was then much more intelligible. It had, like all dreams, a multiplicity of determining factors, and was open to several interpretations. It was a reminiscence of the circumcision at which a portion of the head had been cut off and sewn on again by a doctor. But if this event made such a lasting impression that it was able to form the plastic material of a dream after twenty-five years, the only explanation is that her unconscious thoughts were occupied with the son. In others words, *that repressed incestuous thoughts were the cause of the phobia.* This was actually the case. She was secretly obsessed with the fear that her son should contract some sexual disease which would eat away the member, as she had seen it depicted in a medical atlas of a lodger. He would then be obliged " to live without a " tail." On the other hand she had heard that diseases of this nature were now very easily cured if a doctor were consulted in time.

This case throws a remarkable light on the peculiar train of thought of an hysteric. Her husband had neglected her for years, spending his time in restaurants or tea-shops without giving much consideration to her. She now revenges herself for this treatment on her son, whom she loved just as passionately as she once loved her husband. Her husband had always left her at home and gone out alone. She now forced her son to remain with her continually so that he could not frequent restaurants and tea shops. If he went away she had an attack of anxiety. This phobia presents a bad outlook for therapy. If the patient's wish encounters such powerful needs, if her illness can be proved to be of exceptional service in the economy of life, she will strenuously oppose all efforts to induce her to betray her secret and restore her health. *She lacks the will to health, for she can obtain through her illness all that love she desires from her son.*

We find in all phobias connections between anxiety and the problem of death (" The death-clause.") All anxiety has a certain amount of " fear-of-death " attached to it. It is that component of anxiety which arises from the instinct of self-preservation. In dealing symbolically with " places " careful analysis will always find, standing at the end of the road that seems too long, the figure of His Majesty, Death. A neurotic is unable to cross a bridge. Why ? Because a bridge not only symbolises the way to forbidden things, but also the way to the other shore, the hereafter. (*Kleinpaul*) Death stands on the other side of the bridge and is waiting for us. To all topophobists the roads seem endlessly long. " Neurosis is the tyrant of symbolism." The road becomes the road of life ; the patient sees his whole life dramatised. And again at the end of the road lurks death. The inexorable Judge is waiting. The neurotic trembles at the thought of the last reckoning. It is quite superfluous to search for any root of anxiety other than a purely psychological one.

Abraham (über eine konstitutionelle Grundlage der lokomotorischen Angst Int. Z. f. ærztl. Psychoanalyse. Bd. II., 1914, S 143) traces the anxiety of movement—*i.e.*, every form of Topophobia— to an originally over-powerful desire for movement and *Reik*, in his essay on "Zur lokomotorischen Angst " (*ibidem*) confirms this hypothesis. I have repeatedly pointed out that even in speech the act of walking (Gehen = co-ire) represents a sexual act which accounts for the symbolic construction of topophobias. But experience does not confirm the part played by muscle erotism (*Sadger*) in the sense accorded it by *Abraham* and *Reik*. There are people who masturbate while walking, especially women, who have emissions, and even reach the stage of orgasm, and despite the repression of this form of auto-erotism are not afflicted by topophobia. On the other hand we often come across cases of topophobia which are entirely lacking in these constitutional components. *Abraham* describes the case of a girl who could only walk with her father. Why did not the inhibition of the incestuous impulse render her, by anxiety, incapable of walking ? I know other girls who are overcome with certain forms of anxiety whenever their fathers enter the room. It is quite certain that psychic determining factors are always at work. The so-called constitutional basis of *Abraham* (it is at most a " conditional " one in *Tandler's* sense) is merely a proof that this type of patient has sexualised the act of walking. But this is only a paraphrase of the facts which I have already dealt with in the first edition of my " Anxiety Conditions."

The meaning of disease without constitutional foundation, in *Abraham's* sense, is illustrated by the following observations :

No. 105.—Mrs. L. K., a lady of thirty-nine had been bedridden for ten years. She was afraid of getting up and going about. When an attempt was made to get her out of bed and place her comfortably on a chair she was seized with a fit of anxiety, protested that she would never survive this moving about and that she would die of a heart attack. When, however, we know the psychic source of this illness it does not surprise us that she strenuously opposed all therapeutic endeavours. The whole illness consisted, as in the foregoing case, in a reaction to the ill-treatment of her husband. She first of all punished him for his rough, tyrannical behaviour by means of her illness, and secondly, she compelled thereby his loving attentions. For her husband was only affectionate and attentive when she was ill. Concealed behind this form of anxiety were also various sexual motifs of an auto-erotic nature which I will not enter into further. I have mentioned this case only as an example of the way in which patients prefer to *take refuge in illness* with the object of procuring for themselves certain advantages in life, and are therefore much more difficult to cure and need a longer treatment whereby the error of thought in the patient has to be corrected by the personal influence of the doctor.

" *The refuge in illness* " is a frequent motif of phobia. Phobia is always the patient's means of escape from severe psychic conflict, and the anxiety ideas which appear so absurd on the surface prove themselves to be psychically well-founded.

The following observation points to a case of parapathia developed on the grounds of severe psychic conflict.

No. 106.—Mr. S. V., a forty-four year old postman, employed in carrying letters containing money, of perfectly healthy parentage, came to consult me about agoraphobia. The trouble had begun about two years previously with an almost imperceptible psychic depression. He became dejected, showed little energy and began to be troubled with vague feelings of anxiety. If there were many people in a room he felt a strange sense of uneasiness. He was obliged to go outside lest he should suffocate. He ceased to attend the theatres or church. On one occasion he had to cross a narrow bridge that spanned a little brook. He was seized with a violent fit of anxiety and giddiness and could not go across. From that day he also suffered from agoraphobia.

The condition grew worse and worse. He lost his appetite. His sleep became restless and haunted by horrible anxiety dreams. He lay for hours with palpitating heart, tossing from side to side without being able to sleep. In the street he was afflicted with a variety of unpleasant sensations, so that he would have preferred to remain at home. He only went out when necessary to his occupation. He had anxiety ideas. Something was the matter with his clothes and everybody was laughing at him. He lived on the fourth floor, and could no longer approach the window because it at once made him giddy. There was a little window in his office through which one of his colleagues was accustomed to pass him letters. He felt incapable of opening this window and was obliged to report himself ill.

He was allowed temporary leave for " neurasthenia," and underwent the usual treatment, without success.

Psychanalysis provided a complete explanation of this obscure case. He had practised coitus interruptus for fourteen years. Slight symptoms of an anxiety neurosis had been already manifest for eight years (irritability, diarrhœa, anxiety dreams, nervous asthma !) Two years previously his only son had died suddenly. He reproached himself with not having done everything that lay in his power to save him. He had been too strict with him, had thrashed him repeatedly without cause, etc.

But there was a much deeper reproach behind these reproaches. He had made the acquaintance, at that time, of a pretty young girl and had fallen in love with her. He pondered on ways and means wherewith to free himself from his wife. Then his son fell ill. *For just one moment he had played with the thought " What is there to bind you to your wife if the boy were to die now ? Then you would be free and could marry the other girl."* In addition to this there was a good deal of psychic conflict. The girl's guardian had been in his office and had complained about him to the director. The director had spoken seriously to him. He was no longer a young man and ought not to make the girl unhappy. He was ashamed, therefore, to go to the office and kept repeating to himself the words of his superior. But of what avail were argument and logic against the force of his passion ? He began to wonder whether it would not be better to elope with the girl. He was a " money-postman " and often carried large sums in his hands. Supposing he were to go off with a few thousand gulden ? (Cp. Case No. 1.) But— he was too weak for such a crime. It got no further than phantasy with him. A phantasy which he strenuously repressed.

Nor was there any possibility of marriage after the separation from his wife. He was a Catholic. It was a sad love-affair, full of wretched hours without prospect of their passionate longing ever being satisfied. Their passion was gradually overwhelming them.

One day the girl wanted to yield to him altogether. But he was so excited that he was completely impotent. (He could not open the window—symbol for vagina). He became weary of life, and for a time contemplated throwing himself from the fourth floor on to the pavement. His dread of going to the window, his giddiness, his anxiety that people would notice something, all these conditions were, as one could see at a glance, of psychic origin. The giddiness on the bridge attacked him on the day when he had made up his mind to possess the girl at all costs.

The man was a criminal without the courage to commit a crime. His phobia was the symbolic representation of a severe psychic conflict between impulse and duty.

After psychanalysis his condition improved rapidly. On my advice the girl left Vienna. He took up his occupation once more and managed to lead a tolerable existence with his wife.

The criminal root is still more clearly evident in the next case.

No. 107.—A clerk, suffering from insomnia, inability to work and severe mental depression. He had a somewhat responsible position to which he no longer felt equal. In consequence he was worried by the thought that he would soon lose his position ; his wife and only child would then starve, etc. He found it impossible to finish writing a business letter, or add up a column of figures. At home he had not spoken a word for weeks, was very ill-humoured and used to sit and brood by the hour ; he was very irritable, flew into a rage at the slightest provocation, assaulted his wife and then regretted it afterwards and wept just as immoderately as he did at the smallest other provocation. I will not enter into the whole psychanalysis of the case. It was not of long duration. After a fortnight I discovered the cause of the malady. Years of association with these patients gives one a certain insight, which in this instance was not even particularly difficult. The man had married a woman (who had been living with him for some years previously), because she had become pregnant. He felt honour bound to take this step. The girl was poor, and brought him nothing but debts for the trousseau and furniture ; he was ambitious and was always making plans to become independent. He was now obliged to renounce all these plans. Immediately after the marriage he had violent rows with his wife, in which he even assaulted her. He had been suffering for three months from depression, which rendered him incapable of work. I arrived at the cause of this depression through a stereotyped dream, which repeated itself several times during his illness. He was continually dreaming that his wife and child were being poisoned by gas ; in his dream he had forgotten to turn the gas-tap off. He then awoke (in his dream)[1] and found his wife and child unconscious

[1] The explanation of this interesting psychic phenomenon of dreaming

and dying ; he cried out and then awoke in reality with palpitation and a feeling of deep depression. It was easy to recognise that this man's criminal thoughts took the form of getting rid of his wife by gas-poisoning. They had no gas in their flat, but his wife informed me later on that he had been talking for months of having gas laid on, and they had often discussed the " pros and cons." The thought of recovering his lost freedom by this means was obviously a compulsion idea. (These compulsion ideas frequently reach consciousness in the form of a stereotyped dream). In short, the patient admitted to me frankly, that he thought how, if his wife and child were dead, he would be a free man, and would be able to exchange his position with which he was dissatisfied for another, with the help of the gas. And when I drew his attention to the criminal phantasies which he must be harbouring, he confessed, after some hesitation, that he had even consciously given way to criminal phantasies against which he had energetically guarded himself. Other criminal phantasies of this man took the form of poisoning his family. These phantasies however only flashed like lightning through his consciousness, and were completely repressed.[2] He was not conscious of them any more. The success of the disclosure of these plans was nothing short of amazing. He was able to sleep and work again and the remorse which his evil thoughts had occasioned was productive of an entire change in his attitude towards his family. He became tender and considerate ; his wife, who visited me some weeks later to express her gratitude, assured me she would never have believed that such a change could take place in any human being. It was the revelation of the various criminal phantasies, of which I have only mentioned one, which had produced such a wonderful effect. I could multiply examples of this kind. As I have already said, I consider that all neurotics are, in a sense, criminals without the courage to commit a crime.

The description of these maladies affords us a deep insight into the psychogenesis of phobias. In all the cases there is psychic conflict, the struggle between impulse and morality. Phobias are the outcome of a guilty conscience. And all these patients were acting a part to themselves. They were unaware that they had been repressing criminal desires.

Our wishes are like " revenants." Hopes are buried, and with them the unspoken wishes, under the threshold of consciousness. But they are for ever knocking on the door of their prison craving to be released. When we hear the knocking of these subterranean desires, we are seized with sinking anxiety. We are really afraid of ourselves.

In the next chapters I shall introduce a strange assortment of patients. We shall be permitted to see *men as they really are and not as they appear to be.* If we open the graves of buried desires out will spring wild passions as from Pandora's box. But they cannot bear the light of day. They fade and die, never to appear again. It is only the repressed thought that can, as *revenant,* lastingly disturb the equilibrium of our soul.

that one is awake, together with particulars of the so-called " dream within a dream," may be found in my work, " Die Sprache des Traumes." (*J. F. Bergmann,* Second Edition, Munich, 1921.)

[2] The original criminal wish is repressed and replaced by a more harmless compulsion idea or doubt. In this case the substitute was the unimportant question : Shall I have gas laid on or not ? (For further particulars see my treatise, " Zwangszustände, ihre psychischen Wurzeln und ihre Heilung." (Mediz. Klinik, 1910, No. 5-7.)

CHAPTER XVII

ANALYSIS OF A HEART NEUROSIS

NO. 108.—A " nervous " lady, with no hereditary taint, came to consult me about a " heart-affection." She suffered from attacks of violent palpitation, which lasted for hours and were accompanied by painful anxiety ; several times in the course of the year she experienced threatening symptoms of heart weakness at which the pulse ceased and she was only revived with the help of camphor injections, black coffee and champagne. On the previous day she had had another serious attack. She did not wish to call her family doctor because she felt dissatisfied with him. He had become " casual " of late and took no trouble. She now turned to me, and requested me to undertake her treatment. This thirty year old woman, somewhat pale but well nourished, proved, under examination, to be organically perfectly sound ; nor was there anything of a pathologic nature to be detected in the alleged diseased heart, beyond a slight irregularity and acceleration of the pulse. There was a scarcely perceptible struma parenchymatosa.

A more detailed description of the heart attacks at once betrayed the neuropathic character of this affection. Just before the commencement of the attack she was conscious of an aura which produced a pleasurable sensation. It was a " pleasant dying." This was succeeded by anxiety which increased in intensity until she was convinced that " her last hour had come." I suggested a psychic cure to which she was all the more ready to agree, having obtained no relief from all her water-cures, strophantus, digitalis, and caffein.

I requested the patient first of all to give me an exact account of her life. People have such a curious way of beginning, when we ask them for their life-history. They generally make false statements, either intentionally or unconsciously, which are often not corrected until weeks later. When we draw their attention to the contradiction they maintain that they do not remember having said anything different before. My patient related a harmless and uneventful youth. She had been brought up with several brothers and sisters in her parents' house, had known no particular trouble, and could not remember any sexual factor which might have been instrumental in disturbing her mental balance. At the age of twenty-two she had married, for love, a man who proved to be a model husband. About four years after the marriage the nervous condition began. She felt sexually perfectly satisfied, loved and respected her husband beyond anything, and was the mother of three children. She considered her illness to be due to continual vexation and the fact that she had the whole responsibility of the household. Her husband earned very little. She carried on a large business the responsibility of which rested on her shoulders. "I have simply overworked myself; I am not fit to cope with all this trouble and exertion. First I have to pay heavy taxes, then to meet the demands of my various creditors, then the customers become dissatisfied; one thing comes on the top of another until my head is sometimes in a whirl."

Now let us put ourselves in the position of the doctor who listens to this anamnesis and deduces the nature of the illness therefrom. He will come to the conclusion that cares, anxiety, worry, over-exertion, and overwork are accountable for the terrors of the neurosis.

I have repeatedly found, and I will refer to these cases again later, that patients during eight to fourteen days, have enumerated all their psychic emotions and persistently denied the sexual ones.[1]

For the first day I let this suffice and strove to win the patient's confidence. I devoted the second interview to the genesis of the attacks: "How did the attacks originate? On what occasion did they break out? You will remember the last attack best, tell me something about it."

"Oh, I remember that one very well. It was on my wedding day. A married couple we know came to visit us and enacted a dramatic scene before us. I was terribly excited. Mr. X. violently reproached his wife for coquetting with Dr. W.; in fact, he even maintained that she had had an affair with him."

"But why did this excite you so much?"

"Because—" and here the patient hesitated a moment—"because the doctor whom he accused used to be our family doctor."

"Whom you gave up because he became casual?"

"Yes, that was the man."

"That does not yet explain your great agitation."

"Yes, it concerned a near relative! Mrs. X. is my husband's sister."

On enquiry I learned that a certain rivalry existed between her and the lady who was accused of adultery and I also found that she was distinctly fond of the family doctor, concerning whom she had heard, before her attack, that he had been to a certain extent "*unfaithful*" to her. Not that she had had any affair with him!—Never had an unseemly word been uttered; but a

---

[1] "Excitement" is a favourite scape-goat for the various neuroses. But in reality people rather fall ill from lack of excitement. Excitements are generally stimulating and nervous people cannot live without excitement.

silent sympathy had united them and he had quite openly paid her attentions. She had long been jealous of her sister-in-law. On that night she realized that he had been having an illicit love affair with her. No sooner had their friends stopped quarrelling, than she fell down with a loud cry[1] and was shaken with convulsions. This was the worst attack she had ever had. They had to call in a strange Doctor who lived near by and who took half an hour ro restore her to life.

On further enquiry it transpired that she had had three similar attacks, also on *wedding days*, once on her own and twice on her friends' wedding days. She evaded all closer information and went into details about her youth, about numerous men who had courted her, how beautiful she had been and how much sought after, and so forth. A typical trait in women who are not satisfied in the choice of a husband. They always indulge in flights of fancy depicting a procession of men whom they could have had. . . . .

It took three more interviews to penetrate a little further into her psychic life, after the removal of superficial layers. This was achieved by the aid of a dream. It is a curious fact that every time patients come up against an inner resistance, they then have a pretty vivid dream which affords the doctor a clear insight into everything that they wish to conceal from him. The dream certainly speaks its own curiously distorted symbolical language, which must first be translated with the help of dream interpretation.

She saw the Kaiser in his palace, mounting two horses alternately, a large black one and a small white one. "*Kaiser*" is one of the most familiar symbols and in dreams nearly always signifies *father*. I saw through the dream fabric at the first glance and understood that it concerned a sexual scene between her father and mother, which had assumed still larger proportions in her imagination. It seemed to be a combination of a fact and a fancy. But I took good care not to betray any knowledge of the dream and began the interpretation: I asked the patient what thoughts the dream called forth in her mind, whereupon she promptly began to tell of family scenes, until she finally got to the core of the matter. As a small child she had repeatedly listened to the conjugal intercourse of her parents and this used to excite her very much, although she did not rightly know what it was all about. The dream was easily interpreted as the fulfilment of an infantile desire, that the "riding exercise" should be practised with her too. The big black horse represented the mother, the small white one the child herself. (The mother was tall and dark. Since then she envied her mother and wished that she could be in her place.[2]).

---

[1] The cry was not the well-known cry of fear and horror. It was the cry of rage which could be discharged in this masked manner.

[2] A different interpretation of the dream in a functional sense (*Silberer*)

Now the flood-gates were open and a sea of memories irresistibly arose within her. My interpretation was not denied but was, on the contrary, confirmed and supplemented with a host of memories. Though she used to disclaim any attempt at masturbation, she now admitted it and also confessed to having practised it mutually with a woman friend. (Homosexual components of her neurosis ; this is never lacking, as we shall see.)

The whole fabric of repressed erotism, woven partly of truth and partly of fancy, was slowly unravelled. She felt better and freer every day. But she still complained of palpitations now and again. We had not yet penetrated to the deepest origin of the illness.

A number of other dreams carried us a little further. The next one was as follows :—

" *Three old Jews danced about in the meat market, and I became so furious about it that I awoke with palpitations.*" The three old Jews, representing in reality three young Christians, were her husband and his two brothers. One of these always bargained like a Jew ! A few days previously they had all gone to a party and she went home by herself as her husband had wished to accompany his brothers and have a little more gaiety. The thought had then come to her that those three had some wickedness up their sleeves and would probably go to a bad house (meat market). During the day-time she had always repressed this thought. The dream was to bring her certainty. She was jealous. The typical jealousy of unsatisfied women. She got too little because her husband spent himself elsewhere. Thoughts of incest were, moreover, revealed concerning her brothers-in-law.

And then all the unspoken enmity (sexual aversion) which existed between husband and wife was discharged on to the head of her husband. She called him frivolous ; he had lost a good post ; she had to keep the whole house ; he was passionate and easily roused to anger and did not know how to treat her properly. He had no appreciation for her thoroughness, her individuality and her peculiar nature. And she finally admitted that of late she had often been sexually unsatisfied. The husband suffered from ejaculatio præcox. The heart attacks were equivalents of an anxiety attack.

We continued our work. She went on about her husband for a whole week. The whole of her suppressed hate, the suppressed torture of an unhappy choice, disburdened itself. The next dream was as follows :

" *I came into the street and saw a bed standing there. In the bed lay a dark person who was very amorous with my husband. I was very angry and said : ' Wait, if you are like that, then I shall show*

admits of the following conclusion : The *Kaiser* always represents the ruling idea. She wavers between two passions, a big dangerous one and a small harmless one. Expression of her split personality (dissociation).

you'—*and I ran away, furious, and a tall dark man with a black beard ran after me up the stairs and followed me into the room.* He *tried to kiss me and make love to me, but I did not allow it and just had enough strength to push him out of the door and lock it after him."*

The analysis of this dream was very simple. The "bed in the street" represents the prostitute in dreams. This dream revealed that part of her thoughts which concerned her husband's supposed unfaithfulness. For it was he with whom the woman had played in bed. She had caught him and wished to revenge herself. She then sought a legitimate means of revenge in the sexual sphere. (German: Zimmer = Frauenzimmer—door = vagina.) The analysis of the dream revealed furthermore that I, her doctor, was meant for the man who followed her. The transference had begun. Besides this there was also the reminiscence of a sexual attack, an attempt at rape, to which she had almost succumbed two years previously. ("I just had enough strength to push him out of the door.")

What was said about the husband during the following days was not exactly flattering; whereas she had previously described herself as the happiest of women, who had the best of husbands, she now tried in every way to show that it would really be no wonder if she should become unfaithful to him. This theme worked itself out logically and in the following dreams and analyses every single admirer that she had hitherto had made his appearance. Her previous doctor was, of course, one of them, and she now admitted a great liking for him, a fact which we had already recognized as having been the cause of her last attack. A further analysis revealed that the attacks took place on her friends' wedding days and were always accompanied by feelings of jealousy and envy. *It was as though a great disappointment had occurred on her own wedding day and had continued to this day,* and which, operating through the unconscious, evoked the attacks at such critical times.

Finally she confessed that she had not really married her husband for love ; her love had belonged to another. He too was, curiously enough, a medical man who had courted her for some years, during which time they had repeatedly embraced and kissed one another. She had been dreadfully agitated after such embraces, could not sleep for nights and indulged in sexual fancies. One day the medical student, who had in the meantime become a doctor, explained to her that he had fully considered the matter, they were both poor and would not make a success of it, therefore it would be best to give up the idea. She had been very unhappy about it and was for a long time inconsolable.

I had to listen to this story in all its details for three days in succession and was spared no item. In such cases patience is essential and we must wait until fresh clues are brought to light. Again we struck the new track by means of a dream,

"*Last night I had a bath in my room and Mrs. N. came in and* said : ' *Oh, you are having a bath now, that is splendid. I will come and have one with you.*' *She got into the bath with me and paid me compliments all the time :* ' *You have a beautiful body, as white as marble.*'[1] *What happened then I do not know.*''

The conclusion of the dream could, of course, have provided valuable elucidation. But most erotic dreams are so concealed that they never produce the actual scene, the final act. This is only the case in dreams of pollution, where sexuality manifests itself undisguised. In these cases of " repressed sexuality " we always get the typical refrain : " What happened then I do not know," or " I cannot remember the end." Of course not ! Otherwise the whole disguise of sexuality would be superfluous. It was a great pity in this case, for it was just the continuation of this dream that would have interested us ; it obviously concerned a homosexual phantasy.

" What do you know of this woman ? " I asked.

" She often comes to see me and is strikingly beautiful. I like her very much."

We pursued this trail with the result that a number of women appeared on the scene with whom she had lived in friendship ; amongst others was the girl with whom she had mutually practised masturbation, and finally her mother. It was clearly proved that it was her mother who had aroused in her the first sexual tendencies. It had always pleased her immensely when her mother undressed, and as a baby she howled lustily whenever she was taken out of the room while her mother was dressing. She pretended to be ill so that her mother should take her into her own bed at night, which always gave her great pleasure. Even now her love for her mother was exceptionally deep and strong. I explained to her that everybody was inclined to be bisexual, some were more so and some less, and that evidently there was a homosexual component operating in her, which was perhaps the reason for her marriage having hitherto been an unhappy one.

But here was a curious fact : Amongst the women of whom she was very fond, was also the sister of her present husband, the same sister-in-law who played such a large part in her last attack. Shortly after the break with her first fiancé she went into the country to rest her nerves and was kindly received by her husband's family. The sister-in-law was a friend of her youth. She missed no opportunity of passionately embracing and kissing her. " We lived like turtle-doves." In the country she had often shared a bed with his sister. She denied mutual masturbation ; they had always lain in each other's arms and kissed ; they had envied each other the beauty of their bodies and praised them, etc., until, after endless caressing, they fell asleep. . . . . . .

The scene of the last attack caused excitement for two reasons.

[1] Here the pronounced self-love (narcissism) of the patient is betrayed.

She was jealous of Dr. W.[1]   But just as jealous of her sister-in-law. This love for the beautiful girl played an important part in bringing about her marriage.

Once it happened that her present husband was forced to sleep in the same room.   They had hardly got to bed when the brother came into the room and undressed in the dark.   But when the sister was asleep—and she always slept very heavily—he came up to their bed and from behind, without his sister noticing anything, quite quietly but persistently kissed her on her brows and eyes. That had excited her very much and when, two days later, he proposed to her, she was quite unable to refuse him.

We here have an occurrence that is frequently to be met with in life,—the indirect course of passion through a second person. Her husband's sister had powerfully aroused the homosexual component in her and greatly excited her sexuality.   This is an example of the transference of the libido from the homosexual to the heterosexual, an occurrence that also comes into consideration with the fixation of homosexuality.   In this condition she was, of course, more responsive to the man's desire and allowed herself the more easily to be enticed into love-play ; she could easily make herself believe that she had a great "penchant" for the brother. And in her subconscious mind the thought may have arisen : "If you marry the brother, the sister will be still nearer to you and will remain yours."   His close resemblance to her friend was an additional reason.

I have often observed similar cases.   We shall later on hear of a male counterpart to this.

Such homosexual desires obtaining indirect satisfaction mislead the inexperienced and easily deceive them concerning their own individual passions.

Several interviews were then devoted to memories of those days, with women friends and with various other admirers of both sexes and each time she impressed upon me how great her disappointment had been when the man's affectionate manner so soon gave way to inconsiderate brutality.   The patient, who had felt very well during the analysis, now grew agitated again and it was evident that a knotty point was before us.   Various recollections of an exhibitionistic nature came to the surface.   Once while dressing she had been taken unawares ; she had herself watched all kinds of things through the keyhole.   They used to live in a suburb where they could observe the life and habits of prostitutes.   She had seen gentlemen go in and out and had discussed it exhaustively with other *children*.

At last there came a dream : "*She was in a salon, where she was selling overcoats and umbrellas.*"   The dream could easily be inter-

---

[1] This homosexual root is always to be found in jealousy.   We are only jealous of such people whom we ourselves find loveable and worthy of love. (See the chapter on "Eifersucht," Vol. II, Chapter X, Second Edition, *p.* 379.)

preted as a sexual phantasy. As a child she had a wish to be a prostitute too. " Overcoat " is too palpable to need an explanation. This led again to a number of fresh themes. She was suspicious of her husband because she had found several condoms in his pockets. Why did he carry these about with him if he did not want to use them elsewhere. He could just as well leave them in a drawer. She was certain he was deceiving her. Umbrella, an object that can be erected, is frequently a phallic symbol. In her dream she was a prostitute. For years she had had business relations with a so-called " salon," where " umbrellas and overcoats " were used.

Dream followed dream. The last one was an undisguised sexual phantasy, no longer concealed by images. " *She was in the street ; a gentleman accosted her. In his buttonhole he wore, instead of a rose, an expedient that was otherwise used as a contraceptive. Suddenly she felt a congressus a posteriori.* Further revelations of unfulfilled sexual phantasies followed in rapid succession, until finally, amid great agitation, the most important sexual trauma of her youth came to light. *Suddenly she remembered it, she could not understand how it was that she had hitherto forgotten it.* She was only a little school-girl (six or seven years old), when the lodger who lived with them called her into his room, unbuttoned his trousers and showed her his erect penis. As soon as this recollection came back to her an attack of palpitations, anxiety and spasms occurred with the most violent emotion, and we were obliged to put an end to the interview.

On the following day the patient received me with a beaming smile. She felt as if a weight had been removed ; she was supremely relieved. Further analysis showed that she had been controlled by this experience of childhood ever since. The immense size of the phallus, which had increased in her imagination year by year, had especially struck her. In her embraces with the medical student she had also felt an exceedingly large phallus. On her wedding night she had remarked with horror that the phallus that was destined for her did not in any way approach the enormous dimensions of the one in her imagination. (Her husband, by the way, possessed a normally developed penis, rather large if anything.) The anticipated pleasures of the wedding night were also lacking —she was anæsthetic on account of her masturbatory practises,[1] —and she wept for hours with excitement. She then already had feelings of anxiety and palpitations.

The attacks evidently had a two-fold origin. One root went down to her earliest childhood and reproduced the experience with the student, which was completed in her imagination as far as was possible. On the other hand, the disappointments concerning her husband's small phallus, which had remained in the unconscious, manifested themselves on wedding days when the big attacks took

---

[1] A part of the anæsthesia must be attributed to her homosexuality.

place. As a substitute there occurred loss of consciousness, palpitations and that attack which through its whole course gave a clear, imitative picture of sexual union. Every attack was the fulfilment of a wish, wherein she compensated herself to a certain extent, in that moment, for all that life had withheld from her. *It was a wedding night after her own heart.* The anxiety served on the one hand to cover the sexual agitation and on the other hand it was the expression of her moral ego.

The analysis continued to take its course. A host of erotic experiences of her early childhood, which had been repressed and forgotten, came to light.

After that she felt considerably better, but there remained a big task to be performed. *The paient had still to be educated and her marriage to be made a happy one.* This, too, was an unqualified success. First of all I cleared up her misunderstanding and taught her to reduce her demands to a natural, modest degree ; secondly, I was successful in correcting various points in her behaviour towards her husband. She had hitherto been shy, cold and reserved and had always expected the husband to take the initiative. He was one of those who always had to be lured, stimulated, to erotism, who responded gladly to it and who had for this reason only preferred the marketable charms of prostitutes to those of his beautiful wife. She had to learn that it was absurd for a woman to think that the conquest of the husband was accomplished as soon as she was married. That was just the time when she must daily set to work to win him anew.

I enlightened her a little concerning the necessary coquetterie and subtleties of married life. On the other hand I gave the husband to understand that he could never count on a healthy wife if he satisfied his sexual needs elsewhere and did not approach his wife with kindness and consideration. A new epoch of love commenced for them both. She blossomed forth, rejuvenated, and was brimming with happiness ; he became the most faithful and satisfied husband imaginable and could not understand how he could ever have been untrue to his wife. He found it difficult to realise how she had changed and that she was no longer so nervous and irritable.

After six months, during which period I received a little confession and gave absolution at intervals, the wife had to face a severe psychic shock (business bankruptcy) which she bore so well that it was impossible to remain in doubt about her complete recovery. This cure took place six years ago. The attacks and palpitations have entirely ceased. She went through two confinements easily. The marriage is in every sense of the word a perfect and happy one.

Let us reconsider the whole history of the illness. On the foundation of an anxiety neurosis, which came to the surface shortly after the wedding, a heart neurosis developed, the causes of which were traced back to her childhood. All the characteristic symptoms of a severe parapathia were to be found here : infantile traumas, repressions, tendencies to sexual perversions, an overflowing erotic imagination and an unfortunate attachment to her family doctor. The psychogenesis of the violent attacks with loss of consciousness was interesting ; they were erroneously taken for fainting fits resulting from cardiac weakness. The phantasy of the gigantic phallus is also characteristic. We shall come across this again. But we miss, on the other hand, the characteristic thoughts on the death of some individual dear to her. This woman loved her husband on the whole much more than she hated him and that made the complete cure possible.

H

CHAPTER XVIII

THE FEAR OF INSANITY

ACCORDING to *Freud*, hysteria invariably manifests itself when an insupportable idea sinks into the unconscious. The ego is roused to defence and summoned to use repression. He writes (Zur atiologie der Hysterie, Wiener klin. Rundschau, 1896. Nr. 22-26) : " The resistance then fulfils its purpose of forcing the insupportable conception out of the conscious mind, when infantile sexual scenes manifest themselves in the patient—hitherto in good health—and if the conceptions that are to be repressed can be brought into logical associative connection with this infantile experience."[1]

A repression of this kind either leads to a conversion hysteria, *i.e.*, to the transference of the psychic symptoms into the physical realm, or to an anxiety hysteria. In place of the repressed thoughts we have pains, paralysis, paræsthesias, which stand in a certain psychological causal nexus with the repressed thought, or else a phobia is developed which reveals a similar association. Neuroses that have originated as a result of the repulsion of unbearable conceptions are called by *Freud*, " Abwehrneurosen." (Die Abwehr-Psychoneurosen, Neurolog. Zentralblatt, 1894. Nr. 10 and 11.)

" When the tendency to defence dominates a person, and when to drive away an unbearable idea it has been separated from its affect, then this affect must remain in the psychic realm. The conception, which has now grown weaker, remains in the conscious mind free of all associations, but the liberated affect becomes attached to other conceptions, unbearable in themselves, which then, through this false combination, become compulsion ideas."

While the compulsion *neurosis* is a sharply characterized psychoneurosis, obsessions (compulsion *ideas*) can be traced in many phobias. But we must strictly differentiate between the meaning of " compulsion ideas " and " compulsion neurosis." Every compulsion neurosis produces numerous compulsion ideas. But not everybody is a compulsion neurotic who suffers from a compulsion phenomenon. We only have a right to speak of a compulsion neurosis if the compulsion is in the centre of the clinical picture.

[1] In this context the sentence is not correct. The resistance is not by any means invariably directed against the bringing into consciousness of " infantile sexual scenes." Every painful thought, every humiliating experience, every criminal desire, in short, everything that does not suit our ego can be repressed and become the cause of a neurosis.

Every suppression of a painful thought, every repression,[1] can produce a form of compulsion idea which we shall call " obesssion " in order to draw a sharper distinction. We now come to a confirmatory observation.

No. 109.—Mr. Z., a very strong, organically healthy man of fifty, suffered for three years from violent attacks of vertigo and anxiety feelings. The first attack of vertigo took place in church. He was an extremely religious man, a fanatical upholder of the clergy, who went to church every day, and also did political work. One Sunday morning he had a very nasty attack of vertigo and nearly fell over.[2] He also suffered from harassing anxiety feelings in church. The blood rushed to his head, his temples throbbed and he felt a horrible anxiety. Topophobic symptoms were not lacking either. If he only went a few steps away from his house, he had a feeling as though something terrible might occur in his absence. He had not left his district for three years. His condition had grown considerably worse during the last few months. There were only a few roads left through which he could walk without anxiety feelings. For some days he had been unable to go beyond No. 40 in the Mariahilfestrasse. Further he could not go. He had tried all kinds of treatments. All internal remedies, water cures, electricity, were powerless to influence his anxiety feelings. They were increasing and taking the form of more serious ailments. In spite of his great piety he had not been to confession for some years. He told his priest in the suburban parish that he went to confession in " the city."

I worried over this patient for some days without finding any clue that could assist me to an understanding of his phobia. He had masturbated moderately in his youth, had never experienced anything out of the ordinary and had a normal " vita sexualis." He would hear nothing of a psychic conflict.

Then one day he told me about an obsession. His coachman had given him notice because he had got a permanent situation at the G. Asylum. Mr. Z. said to him : " I cannot keep you back, I realize that you will have a life-long post there and that you will qualify for a pension, which I, of course, cannot offer you." Since then he was obsessed with the idea *that this coachman would be certain to drive him to the asylum at G. some day.* He could see the carriage before him in which the coachman would drive him, and could not rid himself of the thought by day or night ; even in dreams he was still obsessed by this tormenting idea.

I began with the analysis :

" What comes first into your mind when you think of this drive ? "

" That the coachman will stop at Kahlenbergerdorf."

" But why at Kahlenbergerdorf ? "

" Because that is on the way."

" But there are other inns between Vienna and Gugging. Must it just be Kahlenbergerdorf ? Haven't you a special reason for thinking of Kahlenbergerdorf ? "

" No."

" What will the coachman do at Kahlenbergerdorf ? "

" He will dismount, drink a glass of wine, and tell the innkeeper : ' I am now driving Mr. Z. to G., he has gone mad.' But stop ! Now I remember that my parents once drove to Kahlenbergerdorf when they were engaged and that they came home very late. My father told his parents-in-law as

---

[1] " Wherever neurotic compulsion is manifested psychically, it springs from repressions." (*Freud*, Sammlung kleiner Schriften zur Neurosenlehre, S. 120.)

[2] Religion plays a larger part than we had hitherto believed in the psychogenesis of neuroses. For it is religion which proclaims sinful the erotic impulses, and so becomes the foundation of the psychic conflict. *All neurotics are religious people*, however much they may claim to be free-thinkers. Their atheism is only defiance and revolt towards overpowering infantile religious currents.

an excuse that he had missed the train. We often teased my parents about it when we were grown up."

" Then you believe that this excursion was not so innocent and that your father anticipated certain rights before the marriage ? "

" Yes, that is what we believed and we always teased our parents with the phrase : ' The tea-place at Kahlenbergerdorf ! '—This afterwards became a recognized expression for a couple who had a child before marriage."

" It seems as if your childish imagination had dwelt more upon this scene than you have admitted to me. Did not the occurrence, or rather the history of it in your youth, greatly excite you ? "

" Oh, yes ! It was one of the most exciting fancies of my childhood. I often wondered how my mother conducted herself."

" But in saying that you confess that your sexual desires were directed in a sinful way towards your mother."

Mr. Z. was silent ; the subject seemed to be an awkward one. I did not appear to pursue it, but asked : " Did you ever listen to the sexual intercourse of your parents ? "

" Very often ; I was then eleven years old ; the bedrooms were adjacent and I often stayed awake in order to listen."

" Didn't that excite you ? "

" Considerably ; I always masturbated then."

" Really ? You have hitherto concealed that fact : Your thoughts during masturbation were evidently with your mother ? "

Mr. Z. was silent, then he said : " You have reminded me of the fact that even when I was quite a small child I greatly enjoyed watching my mother undress ; I went so far as to take every opportunity to be present whenever she undressed or changed her clothes."

" So you see that the compulsory idea already has a certain reason to be charged with emotion, or in other words : *Because I was sexually roused so early in life, because I masturbated so young, because I directed my thoughts towards my mother in sexual perversion*, I shall lose my reason. This is the reason you are tormented by the thought of the coachman stopping at Kahlenbergerdorf.   But please tell me what else occurs to you concerning this subject."

" The coachman who has left me is very much like another with whom I had a significant experience that I had quite forgotten ; it has suddenly come back to me. I was in the country staying with my aunt, where a little boy taught me masturbation and initiated me into the mysteries of sex life. One day he told me that my aunt's coachman had an enormous penis and advised me to have a look at it. I was not at all shy and ordered the coachman to show me his member, whereupon he replied : ' That is not so cheap, that costs a gulden.' I could get no rest, so I pretended to my mother that my watch was out of order and the clockmaker wanted a Gulden to mend it ; in this way I got the Gulden, which for our circumstances was a large sum. I gave it to the coachman, who led me up to the hay loft, where he showed me the penis and it was, curiously enough, quite erect and certainly unusually big."

" What happened then ? "

" I cannot remember."

" Didn't the coachman demand certain love-services from you ? "

Mr. Z. said nothing for some time and then spoke hesitatingly : " I think we were interrupted then, the coachman was called down."

I noticed that there was more behind that, which Mr. Z. did not want to confide to me, but I concluded from his coughing and choking that the coachman had asked him to put the penis into his mouth, which he did not, strictly speaking, refuse to do ; he could not remember. I gave him to understand that it was quite an exceptional thing for a boy to sacrifice such a large sum for the sight of a male member, a sum for which he could equally well have had the enjoyment of a woman's genitals. This occurrence admitted of a definite inference as to the existence of a homosexual component in his nature.

And then followed a number of homosexual memories : the boy with whom he had masturbated, other friends, until he suddenly remembered that his schoolmaster had once asked him to send his father to speak to him. He then seems to have told the father that he masturbated. For on the same day his father brought the conversation round to masturbation while they were out for a walk, and told him that he would fall seriously ill if he practised that vice and *that he would lose his reason and become insane*, and further similar prophecies.

" Surely you did not believe that ? "

" No, but the other day I met the boy who first masturbated with me."

" Really ? What did he say to you ? "

" He is now a clerk of the magistrate. He confided to me that he had his office between the burgomaster and the councillor. I was quite puzzled and asked him how high his salary was. He said : ' 20,000 Kr.' Then I knew immediately that the man had lost his reason, for a magistrate's clerk gets 2,000 Kr. at the most and is not an intimate chum of the burgomaster and the councillor as he told me he was."

" So that gave you a considerable shock because you thought it was the obvious result of masturbation ? "

" Yes, I thought involuntarily that he had become insane from masturbating."

" Now it is of course quite clear. Behind the coachman who gave you notice is concealed the coachman who reminds you of the time when you practised masturbation and with whom you performed some sexual act or other. Behind Kahlenbergerdorf your father, too, is concealed, who warned you about masturbation and prophesied insanity. Nothing but repressed ideas, which in themselves are enough to create the compulsory ideas. All the same I take it that the secret of this obsession is not yet completely revealed. Have you told me everything that in any way concerns it ? Or can you think of anything else ? "

And now we have the most curious part of the whole story. Mr. Z. related several facts about his father that were most painfully incriminating. After the death of his father, whom he had greatly honoured and regarded almost as a saint, he had heard things about him that were simply incredible. His father had seduced a poor girl and then deserted her, after having given her two children, in order to marry a richer girl. He said he had allowed himself to kick over the traces and made other similar accusations.

In this attempt to accuse his father, whom he looked upon during the analysis with the feelings of a sexual rival where his mother was concerned, he also sought an excuse for his own intentions.

The most important point was revealed at the next interview. He himself had had an affair with a woman for many years and now wished to desert her. He wanted to give her up lightly. Her age was forty. *This was the reason he could not go beyond the No. 40.* A young niece also lived in the house, to whom he was apparently quite indifferent. He was, however, much agitated because some official had proposed to her, a pauper, who had nothing. A miserable wretch. He would never consent to the niece making herself unhappy and marrying " this " man. He did not say that from jealousy, only from a feeling of responsibility as an uncle.

On the following day he confessed to being slightly jealous. The niece slept in the room through which he had to pass in the morning on his way to the office. A few days previously he had seen her uncovered breast and this had greatly excited him. He tried not to think of it but was forced to do so involuntarily. Also at church when, on one occasion, the " immaculate conception " was mentioned, he had wished that he could have intercourse with her without impregnating her.

He had then felt so ill. Now he knew : that was the first attack at church. He would like to have an affair with the girl, who seemed to him very sensual, but the sister-in-law watched him too carefully.

For the first time the name of the sister-in-law, his brother's wife, was mentioned. He at last admitted that this was the woman with whom he had had a love affair for the last ten years.

His brother had died five years ago. He would have liked to marry this woman in order to make amends for his wrong-doing. But he feared that people would say: " Aha, he must have had an affair with her for many years ! " But if he were to marry the young one, gossip would be put to an end once and for all. He had started this affair at forty years of age. Again the important figure, forty !

His attacks at church were now accounted for. He was a religious man ; or had in effect become religious in order to expiate his sins. He did not continue to go to confession because his father confessor had advised him to marry the sister-in-law and convert the sinful intercourse into one legalised by the church.

His heart and his senses belonged to the girl. He was afraid to go away : he might lose her in the meantime. People might learn his secret.

After the analytical elucidation of the case—the treatment lasted two months—the niece was sent away from the house. In a few months' time he married his sister-in-law and was entirely cured. Since then his piety has increased. He makes many pilgrimages and attributes his cure to a pilgrimage he made to Mariazell.

The fear of insanity is one of the most widely spread phobias and has already driven many people to suicide. The malady is especially terrible when it concerns those who have once been cured of syphilis and now fear paralysis. They then undergo the Wassermann test several times a year and ruin their constitutions by undergoing mercury and salvarsan cures with exaggerated frequency. But with these syphilitics the "fear of insanity" also manifests itself as over-determined and arises from the "fear of oneself." All who struggle with forbidden desires suffer from this phobia. They also complain of unbearable head-aches, of feeling as if something would explode in their heads, as if the skull were too small, as if an iron ring clasped the head, as if everything would fall to pieces with a great crash.

Every conception that is unbearable to the "moral ego" continuously endeavours to overpower it in the service of the "instinctive ego." The fear of this overpowering factor also corresponds to a secret desire. Neurotics repeatedly express a wish to be put into a lunatic asylum. ("There I should at last be at peace ! ") He seeks protection from his evil impulses behind the walls of the asylum. There is also a "desire for insanity." The lunatic is not answerable to the law. He cannot help it. ("Pleasure without guilt ! ") He can do all that is forbidden (incest, para-philia, homosexual or criminal actions) and is not treated as a criminal but as a patient.

The more repressed the forbidden tendency, the stronger can be the fear of insanity. In such phobias are to be found the most extreme forms of paraphilia : sadism, nekrophilia, cannibalism, vampirism, all kinds of infantilisms, mysophilia and exceedingly frequently incestuous impulses.

A bad conscience regarding the phantasies connected with masturbation can also—as is proved by the above case—generate a "fear of insanity."

CHAPTER XIX

ANALYSIS OF A DEPRESSION WITH OBSESSION

NO. 110.—Mrs. A. R., a big, strong woman of about thirty-five, was seized with an acute "anxiety neurosis." Violent attacks of anxiety alternated with periodical moods of depression, during which she did not speak a word for days at a time and only stared into a corner. She could give the exact date of the first attack. She was a strictly orthodox Jewess, who, according to their rites, always took a bath after her periods in order to be clean again for her husband, *i.e.*, so that she could again have intercourse with him. Once she took her bath and went home, thinking she had caught cold. As usual her husband practised coitus with her. As happened every time during recent years she grew intensely excited, but without being satisfied. Her husband suffered from ejaculatio præcox. She went to sleep unsatisfied and awoke after a few hours with a feeling of intense anxiety. She was obliged to jump out of bed and burst into tears. She felt that she was dying. After this attack she remained monosyllabic and laconical for a day, and in the depths of melancholy. *One* thought tormented her all the time, repeating itself in the following stereotyped manner : " *My poor children ! What will happen to my poor children ?* " The attacks recurred after this and always took the same course. A state of melancholy depression always followed an attack and it was always accompanied by an anxiety conception regarding the children. Later on the trouble increased and the patient thought incessantly of her children and always with the formula : " What is to become of my children ? " . . . . . . Only during pregnancy (the patient had five children) was a slight improvement apparent, which also lasted during the period of lactation. The *status quo* reappeared immediately after the weaning. This patient, too, had a *slight struma.* Her neck measurement had increased during her illness by about 2 c.m.

The psychanalysis of this case revealed an extremely vivid sexual imagination in the patient, with a tendency to paraphilias (fellatio). As is usual in these cases the dream analysis,—the complete mastery of which is absolutely essential for the execution of an analysis—provided the most valuable revelations as to her unconscious thoughts. The very first dream led us in *medias res. :* " *A hand touched me and I felt a kind of fear. I had quite*

*a normal sensation. Then I was confined and had seven children
at once. The ladies said : ' There is nothing the matter with Mrs.
R., she was only pregnant.' "*
The dreams of every anxiety neurotic betray the deepest meaning
of his anxiety feeling. Here the anxiety feeling was concentrated
on the touch of a hand which she described as *large* and *brown,*
in short, as the hand of a man whom she knew and credited with
great sexual potency, as he once performed coitus seven times
in one night,—so her own husband had told her, as if it were a
miracle. The dream fulfilled her desire for adultery, a desire
that was at the same time her fear. She had (contrary to her
experience of coitus with her husband) the normal feeling. But,
it should be noted, only through contact with the clitoris (infantile type !). The seven children had reference to the seven repeti-
tions of coitus. The dream gave, moreover, an adequate description
of her malady. There was nothing the matter with her, she was
satisfied, she was expecting again, which meant that she was going
through a period in which she always felt much better.
The second dream was short, but full of significance. " *She
saw a procession—not a funeral procession—her husband was not
there. The rector was among the large crowd of people.*"
The interpretation of this dream revealed that it was the funeral
of her husband. Her husband was not there because he lay in
his coffin, *i.e.*, she could not see him. The negations of the dream
only served to emphasize his presence, distorted by the censure
of the pre-conscious (*Freud*). There is no such thing as a negation
in dreams. The evangelical clergyman had lost his wife a few
weeks earlier. He was now to marry again. A proof that her
thoughts were intent upon another.
The patient tearfully admitted that she had had a very bad
day the day before. All at once in her waking hours the thought
had come to her as to what would happen if her husband were
suddenly to fall seriously ill. She kept seeing him in bed and
herself as nurse at the foot of the bed. The thought of nursing
the sick had already come to her in dreams several times. She
had thus had a similar dream concerning her brother a few days
before his marriage. *The brother was her first and greatest love.*
In her dreams she had wished that he might rather die than belong
to another woman. In the same way her dream brought her
the fulfilment of the wish that had already manifested itself in
day-dreams from the unconscious mind and filled her with fear :
" Oh, that my husband would fall seriously ill, so that he would
be dependant upon my nursing. Oh, that he might *die !* "
Hardly any case of anxiety hysteria is lacking this psychic root.
Whatever stands in the way of love is removed in dreams and in
reveries during day-time when the unconscious predominates.
Such patients are much distracted and dream by day. We shall
still have occasion to analyse these day-dreams. The extremely

harassing sensation of *conscious guilt* that is never absent from any neurosis whatever[1] then manifests itself as a reaction to these sinful desires.

Our patient's third dream carried the thought still further : " I saw a young man. I did not know him personally. We were at a large party ; but I did not see my husband. There were some other ladies there. The young man asked how many children each one had. One said three, the other, four. Then the figure seven came to me in my dream. He then asked me : " How many children have you ? " I answered proudly : " I have five children."

The young man was an acquaintance of her youth who married and had no children. Naturally her thoughts turned upon the sexual potency of this man. See the figure *seven* in the first dream. Her ideal was a man who could practise coitus seven times in one night. She would be certain to bear this man children. It was a fact that she had five children. But the supplementary statement, which always reveals the most important fact, proved that the most significant part of the dream had been concealed. It ran : " Then I saw my husband in tears." She awoke with palpitations and an anxiety feeling.[2]

She hereby revealed a new component of her anxiety affect. She played with the idea of getting a divorce from her husband and then marrying the young man. For she had *heard that he was divorcing his wife because she had no children.*

Her obsession, " *What will my children do ?* " was therefore justified. What should happen to the children if she were to get a divorce and if her husband were to die ?

She must free herself from her husband at all costs. The fourth dream suggested a new solution : " *My husband had sold his business. We were all dismayed about it. We protested, until he himself realized what he had done. It meant a hard struggle before he got it back again.*"

Business was here a symbol for her genitalia. (Workshop, shop, are used in a similar way.) Her husband sold her to another. " We were all dismayed about it "—to be interpreted conversely : I was very glad about it. He did it voluntarily. But he loved her all the same. He would not let her go. He wanted to get back his business. She saw herself surrounded by numerous suitors (purchasers) in this dream, the analysis of which goes back to her childhood (she used to play " shop " and " Father and Mother " with her brother) but this is here barely indicated on broad lines. She would not make it so easy for her husband, whose matrimonial faithfulness she had reason to doubt. It would cost a hard struggle.

[1] The *consciousness of guilt* has still deeper reasons. Besides the " passive criminality " (the death wishes) the patient has active criminal thoughts as well.

[2] It would take too long to enlarge upon the details of the dream analyses. I only lay stress on the most important incidents.

The fifth dream revealed her further wishes and disclosed the phenomenon of *transference*. I, the doctor, began to play a part in her dreams. She transferred her affects and wishes to my person. The dream ran thus : "*I turned round in the street and saw Mrs. K., my midwife.* '*Oh,*' *I said,* '*You are here, too.*' " The associations led to me personally ; here again I will only indicate the results. She was again prepared for pregnancy. The child should be mine. For safety's sake, Mrs. K., the midwife, the approved nurse, without whom she would never give birth to a child, appeared in her dream also in Vienna. The emphasis lay on the word " also," besides the allusion to the life of a prostitute ("I see myself in the '*street.*' ")

If this transference is not broken up the analysis is often checked and no further progress made. I informed the patient that it was a case of sexual desires concerning me personally. She admitted that she immediately looked upon every man she met from an erotic point of view. She also confessed to having had such thoughts about me.

The transference stage was easily overcome by candid discussion. In spite of this I found that I still played a certain part in the two following dreams. The *sixth* dream revealed the nature of her paraphilia.

"*There was a large fair in the country. We were there, my husband and a few acquaintances. There were a great many people. But the others were unknown to me. But on the way back I missed my nurse with the two children. (The small child and the big one.) I spoke to the wife of the Rabbi about it and asked her whether she had seen the nurse. She said she had not seen her, she did not know where she was.*"

The interpretation of this dream was very complicated. The beginning represented the contrary, and ran : " There was a small féte in the town. Neither my husband nor any other acquaintance was there. It was a secret (many people often denote a secret) ; nobody noticed anything of it. I was there together with one who is near to me. (The others were unknown to me)." Afterwards she remembered that she had felt very much afraid at the fair. The dream showed a large gap. The most important point had been forgotten. Something was happening in her dream that frightened her. It could be easily guessed : a sexual incident. On the return from the féte she missed her nurse. She had never had a nurse. But the children provided the clue to the dream. The " child " in dreams nearly always signifies the " little one " —*i.e.,* the genitals. The small child and the big one were in this case the normal and the erect penis. And the nurse was no other than the desired man with whom she practised fellatio. (She was still fond of sucking as in childhood.) The Rabbi's wife, the type of a religious woman, represented the reproaches she made herself on account of this phantasy. This Rabbi's wife, whom she knew well, had nine children. In spite of this she knew nothing of all these facts. (She had not seen her, she did not know where she was.) The patient awoke at this stage with violent anxiety feelings. It was significant that she lost her children in her dream. Her death wishes concerned not only her husband, but also her children. The children were the hindrance to a new marriage. If the children did not exist she would leave her husband and marry another. All mothers who tremble for their children (Maternity neurosis, cp. *p*. 86) are inwardly hostile towards them. She was, however, innocent of the loss of the children. The nurse lost them in the crowd.

It must not be thought that this analysis was so simple a matter. I asked the patient to tell me her thoughts concerning this dream, without any influence. Her resistance to the revelation of the secret phantasy took the form of a complete lack of ideas. I made use, in this case, of the trick already mentioned. I got her to recount the nearest associations to the enigmatical word of the dream, *nurse*, and thus in a roundabout way gained access to her concealed trains of thought. This method ("free associations") sometimes leads to the goal in the quickest way. Note, e.g., the associations which follow the words, "Rabbi's wife": *Child, father, parents, house, furniture, life . . . . divan, bed, lamp, flame, stove . . . . fields, agriculture, theatre, actor, singing, illness, doctor, flowers, garden, mirror, curtains, well, river . . . . theory, misanthropist, philanthropist . . . . brother, washstand, business, cellar, tavern, cheerfulness, hotel, coffee house, dwelling house, nursery, temple, prayer, foundation, plough, snow, rough weather, storm, sea, shipwreck, wilderness, lion.*"

One might believe that this represented a list of words chosen just by chance. That is by no means the case. It is evident that important complexes are betrayed in this way and that certain words always recur until the analysis provides a striking solution for them. The laws discovered by Jung (Diagnostische Assoziationsstudien, Leipzig, 1906) also hold good for these free associations. Long pauses occur before the disclosure of significant conceptions. An inner resistance must first be overcome. This was the case in my example with the words "divan," "fields," "theory" and "brother."

My method has great advantages compared with that of Jung. For Jung chooses any kind of stimulus words and it is left to chance as to whether the patient exposes his complexes or not. I let the associations reel off as from a spool from the *one* stimulus word or also from a free choice of a word. This is the psychanalytical method as practised by *Freud*, in which the patients freely produce their thoughts by associations. But I note the key-words which are given me voluntarily and almost without resistance, and then endeavour to decipher the thought behind each word.

Let us analyse the chain of associations before us : The words "*child*," "*father*," "*parents*," refer to domestic scenes which she had observed at home with her religious mother (ironically called the rabbi's wife). This track leads to thoughts of incest. She had heard all kinds of things at home. "*House*," "*furniture*," "*life*" (to live oneself out) lead to "*divan*," a scene during court-ship. "*Bed*," "*lamp*," "*flame*," "*stove*," all sexual symbols which lead, after a long pause, to "*fields*." Here an unpleasant recollec-tion of her youth came to light. As a little girl she was walking home from school with several friends across the fields. A man came towards them with his trousers undone and laughingly showed them an enormous erect penis.

Such recollections are very frequent. In imagination the penis increases in size till it becomes gigantic. The husband's sexual weakness gave rise to the desire for the enormous phallus seen in her childhood. With some patients it is only a question of phan-tasies. In this case the recollection was confirmed by a friend. The word "*agriculture*" also brought to light an infantile experience. She was again walking across the fields with some young girls. In one field a farm-hand helped them to pick flowers. Suddenly he lifted up her frock and touched her indecently. They all fled away screaming and said nothing about it at home. They all of them feigned incredible naïveté. Hence the words "*theatre*," "*actor*," which, by the way, still had the sexual meaning of "play." She acted before me, too. What she said did not ring true, "*singing, illness, doctor*." She would have liked me to behave like the farm-hand in the field. "*Flowers, garden*." The doctor at home had examined her. "*Mirror, curtains*" (so that one should not see that she was undressed), "*well*" (bladder and urethra), "*river*" . . . . (she had suffered from discharge). Again her thoughts turned to me. Would the cure do her any good ? After a long pause the word "*theory*" appears, which contains a reproach against my treatment. (She would have preferred it practical). I am a "*misanthropist*." The "*philanthropist*" is her brother whose "*business*" she had repeatedly seen in front of the "*wash-stand*." She also had a vivid recollection of erotic games in the cellar. In the "*tavern*" a peasant had once asked her if she wanted a "*big one*." The other peasants had all laughed ("*cheerfulness*"). "*Hotel, coffee house, dwelling house*" ; memories of the friend's honeymoon. "*Nursery, temple*"; symbol, like business. Then her thoughts turned to the bath previous to the critical intercourse with her husband. "*Snow, rough weather, storm*"—she caught a chill. "*Sea, ship-wreck*"—an acquaintance had been drowned ; her husband should have travelled on the same boat. The "*wilder-ness*" was as dead as the "*grave*," full of "*stones*." Stones were also erected to the dead. He, the husband, was of the tribe of "*Levi*" : Those were priests. She, too, was practically a priestess. she was the *rabbi's wife* herself. Unfortunately she had seen neither the *big* nor the *little* child of the doctor—for I was the nurse of the dream (from whom she wanted to drink).

I have given this chain of thoughts in detail in order to convey an idea of the difficulty and the lengthiness of a thorough dream analysis. It reveals the unlimited sexual phantasy of the patient, whose anxiety feelings originated in the repression of those conceptions so painful to the conscious mind.

The phantasy of the gigantic phallus is to be found in all unsatisfied women, especially in women of strong homosexual tendencies who only expect to have their own manliness overpowered by a man of superior virility.

The seventh and last dream—she had, in a sense, symbolically presented me with *seven* children—contained the renunciation of my person and the fact of a new birth. No further anxiety affect was to be found in this dream : " *I saw my husband and our doctor turning over the leaves of books. I was standing at another table with another gentleman and was dressing the child. Quite an ordinary lamp was on the table. The burner was taken out and the nurse put the child into the lamp. I cried : ' What have you done there ? ' and tried to take the child out. When I had finished dressing the left side was coloured blue-black.*"

Renunciation of me and her husband, who were heroes out of a book, and were balancing accounts. She did not need us. She *lay* in another bed (separation of table and bed) with another man (a certain man who possessed the sevenfold potency of her ideal husband) and held the penis (child). (She dressed the penis. Reproduction of conjugal facts.) Lamp = vagina. Nurse = wet-nurse = lover. Phantasy of a coitus against which she struggled for the sake of decency. (" What have you done ? ") She was pregnant. She always had varicose veins on the left side during pregnancy.

The analysis further revealed a number of important facts. The dissatisfaction with her husband which was transferred from the sexual to the social and ethical spheres. The harassing thought that her children were actually obstacles and that without them she could marry again. The wish to run away and never to return.

Again we see the same picture. Always unsatisfied on account of her husband's ejaculatio præcox, her sexual needs were directed to imaginative activities. She longs to sin and sought expedients by which she might attain the fulfilment of her wishes in another way. She played with the idea that *her husband and children might die.* Her anxiety was the anxiety of death. Her anxiety was a bad conscience. Repression of the painful idea of her husband's death and transference to the children. Her obsession, " My poor children " had a perfectly logical foundation. " What will happen to my children ? The poor children ! "—meant : " My husband is dead, I have run away with another man. The children are orphans."

We realize what severe psychic conflicts these unfortunate patients inwardly struggle against. It is, as a matter of fact, always virtue that makes them neurotic. An unsatisfied woman has actually only the choice between sin and a neurosis.

If we consider the whole history of the illness once more we shall understand how it was that a severe neurosis arose. Infantile dreams in abundance. Incestuous thoughts concerning the father and brother. A hypocritical repression of a powerful erotism ever since her youth. The beginning of an anxiety neurosis through her husband's ejaculatio præcox.[1] A tormenting jealousy on account of the husband's unfaithfulness. (He had an affair with another woman.) Severe psychic conflicts between desire and duty. A boundless imagination with a tendency towards paraphilia. Active and passive criminal phantasies. An obsession arising from repression. (My poor children!) The result was melancholic depressions of such severity that they feared for her reason and seriously thought of putting her into a lunatic asylum.

The condition speedily improved after treatment. She certainly attributed the improvement to a water cure she underwent during the treatment. That is nothing new to us psychotherapists. *We are our patients' friends as long as they need us.* When they are well again their cure is always due to something else. The patient had in this case undergone several water cures before the analysis, without any success at all. During the analysing of her repressions she reacted to the treatment with great excitement, which gradually wore away by the completion of her cure.

An interesting item : *The struma decreased by three cm. without any local treatment.* That is a fact often observed. The psyche influences the inner secretion. *There are also psychic hormones !* Disturbances of the inner secretions are often originated and relieved by psychic forces.

In this case of anxiety hysteria we also find the characteristic phantasy of the gigantic phallus, the tendency to perversion, the thoughts of the death of someone near to her. Here, too, the unconscious urged her to sin and crime while the conscious mind, summoning all available energy, struggled to overcome these wild impulses. . . . .

[1] Her husband's ejaculatio præcox was a proof that they did not fit in together and that he did not love her. (Cp. Vol. IV. The important chapters: " Psychologie der Ejaculatia Preacose.")

CHAPTER XX

A CASE OF TOPOPHOBIA

NO. III.—Mrs. F. K., aged thirty, of healthy parents, came to me for treatment of "agoraphobia." About ten years previously she had begun to have attacks of anxiety, at first infrequently, in bed at night, and then gradually increasing. One day while crossing a square she had a violent anxiety feeling. Now she was so badly tormented by anxiety that she could not walk a step by herself. She always had to have a companion with her. If she saw a number of people at once she also grew afraid. She therefore never went to a theatre. Shopping was especially painful to her. If she entered a shop she was attacked by such violent anxiety that she could hardly utter the most necessary words. Even when her husband went with her she did not dare to go for a longer walk. Every year her freedom to move diminished. She was now limited to a few roads through which she could pass, accompanied by her companion, her sister, or her husband. Every attempt to go beyond these roads failed. She absolutely could not cross a square. She never went for an excursion or to a theatre or concert. Before her malady had become so bad she had undergone water cures in Gräfenberg, Kaltenleutgeben, Sulz, Purkersdorf, without any success whatever. Massage, electric treatments, bromide, opium, arsenic, a fattening cure, had all been unavailing.

I undertook psychotherapeutic treatment and first got her to tell me the history of her illness. This she did very inadequately ; the patient hardly remembered any important details. Of her childhood she could only relate a few general incidents of an unessential nature. Her resistance to the treatment was extremely great. When she was to impart her ideas to me, she had none. In answer to the enquiry as to her sex life, I learned that she had practised coitus interruptus for about ten years. During recent years she had been almost entirely anæsthetic. She seldom had any kind of feeling during intercourse. She was altogether, she informed me, of a " *cold* " nature and was glad when her husband left her alone.

This treatment lasted a week without our approaching a step nearer to an elucidation of this phobia. She was obstinately silent and always replied to my enquiries : " Nothing at all occurs to me. What am I to say ? You already know everything. All that I had to tell I have told you." Up to the time of her marriage she was apparently in complete ignorance regarding sexual matters ; she had never masturbated and never loved anybody but her husband.

A week later she brought me a dream. There was great resistance with the interpretation and I was frequently obliged to use the association method instead of the. usual one of relying upon her own ideas. I was successful in breaking a part of her resistance through the first dream analysis. She then brought me a new one almost daily, so that I was hardly able to interpret all the dreams in every detail.[1] But in spite of this I was able, with the help of dreams, to penetrate to the core of the phobia and to procure her a striking improvement and relief even during the treatment. Let us therefore take the dream analyses in the order in which they were brought before us.

First Dream :—" *I was at a party and was not quite well, so that I was unable to dance. It was really a social gathering and after that they danced. Later on my two children came in and also danced.*"

The party reminded her of her wedding. She had her period on the day of the wedding and could not take part in the dancing. Her husband, too, was unwell on the evening of the wedding. She therefore stopped a few days longer with her mother, before she was given to her husband for—the dance. (Later on my two children came in.) That meant that the result of this love-dance was the birth of the two children. Dancing was used in this dream for coitus. In this sense the first part of the dream would be intelligible. Translated from the language of symbols it ran as follows (" Kränzchen "—wreath[2]—was chosen with reference to the bridal wreath) : I was unwell at my wedding and there could be no sexual union with my husband. It was a harmless intercourse, coitus only took place later. The result was my two children.

It must be admitted that the dream picture of the two children dancing still remained a puzzle. The puzzle is easily solved when one has, after many dream analyses, acquired the knowledge that in dreams children (" the little one "), are genital symbols. The " little one " (masc.)—(so called in the vernacular) very often means the penis, as also does the " boy " ; the " little one " (fem.), the " daughter," means the vagina. It is a fact that these two expressions proved to be the issue of a long string of associations. The phrase, " the children also danced," refers to the claim made

---

[1] This is one of the forms by which inner resistances reveal themselves. Through the over-production of dream pictures, a thorough analysis that should penetrate to the innermost depths is rendered impossible. It is, however, not at all necessary to follow up a dream analysis to the end. The patients bring new dreams that treat of the undischarged material. (Cp. *Freud*, " Die Traumdeutung in der Psychoanalyse." Zentralblatt für Psychoanalyse. Bd. II. H. 3).

[2] Also meaning small " party " or " gathering."

on the genitals during coitus (come-in =come out). Besides this, two ideas arose in her mind concerning her children. Her boy of eleven years—he slept in his parents' room—had erections and suffered from sleeplessness. A few weeks previously he had asked her : "Mother, what shall I do ? My little one stands up so high." The daughter tended to masturbate. The patient worried a great deal about her boy's erections. She seemed to be forcibly suppressing incestuous thoughts. She was jealous. A few days before she had come upon the boy as he was kissing his governess's bare arm several times in succession. She took a stick and whipped him. Obviously the educational intention was supported by jealousy.

The dream was still, however, distinctly overdetermined. When a girl she was at a party that proved to be of great significance to her. She there got to know a young man who made such an impression on her that she fell in love with him. They often arranged rendezvous and used to meet by chance, especially when she went to market shopping. The parents got wind of their attachment and did all in their power to prevent any further meeting. Two years later her mother introduced her present husband to her, whom she married as an obedient daughter according to the wish of her parents, but without love.

But the dream also revealed a further fact. For many years her husband had practised coitus interruptus and this was injurious to her. This fact was expressed thus : *She was not quite well and could not dance.* The dance in question was also not after her own heart. She would have liked longer intercourse before coitus, a kind of courtship. But her husband conducted his conjugal duties like a business transaction. This wish was fulfilled in her dream. *There was intercourse first and the dancing began after that.* Her dream revealed moreover, one of her strongest perversions : her tendency to exhibitionism. And that by means of an inversion of the facts, which so often occurs in dreams. "After that my two children came in" means : Before that the two children came out, and refers to the uncovering of the genitals. The patient emphatically denied this last part of the interpretation. She had never had an idea of that sort and in any case never thought of sexual matters. She was not like other women who liked hearing indecent jokes, etc.

The following day she brought me a second dream, and said : "Now you will not be able to find anything insidious in this dream. This is a *harmless* dream. I wonder what explanation you will find for it."

This "harmless" dream was as follows :—"*I was shopping with my mother in the square. I bought apples and oranges. There was also a packet of sugar in the bag. The woman said I should not buy so much as the bag was already full, the sugar might fall out, somebody might throw a lighted match on it and the sugar would burn. She asked if the bag was not torn.   I also wanted to buy cauliflower, but there was no more room in the bag."*

Afterwards, while we were reading the dream through again, she thought of some more : " *A policeman stood next to us.   The woman said to me :* ' *The policeman will report you if he sees that you carry your bag so wide open and buy so much."*

These after thoughts to dreams generally contain the most important facts.   This dieam seemed to me of importance because she told me that she had had an *anxiety feeling* in that square, fearing that the policeman would really lock her up.   Only then did she wake up, with palpitations and bathed in perspiration. The patient had, moreover, admitted to attacks of anxiety while shopping.   It was therefore probable that this dream would provide an explanation concerning the agoraphobia and that part of the phobia which had to do with shopping.   But after the interpretation of the first dream the patient was not to be persuaded to tell me any of her thoughts concerning this one.   She repeatedly said : " I can think of nothing," so that I was forced to interpret the dream by means of a trick, which is, however, only permissible after much practice.   Through the experience of previous analyses I knew that apples, oranges, matches, cauliflower, were very often used as male sexual symbols, while sugar (sexual sweets), and especially bag, represent pronounced female symbols.   In the dream the question arose as to whether the bag was not torn. I asked at random : " Have you not had a ruptured perinæum ? "

" That is so," assented the patient : " they put eight stitches in me, and now I am to have another operation."

" So now you see what the torn bag means."

All opposition was then happily overcome.   One idea after another occurred to her and the interpretation was no very difficult matter.   The first portion of the dream lead back to Graz ; here the scene was laid where, as a girl, she used to go shopping and where she met her lover.   Although in reality she used to do this secretly and *alone*, in her dream *her mother* accompanied her on the shopping expedition.   The mother, who had prevented her marriage with her lover, was now present at the sexual incident. In her first sentence she annulled the whole of her marriage.   " *I bought apples and oranges,*" referring thereby to the male sexual organs.   " *There was also a packet of sugar in the bag.*"   Her husband was continually telling her that she was sweet and tasted nice.   " *The woman said I ought not to buy so much, as the bag was already full* " ; this meant that her bag was already bestowed, she was already possessed by her husband, and had no longer any right to make purchases in the love-market.   And then anxiety made its appearance and we can conceive on what her anxiety is centred.   " *The sugar may fall out, someone may throw a lighted match on it and it may be burned.*"   She was afraid of catching fire. She was worried about the ruptured perinæum.   She wanted to buy a cauliflower (the most frequent symbol for a very large penis), but there was no more room in the bag. On the one hand a wish for a very narrow little virginal vagina which despite the torn bag will not hold a cauliflower, is fulfilled, but associated therewith is a regret that the bag is occupied by other inferior purchases so that there is no room for the cauliflower.

The most essential factor for the comprehension of the whole of her anxiety is found in the sequel. She imagined her own husband as a " watchman," and, as a matter of fact, one might have guessed that before. The watchman is often the symbol for the wife or husband in dreams, is, in short, the one whose business it is to watch over the faithfulness of the other. (Watchman may also mean, among other things, fear of a law-suit, or it may represent the symbol of " consciousness " as guardian of the moral ego). In this case, watchman signifies " husband," and, when interpreted means as if the woman of whom she wished to make her purchases (her lover) were to say : " Your husband will have you locked up when he finds out how shameless you are and that you are carrying on with other men." (*When he sees that you are carrying your bag so wide open and buying so much.*)

This dream accounts for her anxiety thus : She was unhappy in her marriage and sexually unsatisfied. She yearned to commit a sin, to meet with a large penis (cauliflower) and enjoy love to the full. But she was afraid of being found out by her husband. On the other hand, the dream reveals her strong tendency to exhibitionism : she carries her bag open to market despite the fact that it is torn.

Her dread of going out alone is, to a certain extent, justified by this dream. She had indeed some cause to be afraid of herself.

The third dream appeared equally harmless and unimportant to the patient. It was this :—" *Opposite to us there is a greengrocer's.*[1] *I went to her to buy a cauliflower, and met there a woman of my acquaintance who was also buying a cauliflower. It was too dear for me, but the greengrocer took off twopence and so I bought it after all.*"

The acquaintance, a neighbour of hers, had a very bad reputation. She was said to have not only one liaison but several. The greengrocer who lived opposite was my unworthy self. I live diagonally opposite, as the crow flies. It was curious why I should have been represented as a greengrocer. She then remembered that the Mayor, Dr. Lueger, had once said he preferred herbalist-women to doctors as they understood more about medicine. The phenomenon of transference discovered by *Freud* had begun to operate, with a resistance to it at the same time. The patient began to occupy herself with my personality ; the increasing regard and confidence struggled with unconscious resistance. This trans-

[1] In Vienna vegetables and medicinal herbs are sold in the same shop, generally by old women.

ference is absolutely essential for the completion of the cure. To put it frankly : the patient falls in love with the doctor who is treating her. But he must know how to inform her opportunely of the fact that this transference is a phenomenon intrinsic to every cure and that this love is not " real " but merely a resistance phenomenon ; failing such information the cure could not be completed. In this dream she begins an intrigue with me. Her doubts as to whether I was the sort of man to enter into relations with her were removed when she saw the ill-reputed neighbour with me. If I could have anything to do with that woman, I should also be available for her. " *It was too dear for me* " referred to the great expense of the cure. I shall have to make a reduction otherwise she could not buy any cauliflower from me. " *She then took off twopence,*" referred to a reminiscence. As a little girl she used daily to meet a handsome old man on her way to school, and asked him every time, " for fun," what time it was. Once he gave her twopence, and said : " You are a pretty girl." She also remembered once seeing him urinate, when she was especially struck with the size of his penis. " *She then took off twopence so I bought it after all,*" meant : If I were like that handsome gentleman who had given her twopence she would purchase of me after all. This dream was really a declaration of love, with which was associated some consideration as to the cost of the cure, as I informed her. She wanted to pay with love. She wanted to give herself to me, and naturally expected me in return to renounce all claims to a fee. She wanted to be cured " physically," not " psychically."

At the next consultation already she brought me a dream in which the play of her phantasy on myself was apparent in a somewhat disguised form.

" *I was at a doctor's and was about to leave. As I was putting on my clothes I found that I had in my hand a piece of paper with a liquid glue on it. I wanted at first to take it home with me, but I was afraid of dirtying myself, and looked round to see where I could throw it. At last I threw it in the stove, dropping some on to the floor and carpet. I also made my hands sticky. I saw an open wash-stand and went to it to wash my hands. But it was difficult to get off with soap. There was a towel hanging on the wash stand.*"

Of course the doctor was myself. During the treatment she lay on a sofa and when the hour was over she had to get up. But she dreamed of a different termination. " I was at a doctor's and was about to leave. But when I was putting on my clothes (which should be reversed to " taking them off ") I found a paper with a liquid glue on it in my hand." She described the glue : It was on a circular piece of paper exactly in the centre. " I wanted at first to take it home, but was afraid of soiling myself " concealed an important component of her anxiety. The liquid glue was semen. It was a question of coitus. But she was afraid of soiling her honour. Although in the first dream she was afraid

of the watchman and her anxiety, translated into fear, reads :
My husband might find it out, the second constituent of her anxiety
was formed from ethical inhibitions : *She was afraid of soiling
herself.* This was a moral stain which could not be cleansed with
soap. " Stove " is a frequent symbol for vagina. Naturally the
stove was the place for the semen. All the rest referred to reminiscences of intimate domestic scenes. Her husband had on one
occasion soiled the carpet with semen during coitus interruptus,
in the day-time. He was accustomed to wash his hands after
coitus. She had seen the towel hanging on my wash stand the
day before. She had therefore transferred the whole episode to
my house.

Fifth dream :—" *I was at the second-hand market with my mother,
and wanted to buy some bread and a children's bath there. I saw,
not far from there, a smoked-meat shop. Mother went there to get
some cut sausage. The shop-woman said that her eldest daughter
played the piano and was going to take part in a concert.*

" *Mother replied that her daughter had also played at a concert
and was very much applauded. Mother sent me to buy the bath alone,
but on the way I was seized with anxiety and went back to the shop.*

" *Sequel.—Mother said to the shop-woman : ' Do not give me such
small pieces. You will cut your finger.' *"

This dream is significant for two reasons : it is an anxiety dream
revealing her anxiety to us, and secondly it holds her husband
up to ridicule. The first sentence : " Bread and a children's bath,"
signifies what marriage provides for her. Her husband was embittered, found no more pleasure in life, and already belonged to
the category of " old iron " (second-hand market). The mother
likewise reproaches the husband for his sexual abstemiousness ;
cut sausage for circumcised penis. The pieces are too small for
the wife. We shall see presently that she again makes fun of the
smallness of her husband's penis. The scene at the concert at
which she is so much applauded is her bridal night. In this dream
her mother gives her the right to be unfaithful to her husband,
as much as to say : If your husband neglects you to such a degree
and does not satisfy you, you have the right to seek another man
without your mother. " *Mother sent me to buy the bath alone.*"
Then the anxiety returns and she goes back to the shop, i.e., to
that man who, as revealed in the first dream, puts the whole thing
on too business-like a footing. These are only a few significant
passages in the dream.

Sixth dream :—" *Mrs. Angel, her little girl, my sister and I were
going for a walk. There was a gentleman with Mrs. Angel who gave
her violets. I wanted to have my boa renovated but it was not worth
it. The furrier asked too much, so I preferred to buy a new one.
I liked Mrs. Angel's boa. It was in the latest fashion and suited
me very well. I asked the price of it. She said ' Thirty-five gulden.'
We came to an open pit, which had boards laid across it to step on.*

I went first. A man helped me so that I should not fall. When I was across I saw that Mrs. Angel and my sister were already there. But they had both made themselves dirty. Mrs. Angel's little girl kept hiding." This dream also contains important references to myself. Mrs. Angel, a widow, stands for my wife. The fact that she had turned my wife into an angel signifies in the language of dreams that she consigned her to death.[1] She also converted her rival and her own sister into bad women. *" They had both made themselves dirty."* Thus a homosexual tendency makes its first appearance. She thinks of Mrs. Angel's child. The significance is apparent from the earlier dreams. The furrier is myself. The treatment is too expensive for her. She wanted Mrs. Angel's boa. The price of thirty-five gulden has several interpretations. She had up to then paid me 350 gulden—10 × 35). Her old boa had cost thirty-five gulden too. Her parents had been married for thirty-five years, and in the last sanatorium to which her thoughts turn when she feels dissatisfied with the treatment, she occupied Room 35. The part of Mrs. Angel's companion is played by her own husband.[2] It is as if she wanted to make an exchange with my wife. She gives her husband away, but demands in exchange me and the boa. The word " boa " produces the following association : wide walls above, narrow walls below ; well ; boa constrictor ; giant strength ; embrace ; suffocation (!) The open pit refers to her bag.

It afterwards occurs to her that two workmen were standing there shovelling earth into the pit. The earth was of a grey-greenish colour. The word " workmen " brings to her mind a *baker* and a *greengrocer.* The baker who provides the rolls and family bread, is not very prepossessing (her husband). The greengrocer, a rough, very powerful fellow (myself). She had therefore, in her dream, entrusted two men with the fulfilment of her desires (filling in the open pit !) " Boards " is a frequent symbol for woman. " The man helped me so that I should not fall," is the kernel of the dream. This is her husband, who is guarding her against sin. And she did not soil herself, whereas Mrs. Angel and her sister made themselves dirty, whereby Mrs. Angel evinced all those vices which I pointed out to her in the second dream. She revenges herself on my interpretation by disparaging my wife.

The various death symbols are transparent. A grave is being dug. To whom do her death wishes apply ? Firstly to her husband, then to her own children and all rivals. (My wife, her sister, etc.). She disposes of all obstacles in order to obtain a new boa (snake as phallic symbol).

Seventh dream.—" *An ugly old woman, of whom I once bought some jam, came to see me. My husband would not allow me to buy*

---

[1] Compare the chapter on " Todessymbolik " (Die Sprache des Traumes).

[2] Let her husband go and join the angels, i.e., die.

anything from her and called out from his room : ' *She is very dishonest and cunning and you are not to buy anything from her.*' *I sent her to a lady of my acquaintance and said to her that she will buy of her. She presented me with a photograph, wherein three people and herself are depicted. On the picture she was wearing a Girardi hat and asked me how it suited her. As she was leaving she said :* ' *I have given you the photo because, after Mrs. Angel, I like you best.*' "

A most transparent dream showing every evidence of transference. Woman, old, little, ugly, may, by inversion, be recognised as a young man, tall and handsome, with which attributes my patient has invested my person in her dream. The dream at all events suggests that she had already bought sweets from me. The husband is again represented as an obstacle, drawing her attention to my cunning and dishonesty, and warning her not to buy anything from me. He had, indeed, already at the outset, expressed his opposition to the cure and complained of the high fees. She had seen in my waiting room the photographs of the three people in which I also appear. It is my family. Finally, I make her a direct declaration of love by telling her that after my wife (angel) I love her best. The Girardi hat has its special significance. It produces the following associations in her mind : straw hat ; easily inflammable ; stiff hat ; band ; fish ; letter case ; condom (she had found a condom in her husband's letter case which had made her very uneasy ; was he being unfaithful to her ?) The condom had looked so funny—like a Girardi hat.[1] Her thoughts therefore are already concerned with the means I shall employ to prevent our union being blessed with children.

At this stage it is of the utmost importance emphatically to decline the transference, while at the same time retaining the dependance until the patient is past the resistance stage of the cure.

The eighth dream already shows that I have partially checked the transference.

" *I went with my sister to the theatre. Our parents were there too, but were sitting apart from us. There also was an aunt of ours sitting by herself. We were looking for our box and had to go down some dark steps and could see nothing. Then we went down to the box-office and asked the clerk to give us better places. The box was small and dark. The booking-clerk was wearing a fur cap, a long black cloak and had a large moustache. I told my aunt contemptuously that my mother-in-law had given me sardines to eat.*"

The interpretation of the symbol " Box " as female genitals is met with repeatedly in *Freud's* " Interpretation of Dreams." The beginning of the dream is of special importance. " My sister and I went to the theatre." Translated this reads : Something

---

[1] Cp. *Freud* " Nachträge-zur-Traumdeutung," I. The hat as symbol for the man (the male genitals). Zentralblatt für Psychoanalyse, I. Jahrg. H. 5/6. S 187.

happened between my brother and myself when we were children. We did the same as our parents did (my parents were there too). " There was also an aunt of ours sitting by herself," referring to a reminiscence of an aunt who had divorced her husband, because he had got up to various tricks. " *We went down dark steps to look for our box*," obviously the most important infantile reminiscence. With the word "box" she associates: arbour; milk-market; forest; strawberries; brooch; box (receptacle). She has a dim remembrance of "playing" with her brother on the dark steps which lead from the office to their house. They used to play at "Fathers and Mothers." The dream also fulfils a wish in connection with the torn bag. For the "box is dark and small." The box-office official in the fur cape with a long black cloak, etc., is a combination of a number of young people, who have courted her.[1] The most important part of the dream is in the last sentence. She had received sardines from her mother-in-law. "Sardines" bring to her mind: Fish; headless; spoiled; rancid; pickled. Now in dreams, fish is a symbol the main feature of which is the tail. She makes fun of her husband in the presence of her aunt who is divorced. She also had good cause for divorcing her husband for he was a fish without a head. A headless man who is difficult to digest. This dream also contains a most ingenious reference to the limited potency of her own husband, to his small penis. In this dream there appears for the first time an indication of incestuous thoughts connected with the brother, which we shall meet with again later on and which is obviously the central motive in the hysteria. The most important experience of childhood, of great traumatic significance and subject to endless variations through hysterical phantasies, had undoubtedly taken place between her and her brother.[2]

The next is a very amusing dream :—" *I went over to the green-grocer-woman to buy apples. There was a case with two partitions, on one side good apples, and on the other inferior ones. At first I wanted to buy a quarter kilo of the good apples and then half a kilo. My sister helped me to select them. I wanted to get some more apples out of the case. There were two people sitting on it. I managed with difficulty to get a few more apples out. I requested the people to get up.*"

In the light of the foregoing interpretations this is easy to deal with. I asked if her husband had ₍any mal-formation. She acknowledged that one of the testicles was larger than the other. She thought this was the normal condition. This accounts for

---

[1] Cap stands for male genital, whiskers for crines pubis; the stair is a coitus symbol. See *Freud*, " Die zukünftigen Chancen der Psycho-analytischen Therapie." (Zentralblatt für Psycho-analyse, I. Jahrg. H. ½).

[2] In contrast to her husband who was a circumcised Jew (Fish without a head !) the box office clerk had a long black *mantle*, which often signifies foreskin. The mantle is also a frequent symbol for father.

her having found good apples on one side of the box, and inferior ones on the other. There proved to be fuı ther connections from the association : " Better half." The brother again plays a part therein. The two people who were sitting on the box are identical with the two workmen who were shovelling earth in the pit. The last sentence is very amusing : " I requested the people to get up." A disguise for the difficulty experienced by her husband in producing an erection. The quarter and half kilos signifies the lesser and greater weight ; quarter, of course, refers to domestic matters. The following associations occur to her : Light ; cabbage ; economical kitchener (a jibe at her husband) ; brushes ; soap ; umbrella ; spinach ; towel ; wash stand ; nursery, and lastly, husband : and half kilo reminds her of pudding ; raw meat ; sugar ; blouse (which she tore yesterday) ; letter (received yesterday from her brother), and then brother. In this dream her husband and I are contrasted with the brother, a comparison which is, of course, to our disadvantage.[1]

Tenth dream :—" *Went with my sister and other people to a chapel on a mountain. We remained behind on the way and lost the others. It was dark, and we lit a candle. We saw another candlestick with a candle and appropriated it in case ours should not last out. We were already very high up at the altitude of Stephen's tower. I wanted to turn back, but my sister urged me to go on. At last we saw the chapel —illuminated, the bishop in a long white cloak and the congregation. Grown up people as well as children in the same costumes.*"

Very easy to interpret. And of great importance, as she remembered that when she came to the place at which she wanted to turn back she was seized with violent anxiety. Chapel = vagina. The sister is the brother. Reminiscence of an excursion. The lit candle is a very common symbol for penis in erection. In the dream she has two candles at her disposal. Always one in reserve in case the other should not hold out. She has got as high as the Stephen's Tower. (Her brother is a great climber !) The most important item is : " *I wanted to turn back.*" But the brother urged her to go further. The bishop in a long white mantle[2] and the children and grown-ups in the same costumes : exhibitionist thoughts. Symbolic representation of coitus with a condom. Phantasy of a scene between herself and her brother, besides whom she has one of his friends in reserve. When they were children both boys played with her and touched her. She suddenly remembers that quite clearly the friend's name was Stephen. She does not think that it came to more than a mere touching.

Eleventh dream :—" *My sister and I were going for a walk. Her*

[1] Also homosexual tendencies and death thoughts (case = coffin). She wanted to bring the dead to life : the dead father and the dead brother !

[2] The white mantle appears here in explanation of the black mantle in the eighth dream, and refers to the father. The " *extinguished candle* " a symbol for the dead father.

little girl was at the gate. Her governess came to fetch her and told her to say goodbye. The child did so, ran a second time after us for fun, and stopped at a field near the house. There I saw a cart, the driver engaged in harnessing the horse. There was a second horse standing there, unharnessed. I also saw a bull in the field. The horse ran about in front of the bull, which became enraged, and in the second round it struck the child with its horns. I saw the child fall, and wanted to run for safety to a lavatory in the vicinity, but I did not like to leave the child alone there. No one dared approach."

" My sister and I were going for a walk," infantile reminiscence of an occurrence with her brother. " Her little girl was at the gate " : the penis at the gate of the trousers. " The governess came to fetch her " : the brother was to marry. All sexual phantasies. The bull is the symbol for generative power. Lastly, coitus phantasy : bull and the " little one." Distinct recollection of masturbation in a lavatory, and of scenes in which the brother played a part. " Nobody dared approach " refers to her anxiety. Her anxiety in this dream is the desire for a bull who could thrust his horns in her stomach. The lavatory near the child is the anus. " Nobody dared approach " : the regret that the anus is not being used. And moreover the regret that no one dares approach her. The second perversion in her phantasy life.

Twelfth dream :—A very important dream, for it reveals her pronounced tendency towards perversions.

" I went for an excursion to a castle with some people. There was a large lake in the vicinity. On the way I found some mushrooms, Johannis-bread and chocolate. When we got there my cousin sang a song. My son knew it and sang too. On the way home I said that he was learning French. I also saw a horse, a temple, and a judge."

After thought :—" *The judge had condemned two women but acquitted me.*"

The analysis was effected with difficulty and great opposition was encountered. " Mushrooms " suggested to the patient : Many people have eaten mushrooms.

" What sort of mushrooms ? " I asked.

She replied : " *Herren*pilze, *Stein*pilze " (boleti).

" Johannis bread " (St. John's bread) was associated with a variety of things : they used to be very fond of it as children ; they had it in the " shop." At the last sea-side resort she had seen " St. John's fire " (" looked very pretty in the dark.") One of her acquaintances, whom she disliked, was called Joan. Joan's husband was very congenial to her, she liked him very much, a charming, blonde man. Her husband was a great competitor of his in business. " Chocolate " suggested : I never refuse it ; like it very much ; put it in my mouth and suck it. Further : Piano playing ; larder ; violin ; bow ; buffet ; cup ; letter.

Let us interpret the first part of the dream. The castle near which is a great lake (with the association : Tonight a castle will be imperrilled) symbolises the genitals in the region of the bladder. Mushrooms, *St. John's bread*, chocolate, are symbols for the penis. She hates Joan and gets her revenge in two ways : Her husband deprives her of her bread through competition and she takes posession of the desirable stranger's penis. She thus eats Joan's bread in two senses. The manner of the eating is revealed in the next sentence : the French manner. The son is learning French—it is a question of French love (fellatio). The song that the cousin sang has the refrain : " Tu ne tombes pas " (You will not fall). She had an important experience with this cousin. He went for a walk with her over a field, where they met a man who had his trousers wide open, who frightened them *with the sight of a gigantic penis.* The complete interpretation of this dream would, of course, fill a small volume. The subsequent associations are important : horse, temple and judge. Horse as symbol for the great penis ; temple for vagina ; with " judge " she associates : several people eat mushrooms ; " two were convicted " (two women who were separated from their husbands). " I was acquitted." The whole unbridled sexual phantasy of the patient is expressed in this dream. She practises fellatio, a perversion which is also indicated in later dreams, but is nevertheless acquitted. It was the first sexual dream in which she experienced no anxiety. And in the day time as well she felt somewhat more relieved. She was able to come to me and to go to the baths unattended. The prospects of a favourable termination of the cure were excellent.

But there was a sudden tremendous upheaval from without. Her brother appeared in Vienna for the purpose of meeting a girl who had been " recommended " to him. The old love was obviously reawakened ; she became greatly excited, and her condition began to grow worse again. She brought me dreams in which the phantastic variations of the sexual theme were repeated. After a few days there emerged, under conditions of great anxiety, the dream of her husband's death. Infantile reminiscences of the brother played an important part. The husband came daily to enquire when the treatment would be finished. The expense (to which he had at first made no objection) was too heavy for him.

She came too late to the appointment every day, which augured badly for the continuation of the treatment. In the meanwhile she brought me an interesting dream.

Thirteenth dream :—" *My sister was getting a new maid servant. We went to make enquiries, taking a book with us. On the steps we saw some more people and hurried so that they should not be before us. The woman looked in the book and said that this girl only spoke Bohemian and French. She did not praise the girl, but in reply to our questions said she did her work well. The woman also kept a Registry Office and we asked her if she could not provide us with a suitable girl ; she said she could if we could wait, but she hadn't anyone that day ; my sister said she would engage this girl. Near the house I saw the baths, we were there, and suddenly we heard from the house where we had just made the enquiries, the children weeping bitterly, and father and mother quarrelling. In passing we saw an old woman crying at the window. The attendant at the baths said that information ought to be given."*

A very complicated dream. It deals with the brother, for whom a wife is to be found. Innumerable phantasies in connection with a dentist, alleged to be notorious for his potency. The most important part is the reproduction of a coitus scene between the parents, overheard : the children were crying, the parents were quarrelling and scuffling. Old woman = young man. Give information : reminiscences of a tale told her by a friend, who had confided to her the secrets of her parents' married life. Further recollections of a maid who had told her everything and frequently masturbated with her.

It is thus clearly manifest how sexual symbolism pervades the small cares of everyday life. " Changing a servant " is an important question for a married woman. In this dream the maid servant is the feminine creature who renders sexual service to the brother. This was the part she herself used to play in her youth. This is the part she wants to play once more. " She does her work well " (" She can play at concerts "). She can make love in the Bohemian way (as the maid used to call coitus in anum) and in the French way. The dream fulfils her desire. The brother engages her as his servant. (" My sister said she would engage this girl.") The " book in the dream " deserves special mention. It is the typical prostitute dream—dreamt even by the most respectable women. In order to be respectable in the daytime, they become prostitutes in their dreams. She is therefore a prostitute who possesses a " book." The scene on the steps is repeated in other dreams. There the most important event in her youth took place. She does not yet remember that the boys did more to her than she at first admitted.

The analysis was approaching a critical point. The scuffling parents (Scuffle = infantile impression of a marital scene) provide her with the image which she reproduced when playing " mothers and fathers."

The next dream is much more important.

Fourteenth dream :—" *I went to meet my husband with my little one. On the way I saw a great black bird in the air. I said it was a bird of prey, and explained it to the child. It came nearer to our heads. I gave it a push and it flew up in the air.*"

In her dream she was surprised that the bird flew up in the air so easily. The obvious sexual interpretation, i.e., an erection[1]

[1] Interesting facts about the " Bird " as phallic symbol are found in *A. Maeder's* " Essai d'interpretation de quelques rêves "—Archives de Psychologie, Tome IV, Nr. 24).

corresponds also with the interpretation " the little one " as vagina. It is a question of the phantasy of a gigantic penis, easily elevated, which she encounters before her husband appears. She goes to meet her husband and this happens on the way. But the bird has still another significance. It is the Death-bird.[1] During the evening, before she went to bed, she had been speaking about the death of her friend's husband. Her friend could not get over her husband's death. But the matter seems much easier to her in her dream. The bird ascends with ease. The death thoughts are therefore directed on her own husband. She feels as if she would rather die than go on living thus.

The fact that the bird approaches their heads is a displacement from below, above.[2]

We observe in this case therefore the remarkable coincidence of several factors : coitus interruptus, which releases the anxiety neurosis ; a severe psychic conflict, leading to repression and hysteria ; infantile traumas. Her ideas alternate between death thoughts and passionate love of life; as a symbol of life and pleasure-in-life we have the gigantic penis, but, embodied in the last dream is the thought of death. Eros and Thanatos. There are also further associations with infantile scenes, in which she saw an enormous penis, probably prodigiously magnified in her.phantasy. We see here the suppressed inclination towards perversions (fellatio, exhibitionism, coitus in anum). We see homosexual tendencies, which I have not entered into more closely, and we see the incestuous thoughts in connection with her own brother and father, and even with her mother and sister.

After this dream the patient's resistance increased. She could not think of anything. And she brought me no more dreams. After a few days she expressed the wish to visit some relatives, and thus the cure was discontinued before I was in a position to solve finally the riddle of this phobia, and to release all the repressions. Her dread of going out alone, was dread of her own weakness. She was conscious that she might easily be unfaithful to her husband, and thus anxiety played the important rôle of guarding her virtue in the service of domestic morality.

The greatest repressions—as in all cases of this description— were her feelings against her husband. She wanted him, in reality, to die, so that she might regain her freedom. This " unconscious " cruelty of neurotics should not surprise us. We shall find it typical in all cases. It shows how marriage, when it is not the outcome of, love, may favour the formation of a hysteria. It shows, further, that patients endeavour to transfer their fear of death to some

---

[1] Compare the chapter on " Todessymbolik " in my book, " Die Sprache des Traumes."

[2] The much more important death thoughts against her daughter and desires towards the son, I was at that time unable to interpret, and overlooked them.

other person. If somebody is to die, rather let it be the "other one."

The cause of the relapse and the sudden interruption of the cure was the engagement of the brother. The old love broke out afresh, which she would not relinquish at any price. Her anxiety increased again immeasurably. She accordingly found the treatment of no further use to her. The meanness of her husband accomplished the rest. She went away uncured. At that time she lacked the Will to Health.[1]

[1] I saw her again years afterwards. She had distinctly improved, but was still not cured of her phobia. This unsatisfactory result was undoubtedly due to my lack of experience in those days. I was certainly aware of the homosexual feelings for the sister, but I did not sufficiently analyse them. It was one of my *first* analyses. The phantasy of the enormous penis is found in homosexual women, who want to awaken their femininity by means of an excess of virility. They would only yield to a great, powerful man. I did not at that time clearly recognize the "Fight of the Sexes."

CHAPTER XXI

A VOCATIONAL NEUROSIS

N O. 112.—One day there came into my consulting room a
tall, powerful, robust looking man, who complained of
various anxiety affects. He was a Rabbi by profession,
and did a great deal of mental work. Up to six years
previously he had borne the troubles of his vocation easily. But
about that time he experienced a great shock, and immediately
thereafter his illness commenced. One day he halted in the middle
of a sentence and could not proceed. From that moment he was
overcome with feelings of anxious aversion at every public function.
Before every address, even in the case of the smallest public prayer
he had the most painful feeling of anxiety *that he would not be able
to continue, that he would get stuck.* Even when the prayer-book
was lying open before him he would come to a stop in the *middle*
of reading, if only for a moment. Every Saturday he had to preach
a long extempore sermon. At one time this used to be his greatest
pleasure and his greatest pride. But since the shock he trembled
for a whole week beforehand and was continually thinking he
would get stuck.

All kinds of people used to come to him from far and wide to
ask his counsel in difficult matters. He lost his self-confidence
with these people. He often began to *stutter* and stammer, and
halted in the middle of a sentence. When he was alone he could
repeat the longest prayer without hesitation. It was only before
people that the impediment manifested itself. He sought in vain
a remedy for his affliction in Berlin, Vienna, and Paris. He
went to Scheveningen, Homburg, Wiesbaden, Gainfarn, etc. He
had stayed some months in Wörishofen. All in vain! He complained besides of a burning feeling in his arms and legs. This
feeling increased sometimes till it became like an attack of ague.
(Although his temperature was taken frequently it was never
found to be raised). *For three years his left hand and arm had been
entirely numb.*

On objective examination he was found to be organically absolutely healthy. (It must be added, however, that the anamnesia
disclosed the fact that the man, now forty-two years old, had
suffered in his twenty-first year from tuberculosis of the testicle,
which had been cured after a course of Haller baths and Haller
iodine water). There were still traces of this complaint. Objectively, moreover, there was still complete anæsthesia of the left

upper extremity. Needles could be stuck deeply into it without the patient's feeling anything whatever. But other parts of the left side of the body were distinctly affected by a marked hyperæsthesia. The susceptibility to thermic stimuli was entirely arrested in the left extremity, but otherwise normal. Reflexes easily increased.

I recommended the patient to try a psychic cure. The patient, who as already mentioned, had tried all curative methods in vain, agreed willingly to the proposal. It was with some misgiving then that I commenced the treatment.

The difficulties of a psychanalysis were in this case tremendous. The mental sphere of a rabbi, which was entirely strange to me, the gibberish of German and Jewish words with which I was unacquainted, the natural shyness of such a pious man in revealing his unconscious world of thought, combined at first to form almost insurmountable difficulties.

The great success which I nevertheless achieved is due, on the one hand to my own energy, and on the other to the high intelligence of the patient, who was accustomed to mental work, and was able later on more easily to grasp my purpose.

It was necessary first of all to enlighten the patient as to the nature of a psychanalytic cure. Various—one might say—pathogenic ideas were completely buried in his unconscious where they had formed a tangled skein. It was these repressed thoughts which had caused the anxiety affects. These repressed thoughts were also responsible for the numbness of the left hand.

" How can thoughts produce a severe bodily disease ? *How can mental things be transformed into physical ones ?*" asked the astonished patient.

" We do not know yet how this is brought about. But the facts as such are indisputable."

We began the cure. Let me be spared the description of the toilsome roundabout ways by which I arrived at my results. The conversations at our sittings would fill volumes. I will confine myself to the most important events, whereby I shall be obliged to fuse the incidents of several meetings into one description.

The patient was to give me the history of his whole life. There was little of interest therein.

At the age of five he began to study, and married at eighteen.

" Have you masturbated ? "

I was obliged to give the patient a clearer definition of the meaning of masturbation, at which with every sign of indignation, he exclaimed : " *No, I never had anything to do with ' such things.' It was not until the day of my marriage that I learned of the existence of such things* " . . . .

The patient then recounted a number of unimportant incidents. The story of his tuberculosis, his journeys, etc., until he came to the great shock which was alleged to have caused his illness.

He had had a violent quarrel with his elder brother. The latter had inherited the money on the death of the father, while he had received the collection of historic, valuable books. Then the brother returned, after some years, having lost the money, and blusteringly demanded a share of the books. The books had been written by the father's, grandfather's and great grandfather's own hands, family records which went back three hundred years. All the thoughts of his ancestors, who had likewise been rabbis, were recorded in these books. There was a violent scene between the two excited brothers. The Rabbi stood before the book-case and shouted in the greatest agitation : " I will not let the books out of my hands, *rather would I be taken from the books myself.*"

He had subsequently bitterly regretted this last sentence. It had caused him many oppressive hours of remorse, because he regarded it as a sin against God. He feared that God would take him at his word, and *take him away from his books.*

The patient endeavoured therefore to make me understand his agitation, and to explain the severe conflict to me. But I still lacked the underlying motives. A quarrel of this description could not make one ill unless the deeper emotional zones were involved. I therefore let the matter rest for the present. And that was the end of the first sitting. . . . .

The following sittings took place under such extreme resistance on the part of the patient that I repeatedly resolved to discontinue the cure. He had nothing more to tell me, he had finished his confessions. What could he tell me that I did not already know ?

In those difficult days, however, I had a great ally : the work of the unconscious. While he denied all knowledge of sexual deviations from the normal, i.e., masturbation, and professed never to have even *seen* other women, his hesitating mode of expression said : It is not true.

If I had let him go, then I might have maintained, like so many other investigators : " I have thoroughly examined a patient who related to me his anamnesia for fourteen days and could not find a trace of sexual trauma, let alone discover a sexually abnormal life." But I would not be diverted from my conviction, and thought of *Freud's* theory that the art of psycho-therapy consists in ignoring the persistent " No " of the patient with equal persistence. I stuck firmly to my stand-point. There must have been other causes of the disease, which he would not admit for lack of confidence.

" Had he never masturbated ? " " No ! " " Had he never suffered from an excess of sexual phantasy ? " " No ! " " Had nothing else passed between him and his brother besides the dispute about the books ? " " Nothing whatever."

Until the day of his marriage he had lived in complete ignorance of sexual matters. On the marriage night his mother came into his room and gave the young couple the necessary instructions.

Since then he had lived happily and peacefully with his wife and had never—never in his life—had a sinful thought.

How was I to reconcile this information with my pre-conceived notions? It was my *first* important analysis. I already thought of giving up my exertions on behalf of this pious holy man. The first step towards understanding the malady was made through the medium of a dream, which had a double result. Firstly, it won me the patient's confidence, and secondly, it broke his resistance, and at one stroke tore away the veil from his unconscious psychic life.

It was a dream in which there was a good deal about soldiers, who, adopting a curious position, bending backwards, stretched their bayonets forwards towards the enemy and laughed in a strange manner. The leader of these soldiers seized him by the beard and said to him : " Why have you become so proud and will not have anything to do with me ? " I cannot enter into the whole analysis of this dream, it would take too long. It was a homosexual dream, which reproduced a pornographic photograph he had seen, in which a bayonet was planted on the penis. The leader, whom he described more fully to me, was a " condensation " figure formed of his brother, a friend, and a man-servant in the house. The servant, now an old man, had looked after him in his boyhood. I pointed out to him that the dream gave one to surmise that there must have been some kind of sexual relations between this servant, his friend and himself. The patient emphatically denied this, was somewhat offended, and said that we should make no progress by this means ; there was nothing to be gained thereby, the cure did not help him in the least, he felt distinctly worse. He would rather go away.

Nevertheless he appeared the next day at the appointed hour and began : he now realised that denial was of no avail, he would tell me the history of his youth frankly and without reservation.

He was a boy of five or six, when the man-servant alluded to in the dream, came to his bed one night, began to play with his penis and performed fellatio with him. This went on for some time ; he himself had remained passive and done nothing except hold the servant's penis. While saying these words he began to cough violently, became purple in the face, and it was clearly apparent to me that he was not telling the truth, but that he must have gone through a similar process with the servant himself. The servant still lived in the house, and he was still very fond of him, although since his marriage " such things " were, of course, never discussed. His great attachment to the servant is accounted for by the fixation of the first sexual influence. From subsequent analysis it transpired that the servant was frequently rude and impertinent to him, and gave him every cause for dissatisfaction, but that he had not the heart to be severe with him, still less could he give him notice.

This was followed by such an abundant supply of material facts that there was not sufficient time to discuss and deal with them all. He had masturbated himself since his earliest childhood, and practised masturbation with his brother ; it is true that he had never been unfaithful to his wife, but was tormented day and night by the most unbridled phantasies. Everything he saw, heard, read, felt, assumed the shape of sexual pictures, which he could not control or banish, and from which he was unable to escape.

A second fact came to light, namely, that his anger against his brother had a somewhat deeper cause. His brother who was a man of the world, and addicted to women, had paid conspicuous court to his wife ; on one occasion he had surprised them both coming out of the cellar, where they had gone ostensibly to look for something. He could not accuse them of anything definite, and was, in fact, prepared to swear to his wife's fidelity, but he nevertheless reproached his brother severely at the time for having endangered his wife's reputation. But the motivation for his jealousy of his brother went still deeper. The latter, who had married before him, was continually taking him into his wife's bedroom, where he had once shown her to him in a very scanty attire, with the idea of exciting his feelings, and to hold his wife's beauty before his eyes, as much as to say : " Look, all that is my property, while you have nothing." He was accustomed also, in his brother's absence, to stay with his sister-in-law, when he used to play with her, and " have fun," without going to extremities. They were all children in those days. . . . .

Amongst other reminiscences there was one of a seaside resort, where he and his young wife once passed a whole summer. This was the happiest time of his life ; he was always in a state of intense sexual excitement, and felt that he was satisfying his wife, which was otherwise not always the case. The genesis of this potency is easily accounted for. The friend who had played the third part in the condensation of the dream, was again present as the third person, and managed to increase his passion by innuendoes. They used to have wrestling matches in the wife's presence, in which he was the winner because he was the stronger. He could throw his opponent to the ground, place his knee upon his chest, and then let him go home in peace. After these wrestling matches he was always very excited, and had coitus immediately. It is very evident that it was the strongly developed homosexual and sadistic components in his nature, which combined with the heterosexual element to increase his passion to the fullest extent. He confessed as much quite candidly. He was subject to frequent homosexual dreams, altogether of a most singular character, which were all variations of the sexual-perversion theme. Thus I came to learn more and more of his psychic life, and recognised that this man who led such a pious, sequestered life, was in phantasy, the greatest Don Juan, whose phantasies would put even those of a

Marquis de Sade in the shade. Despite these disclosures, however, the riddle of his remarkable neurotic symptoms still remained unsolved, his arm continued to be anæsthetic, his stuttering at prayers was not relieved.

One day he brought me a new dream : "*I was standing in a room that was strangely square, or rather oblong, in construction. I was lying in a bed and there was another bed hanging over it, in which there was a woman.*"

This dream solved the greater part of the neurosis. Two of his most important, ever-recurring phantasies came to the surface in the dream. The room, it was easy to interpret, was a sleeping-carriage of a train. He admitted that he knew of two possibilities, by which he could remain true to the tenets of his religion and yet be unfaithful to his wife. *If he were in a sleeping-carriage* (this is one of his most frequent dreams) *and a woman were lying in the berth above him, and if she were to fall upon him, a situation might then arise which would resemble coitus, of which he could avail himself without having taken an active part in its production. It would, in a measure, be sinning against his will.* The second possibility, which he had also mentioned occasionally (one of his most frequent phantasies), was : "He finds himself in a forest, and is attacked by robbers ; the robber-chief holds a pistol to his breast and says : 'You will either have intercourse with the woman who lies before you, or I shall shoot you' (force majeure !) In this case it would also be a sin against his will, which God would surely pardon, for it was only by committing the sin that he could save his life." The interpretation of this dream simultaneously solved one of his obsessions. He suffered, to a certain extent, from travelling neurosis.

After three months at home he was seized with an oppressive restlessness ; he could not work any longer, and decided to go away somewhere to consult some professor, or visit some celebrated health-resort. He always travelled at night, and always in a *wagon-lit ;* obviously with the secret hope that a charming lady would occupy the berth above and fall down on him. He was in search of the fulfilment of his secret desire : *Pleasure without sin.* This example provides us with a very clear demonstration of the mechanism of an obsession. The distinct wish for a sexual experience is repressed into the unconscious, under the mask of various more easily attainable wishes, such as consultations with professors, visits to friends, to health-resorts, etc. The most important, in fact, the only important point about these wishes, is the journey. He could not endure any health-resort for long, he used to lose patience, and travel further, always as far as possible, always at night, and always in a sleeping-compartment.

The second phantasy of the coitus-compelling robbers was also the cause of a compulsory-like action. He used to walk about in the woods for days when he was staying at a health-resort, always in the hope that force of circumstances might put a speedy end to his innocence. He was a religious man, who took the commandments of his faith very seriously. These two phantasies were compromises between the importunities of impulse and the tenets of his belief. Of course there was a strong touch of homosexuality in both phantasies. For in sleeping-compartments only men lie above men. The revolver, moreover, is a well-known phallic symbol. He anticipated a homosexual assault through a robber who stole his honour.

A further analysis of this dream will afford us a closer insight into the case.

"You saw a lady in your dream? Of whom does this lady remind you? "

" Of no one," he replied. He was silent for nearly half-an-hour.

" Surely some name must occur to you if you pull your thoughts together."

" Absolutely nobody ! "[1]

A few minutes passed, then at last he said : " Ah, now it occurs to me. The lady has exactly the same face as my housekeeper, with whom I lodge in the summer."

" What part does the housekeeper play in your life ? "

" I am not intimately acquainted with her."

" Is she young or old ? "

" She is young, strikingly beautiful, and finely built."

" She is, in a measure then, your ideal, such as you have described to me in our conversation ? And you have had nothing to do with her ? Not even in your phantasies ? "

" Well, now I remember something. There was something in connection with her. According to the laws of my religion it is forbidden to give one's hand to a strange woman, and above all to regard a woman with lustful desire. One morning, when we had just arrived in the country, the housekeeper came to meet me and said : ' I am glad to see you here again, and hope that you will have a pleasant summer.' She then held out her hand to me."

" And you ? "

" I forgot myself and gave her my hand which she pressed warmly. A burning fire seemed to run through my hand, and thence throughout my whole body. I had never experienced anything like it."

" And a short time afterwards you lost all feeling in your hand ? "

The patient made a calculation, and then said : " Yes, that is so. But are the two circumstances necessarily connected ? Nevertheless, you may be right ; I reproached myself severely for what

[1] When one meets, in analysis, with such obstinate resistance on the part of the patient, when no associations are forthcoming, one may safely presume that there is something of importance involved which is being repressed from consciousness, the release of which is combined with the strongest aversion. This feeling of aversion is expressed in the cure by obstinate refusal to answer the doctor's questions.

I had done, and was perpetually haunted with the thought that God would punish me for it. And now I recollect that as my hand became weaker and I lost my strength, I thought the punishment of God had already fallen upon me. The image of that woman still haunts me, however. It is she who is the main feature in my phantasies."

" And whom you hope to find in the sleeping-compartments ? "

" Yes ! Every time I get into a train, I think of this woman, and always hope that, by chance, she may one day share a compartment with me."

When the patient came to me on the following day he was very much brighter. *The anaesthesia of his hand and arm had entirely disappeared.*

The work then progressed rapidly. The patient found boundless relief in being able at last to communicate his secret thoughts unconstrainedly. He did not know a soul to whom he could speak about these things.

His glance was freer, his manner unconstrained. The art of psycho-therapy consists not only in releasing repressions but also in revealing how human it all is. All these neurotics regard themselves as criminals whose outward life is a hypocritical contradiction of their real thoughts. The physician has a great educative work to accomplish ; he must sacrifice part of his personality, in that he confides in the patient, and by making, in a sense, confessions of his own, facilitates confession for the patient. The very fact of converting the individual destiny into a universal one, creates a feeling of indescribable relief.

My patient had a happy time ; he felt increasingly better, and endeavoured himself to rid his unconscious of its repressions. The theme turned on his marriage, in which he was obviously unhappy. His sexuality was not gratified. At first there were only slight indications, then his complaints against his wife increased in volume, until they strengthened into accusations. Compare this with other cases. "Marriage and Neurosis" would form an interesting chapter, with which I must not let myself be tempted to deal fully here. I will merely point out that the majority of neuroses owe their development to unhappy marriages.[1]

The period of transference to my own person had also to be undergone ; he had various erotic dreams, in which I played a great part. The analysis of these dreams lead us a step further into his psychic life. Suddenly it became apparent by an almost dramatic climax that the solution was near at hand. The patient became excessively agitated. He occasionally lost his voice. This is the mental travail which precedes the ejection of a psychic foreign body. The solution surprised even me. After the analysis of a dream, which occupied two hours, I repeatedly came upon an old book in his dream-thoughts, with which his whole mind was obsessed. Curiously enough it was the same book that his brother

[1] Specifically dealt with in Vols. III. and IV.

had demanded from him, which had been the cause of the great quarrel. There was a passage in this book dealing with sexual life. The patient admitted that even as a child passages of this description in the Bible and kindred literature in which erotic matters are mentioned used to excite him, and he used to pursue these questions eagerly. The old book (manuscript) in question, however, contained very significant instructions on the symbolism of erotism. This book had always been a source of immense pleasure to him. I suggested that the conflict with his brother appeared to have a deeper motive. Formerly it had only been a question of old books, but now the conflict was revealed in quite a different light.

His brother was his rival in a two-fold sense. Firstly, he had displayed his wife to him, and had practically challenged him to fall in love with her, which was what actually occurred. On the other hand, the brother had made love to his own wife, in fact, the patient struggled for some time with the suspicion that there was " something " between his brother and his wife. Then, the free brother was a Don Juan, whereas his pious calling required him to be an ascetic. Combined with this was the fact that the brother wanted to rob him of this very book to which he owed so much erotic excitation, upon which his sexual phantasy turned, and which was, in a sense, his first love, as well as robbing him of the other two (wife and sister-in-law). This also explains his remorse at the words : *I will never let the books go out of my hands, rather would I be taken from the books myself.*

The anæsthesia of the left hand was also of double origin. First through contact with the housekeeper, and secondly through his oath (which was of the nature of a curse) never to let the books go out of his hand (the hand with which he had masturbated !). It was almost as if he was to be separated from a lover. " Rather would I be taken from the books myself."

All this was confirmed by the patient. I asked him the meaning of some of the symbols in the book, and he suddenly became greatly agitated. He must confess something which was very painful to him even to think of, which had haunted him for years, and which after much striving, he had succeeded in forgetting long ago. In his great-grandfather's book there was an explanation of the Jewish word for " God " (Adonai), the letters of which stood for sexual symbols. The first letter represented a phase of the sexual act, the second another, the third and fourth, man and wife. There followed then important disclosures concerning his relations with his sister. At this juncture the patient was seized with an attack of cramp, he shook all over and began to stammer, whereas during the whole cure he had spoken fluently. Incestuous thoughts in connection with his mother and sister thus came to light.

The whole neurosis is now explained. In praying he had always halted at the words " *The Lord God.*" He stopped at the moment when he was about to speak the words, because the repressed thoughts brought the four letters which were sexual symbols to the surface, out of the unconscious. As a pious and holy man he wanted to repress these painful thoughts. But the repression was only partially successful. The repressive factors were his religious inhibitions. But the repressed matters powerfully forced their way into the repressive factors. His religious acts became interspersed with a secret sexual symbolism. He came to a standstill—not without an underlying determination—*in the middle of his speech*. He halted always at the " Adonai," because this word reminded him not only of his sinful desires but of his inhibitions. For the God of the Jews is a stern, merciless, punishing God. He feared the punishment of his grievous trespasses ; of his masturbation, his sinful desires which hovered about his sister-in-law and all other beautiful women like ravenous vultures, of the sexual excitement which he experienced when fulfilling his holy duties. And he had other serious misdemeanours on his conscience. He had wished his brother dead, and his own wife as well, that all obstacles might be removed from his path. His whole life was one ceaseless conflict with sin. Sexual phantasies pursued him all day long, they permeated his thoughts, his actions, his feelings. There was no escape from them. They had been converted by repression into driving forces in the unconscious. They were never resolved from the individual into the universal human. He looked upon himself as the most abandoned profligate. He, the pious, holy man, the pride of his parish, the descendant of a celebrated rabbi family, who should be preaching the word of God—was more evil and more abandoned than the worst member of his flock. The quarrel with his brother was one of the determining factors of the secret, fixed affects. His psychic balance could not be regained without external aid. All this I explained to this highly intelligent man—he had already realised it in the course of the treatment.

With the above elucidation this memorable case came to an end. If the psycho-therapist has at last after long striving, found the solution to the problem, his work has been richly rewarded. The feeling is akin to that of all intrepid explorers who ultimately succeed in the conversion of their thoughts into deeds. A surgeon must feel the same after successfully carrying through a serious life-saving operation.

The next day the patient said the prayers in a synagogue without distress and without stopping. He suddenly remembered his domestic obligations, whereas at one time he wished to remain under treatment for months ; he felt an urgent desire to return home. After a few more sittings at which we dealt with one or two non-essential matters, and solved certain compulsion-problems, he returned home.

Five years later he sent his daughter to me for psycho-analytic treatment. Since the " psychic cure " he had been perfectly well, and in every way fit to fulfil the duties of his calling.

CHAPTER XXII

NEUROSIS OF A PRIEST

NO. 113.—Mr. J. B., a Roumanian priest, aged forty-three, of healthy parentage, had been suffering for two years from a form of anxiety which rendered him totally unfit for his profession. It was one of those profession-neuroses similar to the foregoing case, and also described by *Bechtereff* (Zentralblatt für Nervenheilkunde, 1903, in "Ueber krankhafte Angst von professionellem Character, Angst des Sakramentstragens bei Priestern "—" Morbid anxiety in connection with the vocation, anxiety of priests while carrying the Sacrament ") certainly without any psychologic motivation. *Bechtereff* states that he has frequently observed this affliction in priests in Russia of late years, and gives a detailed description of a case whose remarkable anxiety is described by the patient as follows : " While carrying the sacrament I have a feeling as if the stole were falling off my shoulders. Or that the small cloth in which the sacrament is folded might fall to the ground. My hands and feet begin to shake, there is something the matter with my arms and legs." Bechtereff also mentions that in this case the neurasthenic symptoms were not of a very pronounced character, and he cannot give us any information as to the psychogenesis of the anxiety. It is easily recognisable that this is a case of parapathia, and moreover of pronounced anxiety hysteria, in which a careful psychanalysis would most certainly have revealed the fact that " the symptoms are indicative of the sexual life of the patient." The analysis of these cases often proves *Freud's* theory :

" Not only that a large proportion of hysterical symptomatology is directly derived from expressions of sexual excitement, not only that, in neurosis, a number of erogenous zones by the accentuation of infantile characteristics, acquire the significance of genitals ; but the complicated symptoms themselves are revealed as the converted representations of phantasies which have a sexual situation as content. When we have learned to interpret the language of hysteria we can understand that the neurosis is only a manifestation of the repressed sexuality of the patient. We need only understand the sexual function in its right sphere, circumscribed by infantile tendencies. When we have to reckon with a banal emotion as the root of a disease, analysis regularly proves

I*

that the inevitable sexual component of the traumatic occurrence is accountable for the pathogenic effect."[1]

But let us return to our case. The priest in question suffered from a similar form of anxiety as that of the Rabbi in the preceding chapter. He could only speak with difficulty in public. His malady presented a number of painful symptoms, which he described as follows :—

"In a small Roumanian community I perform the functions of a Greek-Oriental second priest. When I took this position twenty-three years ago, I was inspired by the teaching of my first master, who had earnestly enjoined us to perform even the smallest duty with devotion, dignity and piety—that is to say, slowly. I soon came to recognize, however, that the congregation only appreciated this form of worship on ceremonial occasions, and that the practice of it at the week-day services, or even in ceremonies in passages to which little importance is attached, was not to their taste on account of the time that it occupied. Our prefects and other dignitaries who found the frequent services irksome, and who as elders of the church give the sign to the priest to " *hurry the service,*" were opposed to my form of delivery. When one considers in addition to this, that my method occupies so much more time, and so is infinitely more trying than the other, it is not surprising that I feel the necessity of relinquishing it. But I cannot change my skin. This conception of delivery has become as a second nature to me, and I have made a great reputation by it. But as I am a very accommodating person, there are often two opposing forces at war within me as I am preaching. On the one hand is the knowledge *that my way is the only right way, that it comes naturally to me,* or has become a habit (I do not know whether I could easily acquire another method of delivery) *and is necessary to my well-being :* the second force is the desire to spare my listeners the frequent repetition of the long, monotonous, uninteresting recitative by curtailing it. I often delete whole paragraphs therefore where practicable, and just mutter them unobserved in my beard. This would not cause me any uneasiness if my theft were confined to these occasions alone. But when, at the next service, I want to give out the complete passage, I am unable to do so. When I come to the passage I become greatly excited, and to avoid speaking while in such a state of agitation, I relapse into the habit of suppression. This impediment which I see before me often makes me uneasy for the whole service. Should other circumstances be unfavourable, matters are much worse. If, for instance, the church is very hot, or very cold, if I have been angry beforehand, circumstances which have an injurious effect on me in my official capacity, my excitement increases.

[1] This sentence is only (conditionally) accurate up to a certain point. There are severe forms of hysteria without sexual components, i.e., war hysteria and accident neurosis.

" Six years ago when I had to conduct a secondary service, I was troubled beforehand by the thought : Shall I have the patience to conduct this service to which the public is indifferent, but which according to my nature and habit, is necessary ? I performed the office, in great excitement, from beginning to end, and showed myself off thereat in order to avoid negligence[1] in my agitation, and this incident in my excited condition made me feel so ill that my heart's action was reduced almost to nil, and I was obliged to retire after the ceremony and leave the rest to my assistant.

" Eighteen months ago I had to give a lecture to my pupils on the story of Ahasuerus and Esther. This function took me an hour, for my elocutionary powers show to advantage in it. But in consequence of previous mental excitement I was in an ill-humour. I gave the lecture from the *outset* in a state of agitation, and the naturally resultant shortness of breath during the lecture again produced a feeling of nausea. I felt extremely ill, the blood receded from my head, and my heart and pulse almost ceased to beat. Since then I never speak in public without having smelling salts at hand. I am always afraid of being taken ill, and had several similar attacks during services, but was able to hold out by smelling vinegar-ether which I carried with me. I would mention that I experienced a similar attack six years ago while reading the chapter of Deborah.

"The question that I would put to science is this : Why do I not possess that inconsiderateness *which enables one to look with indifference upon the unauthorised desires of a few people and quietly to disregard them*, when I see that I cannot comply with those desires and know, as an artist, that they are altogether unjustifiable ? "

This, then, is the anamnesis in the patient's own words. We at once observe that the alleged motives cannot possibly be the only ones, or the most important ones ; that behind these questions there are obviously concealed questions of a very different nature. The excitement cannot possibly be due to the fact that the elder finds the length of the service irksome to him. Is he more of an artist than a priest ? He regards himself as an artist, because he has been musically well-grounded and possesses a very beautiful voice. We enquired of the patient, therefore, as to further symptoms, and asked him whether he did not attribute his affliction to some particular excitement. He could not remember any particular excitements. But he found his profession depressing and uncongenial. He would like to have attended a lay High School and become a scholar, a professor, doctor or singer. Instead of that he was stuck in a small parish with his talents and his beautiful voice. He attached especial importance to the latter. Under favourable circumstances he might certainly have become a celebrated concert singer, or perhaps even an opera singer. He also found the small discomforts of his calling very depressing. There were passages in the Old and New Testaments and prayers which

[1] Literal translation, *neglige—canal*, see also p. 235.

seemed to him simply ridiculous. The eternal repetition of one and the same prayer formulas, and especially several times on the same day was bound to become burdensome to any thinking man. He considered his anxiety feeling to be due to an impediment in the vocal organs. The lips obviously become stiffer and the tongue loses its pliability as the result of fatigue.

He had begun to masturbate at the age of fourteen, and continued the practice until his marriage. He admitted frankly that he still masturbated occasionally. He was happily married, has a very beautiful wife who had borne him four children. His life history is soon told. It is incredible how little people remember when they are asked to tell the story of their life.

The whole hysterical amnesia betrays itself usually by the colossal omissions in this first statement. It is, in fact, the most important task of the mental physician to fill these gaps, to eliminate the hysterical amnesia. The best means, as I have often shown, is dream analysis. As everything which the patient told me before the first dream was of little importance, I will begin the analysis of this case with the analysis of the first dream. The dream was :

" *I saw my grandfather, who has long been dead, and talked with him about various things. What, I do not know. I believe about ' water closet.' My wife was there too. Then I dreamed that on week-days I perform a long function which I never ought to have had to do and that I was afraid.*" As supplement occurs to him : " *The grandfather did something in the pissoir. He wanted to mend something. In the pissoir there were four mouths and it was to these he wanted to do something.*"

The dream is of great importance because it openly reveals the fear which tortures the patient, of performing on week-days a function to which he was not equal " and which he never ought to have had to perform," and we are justified in hoping that through the analysis of the dream we may arrive at a knowledge of this anxiety. So I asked the patient to state the ideas which come to him in connection with each sentence, regardless of whether he thinks them important or not ; and I learn from him the following facts which I repeat only in the most condensed form. The analysis of this dream lasted about fourteen days and if given in detail would occupy the whole of this book. I therefore give the bare facts without the circumlocutions and evasions.

The dream contains chiefly thoughts which concern the grandfather. Also it contains the following : Our priest had already completed his studies at the grammar school (*gymnasium*), when the grandfather who, because of his wealth had to decide everything, spoke the word—he must go into a training college. At first brought up to be very pious, it had happened to him that he had at his school very free-thinking teachers who made it their business to bring before the children the idea of progress and enlightenment. And so the boy learned to look at all ceremonies which, in his parents' house he had considered something sacred and exalted, in another light. The free spirit fought with clericalism. Following rather necessity than his own impulses, he gave up the study of philosophy and entered a training college. But in later life he greatly regretted that he had not continued the study. He considered himself suited for a higher calling. He thinks that he would have been happier as gymnasium professor or philosopher. In this dream he ventured to tell the truth to his grandfather who in his lifetime had been a great authority for him : That forcibly dragging a man into a calling for which he was unsuitable was simply " swinish." To this refers " I have seen my grandfather who has long been dead and spoke with him about a water-closet." The second part of the dream thoughts goes back to that time when he lived with his grandfather. There he learned masturbation. He does not remember through whom. At that time he often went to the closet so that he could masturbate undisturbed. At that time also a certain homosexual tendency had broken out in him. He went to the baths with his grandfather and was much interested in the men whom he saw there naked, and made comparative studies on the size of the penis. Further there occurs in the dream a little sentence which at first seems less comprehensible : " My wife was there too." He is not satisfied with his wife. She is haughty, proud, does not willingly associate with strangers, and that injures him in his calling. And then she jests at his calling and his piety. Also he tried, solely at the instance of his wife, to doff the clerical robe and for two years to earn his living as an author. At this he did not succeed very well, and was therefore obliged nolens volens to return to the clerical profession. This partly accounts for the end of the dream, " In the pissoir were four mouths and the grandfather wanted to do something to them." The four mouths are his four children, whom he must feed.

He had often said to himself : If the children were not there I could persevere, I could succeed ; but I have four mouths to feed." In this dream the grandfather shows himself willing to set him free from his base situation (pissoir, closet). We shall see later that this dream is over-determined, and that the most important meanings only appear later. But already the suspicion forces itself upon us that the sentence : " My wife was there too " must have some other meaning. He sees his wife in his grandfather's company. That is, he throws his wife to the dead. He wishes his wife to be dead. This thought of the death of the spouse is —as I have repeatedly affirmed—never lacking in any anxiety hysteria that one can analyse and is the basis of that oppressive consciousness of guilt that makes these people so sad and so weary of life. But there must be some motive to make him find the presence of his wife so troublesome. This he denies at first confessing only to defensive thoughts in connection with her affairs ;

¹ Cf. die Todessymbolik in " Die Sprache des Traumes."

but we shall learn later that by this conception of the dream we get near the root of his neurosis. This repressed thought must stand in intimate connection with his anxiety. For immediately afterwards in the dream at a long function on week-days which he never performs, he was seized by a violent anxiety attack. We surmise then that this anxiety dream will betray more of his anxiety and proceed with the analysis. He states that it is only during the daily prayers on week days that he is attacked by violent anxiety, especially towards the close, but that on Sundays and feast-days he is free from this fear. Among his recollections appears one which is of great importance for the analysis of this anxiety. Since he can remember *he has masturbated only on week-days.* He did not do it on feast-days because he did not wish to take any sin upon himself and because after masturbating he always felt rather faint and tired and, as he expressed it, he needed " all his powers." Also he is not able to carry out his functions on week-days without a certain erotic stimulation. On Sunday there are many people, including beautiful women, in the church. He feels as if he speaks and sings only for these. On week-days there are fewer men and one or two old women there. Then he helps himself by picturing to himself a young and beautiful woman. A friend once said to him, " by imagining something pleasant, one drives away anxiety thoughts." That is only a supplementary motive, however, for he has practised this stimulation much longer than he has known the friend. On week-days then the function proceeds thus : It begins with the erotic visualisation of the body of a beautiful woman and proceeds as the picture of a spiritual masturbation. As in coitus, the tempo increases towards the close of the prayer and he has a sense of anxiety because it is a sin. Also the fear of the punishment of God plays a great part in this function. He is a blasphemer ! Besides he has the typical fear of the masturbator that he has shortened his life by it. Very early a book came into his hands which uttered an impressive warning against masturbation and prophesied all sorts of evil consequences, such as loss of memory, paralysis, spinal pains, consumption. Since then he has waged violent war against masturbation and has always been vanquished ; for he masturbates even now, although he is married. After every onanistic act he feels violent remorse and fear, because he has brought himself a step nearer the grave. Now we can understand the sentence : " Then I dreamt that on week-days I had a long function to perform, which I never do, *never ought to have done.*" What he dreams is that he masturbates for the first time. In the dream, it is a function which he never performs.

We have yet to explain the " long function." He has always been accustomed to prolong to the utmost both the coitus and the masturbation. With him every act must last a long time. It must be executed with leisure, gradually improving in order to increase the pleasurable feeling. We see the connection with his calling. He says of his mode of address that it proceeds slowly, improving gradually. At the close of a sexual act (masturbation or coitus) he restrains himself in order not to reach a rapid tempo. We again see a hint of his fear of falling into too rapid a tempo at the end of his prayer. But this by no means exhausts the whole content of the dream. It appears to be concerned with a long function with another woman, for this is the sense of the dream. *His own* wife he had got out of the way ; she is where the grandfather is, among the dead, and he carries out the function which he otherwise performs with his wife, with another woman. We shall see that in the next dream a complete confirmation of this view is brought by the patient himself.

Freud maintains that every dream must have a link with the infantile. The analysis as it proceeds does not always admit the possibility of seeking for this link. In this case where the analysis of the dream—for the simple reason that no other succeeded it for some time—was pursued into the minutest ramifications, I came upon the complete solution which the final sentence about the four mouths explains to us in astonishing fashion. It occurred to the patient that he was once bathed by his grandfather's young servant girl who took occasion to play with his genitals (age about four years !) The water-closet is the expression of the great sewer, or the symbol for anus and penis. The child makes no distinction between genitals and anus. All that he uses at the water closet is for him a genital organ. Shame is cultivated in him as much for the hinder function as for that in front, and so it comes about that in later years, through fixation of infantile impressions, the anus plays the part of an erogenic zone. In his childhood our patient was very fond of passing his time in the water-closet. Even now defecation gives him a certain pleasure. Now this servant girl appears to have practised the same abominable manipulation not only with him but with his brothers. For the last sentence of the dream becomes clear if one substitutes the servant girl for the grandfather. The servant girl did something in the pissoir, she wanted to mend something. There were in the pissoir four mouths (four boys), and she wanted to put something right. It is as if he wished to charge the servant with the responsibility for his illness, which in fact was the case, for it was just this early sexual trauma which had directed the boy's thoughts into erotic channels.[1] On the other hand, children retain for such a person something of the attachment which one owes to one's first love. Similarly the woman can never forget the man who has first possessed her. Carpenter says that the man to whom a woman first surrenders her body, be his character what it may, maintains an indefeasible claim upon her heart. Similarly I have never noticed in a case of seduction of a young person or of a child who experienced pleasurable feelings and did not have to endure pain, an emotion simply of hate or

[1] According to the dream she made good the injury.

repulsion without a strong outpouring of love for the seducing person. Another experience occurs as an important recollection to the patient, which sharply defines his attitude to his wife. Originally he had loved another (so loved that he nearly lost his reason) and could not obtain her. He was then too young. He adds a number of allusions and connections which cannot be given here. After this dream a number of experiences occur to the patient, which all relate to conquests. In every little town he had another girl. Everywhere he fancied, now a maiden, now a wife, and sometimes—several of each. And in phantasy every one became his own. He possessed them all in masturbating or he pictured them to himself while praying on week-days.

The second dream brings us yet deeper into the problem of his illness :—" *I wanted to hire lodgings from a Mrs. König. But she was not to be had. She was promised to me for later on. The place is not that where I am staying now but my birthplace.*"

If in a dream we have a lodging with many *rooms* one will make no mistake if one thinks of a *woman*.[1] We proceed, however, without prejudice to the analysis of the dream and ask what was to him the most striking thing in it. He says : " The form of the woman." It was a little old woman who stood with her back to him, and whom therefore he could not see. I thought, as the man lives in Roumania where there is no Kaiser but a King perhaps Mrs. König means here, " the mother." First, naturally, one asks if he knows any Mrs. König. He does know one, but has no relations with her, she has not struck him in any way. He does not know why this particular name occurred to him. To the further question of whom the old woman reminded him, he answered at once, " Of my mother," but says that, as to this, nothing further occurs to him. We do not try to get round this resistance by reckless interpretations and leave him to relate his further recollections. A servant girl occurs to him who had promised him coitus. But when he came to her by night she said she had the " red *König* [King] " and he could not come to her then. But she promised to let him know in a few days when she was well. In the meantime she was sent away. We see then that the lodging which he wanted to hire and which was promised to him for later on, represents in one meaning the vagina. Further, a young woman called Kiraly comes into his head. Kiraly is, as he knows, the Hungarian term for King [*König*]. This woman meets his advances very freely, and he has the impression that it would not be difficult to possess her. But he never has intercourse with a woman when it might have consequences, for a reason which he says is very pertinent. *If this woman had a child by him it might happen that one of his children not knowing the near relationship might commit incest with that child.* This precaution evidently serves to prevent his having intercourse with the many women who excite him. It appears, however,

[1] *Zimmer* = room ; *Frauenzimmer* = woman. Tr.

to be also a defensive idea. A defensive idea against his own incestuous thoughts. In the further analysis of the dream he produces a number of incestuous thoughts. He loved his elder brother's wife, in fact he loves and perhaps lusts after her to-day. To be sure, he has never betrayed his thought, not even by a look. But incestuous thoughts of his mother also come to light. He once lay with her in the same room " when he was already sixteen years old." On that occasion he masturbated and showed himself to his mother while doing it. He remembers too having often watched her when he was a child. Now the dream becomes yet plainer. The last sentence was : " The place was my birthplace." There he had seen his mother. But the birthplace was his mother's womb. To visit one's birthplace means very often, in the language of the dream, to commit incest with the mother. We see through his love to the mother : " But she was not to be had." To seek a lodging means here, in the language of the dream, to seek sexual intercourse. The dream reproduces an incest phantasy of the sixteenth year and one from childhood which is known to us by a masking reminiscence, the analysis of which follows later. This thought was very painful to him and he has done his utmost to repress it. Many of his symptoms are to be interpreted as a compromise between the breaking through and the repression of this incestuous thought.

Herewith, however, the interpretation of the dream is not completed. The most important light on it is contributed by the fact that a woman occurs to him who has played a great part in his life and who is called Regina Kaiser. (Regina = _Königin_ [=Queen]). As a very young girl this woman had frequented his parents' house and had allowed him to steal many a kiss from her. There was love between them—burning with a sort of quiet glow— and neither had said anything about it. After his marriage he saw her again as a full-blown young woman of splendid beauty and sometimes he succeeded in stealing a kiss which she half returned. When he moved into his last parish it was one of the attractions that this girl lived there as a young wife. He was on very friendly terms with her and her husband, until one day the wives began to quarrel. For Mr. K. began to pay court to his own wife. This made Regina so jealous that she picked a quarrel and broke off relations. This woman he now hates and despises. But he admits that he once loved her, nay, that he had often kissed her when she was a married woman. He confesses also that he had often thought how it would be if he could make her his wife. Now we understand why in the first dream he pushes his wife to one side. (She is where the grandfather is.) In the second dream, he is still friends with Regina. She had indeed rejected his suit (as the dream says : " But she was not to be had.") But the dream opens a new perspective to him : he will win her yet. (She was promised to me for later on.) The dream reveals the identification of Mrs. Kaiser with his mother. She is a niece of the mother and very like her. The fulfilment of the wish in the dream lies in the circumstance that she is still attainable and that the quarrel between the women has not diminished her love for him.

We see then that the Mrs. König of the dream represents the condensation of several persons : (1) his mother ; (2) the menstruating servant girl ; (3) Mrs. Kiraly ; (4) Mrs. Regina Kaiser.

In the following days the patient is in a permanent state of high excitement. He is constantly dominated by the thought that Mrs. Kaiser has made him so ill. If he only knew how to avenge himself ! A number of little details clearly shows that he had fallen in love with Mrs. Kaiser, that the little erotic excitements of her society were indispensable for him. The desires which these left unsatisfied were promptly met by the onanistic act and by his praying. For in his praying Regina appeared before him in imagination as a friendly figure. The analysis shows more and more plainly that by this patient prayer is practised as a directly masturbatory act. Before praying (N.B., only on week-days) he has a gloomy feeling of oppression which he says he will drive away by beautiful images. So he imagines a beautiful woman (mostly Mrs. Kaiser) whereupon the excitement somewhat diminishes, but only to increase again violently towards the end of the prayer.

The explanations which he gives of this enable us to understand why on reading the Bible story of Esther he had such a violent anxiety attack that he nearly swooned. This story according to the Bible, was as follows : King Ahasuerus wished to show his peoples and princes the beauty of his wife, Queen Vashti. But the Queen refused to comply with the command, so that the indignant King asked the seven princes of Persia and Media what they thought should be done with such a Queen. The princes advised the King *to put the Queen away and to choose another, the most beautiful in the whole kingdom.* Then all the maidens were brought together and from them he choose the most beautiful, Esther, daughter of Mordecai. This story led along the track of unconscious associations to his own secret thoughts. He too had played with the thought of leaving his wife and choosing another wife and queen (Regina Kaiser). But then the complete breach between them had already occurred. This dream or let us say this unconscious indulgence of the thought was all at once brought to an end. The contrast between the disagreeable present and his secret wishes, the consciousness of guilt towards his wife united to bring about that attack of anxiety which was to be the beginning of his severe neurosis.

In similar fashion is explained the fact that as long as six years ago he suffered a violent attack after reading the story of Deborah. There were two passages which had then greatly excited him and which he wished to omit. The passage where the wife of Heber the Kenite enticed King Sisera into her tent and drove a nail through his temples while he slept, and the passage where the booty was then divided and where it says, " a maiden or several maidens for every man." The first passage was an allusion to a form of perversion which he had often had practised on him (fellatio). Nail is an extremely frequent symbol for penis. Nail in the temples —symbolic picture for " penis in ore."[1] Yet more important was the second passage that every man should receive one or several maidens. He remembers that even in his childhood this passage had made a great impression on him, a sensation as if he envied the conquerors their booty.

In general all erotic passages in the Bible were sources for his phantasies and contributed not a little to advance the amalgamation between religious act and sexuality. An exact analysis of the passages omitted in the prayers (which in praying he had to leave out) gives a similar result. He experiences resistances in all passages of the prayer which speak of love and " conception," or of conception in general. He experiences resistances at all passages of the prayer which speak of the omniscience of God, because of his consciousness of guilt, because he deems himself such a wicked sinner, one who, by dragging sexuality into prayer, has profaned and desecrated the service of God. For this reason he halts at the passages which beg for a gracious reception of the prayer ; for this reason he trembles when he has to speak or sing before the open eye of God. After this explanation the patient wanted to know why of late years he had come to a standstill and experienced anxiety at the prayer for the King also. He shows me the passage. This runs :—

" Kaiser and King ! King of all Kings ! " The explanation now occurs to him himself. Unconsciously he had thought of Regina Kaiser, who to him was the royal ruler, most beautiful of all beauties, the Queen of all queens. He wanted to know also why he had omitted certain passages in the prayer which were quite indifferent. He names one passage : " In thy kingdom shall all on this day devote themselves to enjoyment." Always an allusion to Regina is evident.

After a long interval in which we succeeded in liberating a number of small important reminiscences and repressions, he again brings a dream :—" I tell my prefect that the Rev. X. is suffering from an anxiety neurosis and cannot enter the church any more." He once avenged himself beautifully on this colleague. Now he avenges himself a second time on him, by transferring as it were the whole illness to him. But the dream reveals also thoughts of revenge against Regina. For the continuation of the dream runs :—
" The King orders me to give him a report about it." As if he felt he must cry out in Mrs. Kaiser's face : " You are guilty of my

[1] Yet more important are the criminal phantasies which culminate in a parricide. These indications were not followed up. Also criminal phantasies directed against wife and children were overlooked.

anxiety neurosis. I would have you to know that on your account I can no longer appear in the church!" He wrote Mr. Kaiser a letter containing a clear account of the whole gossip affair, and peppered with unvarnished truths about his doubly guilty wife. His state of mind becomes more tranquil, he already feels more confidence, and hopes for the success of the cure. Association experiments which we undertake, show this progress very plainly. In the first experiments at the word " Regina " there was a long pause and then the association, " ill-will." After " prayer " came, after a long pause, "artificial." Then came two associations which were very significant. " Woman—desirable " ; " married woman —honourable," Therewith he really confessed the deepest reason for his conflict. " Reproaches " brought the association, " justified." Some days before the close of the cure there came after the word " Regina," the association " sympathy " ; after " calling," the association " bread," whereas formerly it was " unbearable." After " girl," the association " putting one in a good humour " ; after " vice," " very pleasant." After " anxiety " the association " away with it " and after " cure," " certain."

Also the series of words which freely come into his mind, and which I asked him to tell me, showed the complete alteration in the patient's state of mind ; he finds himself in a visibly freer and better humour after liberation of all repressions.

One masking reminiscence is still to be explained. He sees himself and his brother standing half naked in white knickers. He thinks the recollection dates from his second or third year. It is his earliest recollection. In reality the investigation shows that this recollection appeared much later. It was only in his twentieth year that he began to reproduce this recollection, undoubtedly a masking reminiscence in *Freud's* sense. (Psychopathology of Everyday Life, Berlin, 1907). These masking memories preserve indifferent and trifling sensations while the impressive and stirring ones concealed among them have vanished. *Freud* says :

"Since it is known that the memory makes a choice[1] among the impressions offered to it, it would seem that we must assume that this choice is made in childhood on principles other than those that rule in the period of intellectual maturity. Detailed investigations prove, however, that this assumption is superfluous. The indifferent childhood memories owe their existence to a process of displacement. In the reproduction they are the substitute for really important impressions, the recollection of which may be developed from them by psychanalysis, but whose direct reproduction is hindered by a resistance. As they owe their preservation, not to their own content but to an associative relation of their

[1] A similar thought occurs in Nietsche : " I did that," says my memory. " I cannot have done that," says my pride, and remains inexorable. Finally —memory yields. (*Beyond Good and Evil.*)

content to another repressed one, they have a well-founded claim to the name I have given them, masking memories."

Thus our masking memory, also, represses the most important thing and betrays only a falsified detail. For later it occurs to the patient : He sees his mother looking at the two children and laughing. And as a further detail it occurs to him that his father repeatedly went about the room with his trousers open, so that he could see his penis. That at this time his younger brother could not wear any knickers but only a little dress did not occur to him till afterwards. But if one tries to interpret these masking memories with the key of the dream interpretation, we find that his mother sees the two " little ones "[1] and these two are himself and his father, beside whom he places himself in this dream as rival on an equal footing. In the second dream indeed, he had uttered the same thought. Now it occurs to him too that his father was often very hard-hearted with him, and thrashed him severely without reason for slight oversights. In such moments a feeling of hatred against the father overcame him.[2] This is a typical experience. *Muthmann* points out that a passage dealing with the love of a child for his mother occurs in Stendhal,[3] who in the reminiscenses of his youth relates the following :—

" I was always in love with my mother. I always wanted to kiss my mother, and wished that there were no such things as clothes. She loved me passionately and often clasped me in her arms. I kissed her with such ardour that she felt it her duty, as it were, to go away. I detested my father if he came upon us and interrupted our kisses. I wanted to give them to her always on the breast. And please realise that I lost her when I was scarcely seven years old. She died in the bloom and beauty of her youth. Thus forty-five years ago I lost that which I most loved on earth."[4]

With the solution of this masking memory and the discovery of the incest thoughts, the gravest repression is done away with. The patient feels better from day to day, and two days before his departure brings me another dream :—

" *On the recommendation of my friend Weiser, I received from an assistant Jungmann (who is now dead—naturally) a testimonial as to my learning. When I got home I noticed that the testimonial did not contain my name. Later I met the assistant and told him, and he promised to write me another testimonial, and to send it on. At the close of the dream I was at the theatre and saw Kainz in Tartuffe.*"

The dream is easy to interpret. The patient undertakes the interpretation himself. Jungmann was one of his teachers and as

[1] The little one = the child = a phallus symbol.
[2] Consider the passage about murdering King Sisera with a nail.
[3] Or Stendhal, Henry Beyle, " Confessions of an Egoist."
[4] Abundant information as to incest tendencies is to be found in the Centralblatt für Psychoanalyse (Vols. I. to IV.). Further in the books of Max Marcuse *Uber den Inzest* (Verlag Marhold, Halle, a.s.) and Otto Rank : *Das Inzes.' Motiv in Sage and Dichtung* (Franz Deutuke, Leipzig and Vienna, 1912).

the professor's assistant once gave him a very good testimonial for a colloquium. Later he met the teacher, when he was visiting his father's grave. The man had a neglected appearance, and told him he was in need, as if he wished to beg help from him. But he gave him nothing, being ashamed to give alms to his teacher, and for this he reproached himself[1] for many years afterwards. Weiser was one of his colleagues, one of the best heads and the clearest, his intimate friend, a splendid speaker, once his beau ideal. When I asked him to mention a series of names beginning with Jungmann, he came (after a few other teachers) to me, as I knew from the beginning he would. Weiser, his ideal, is Professor *Freud*, who sent him to the assistant Jungmann—that is myself. While he emphasizes the wisdom of the professor by the association Weiser,[2] he is rather making merry over my youth. On the other hand the dream shows regret for the great expense of the cure. Also a little fear lest I should reveal some of the facts he has confided to me ; I am for him superfluous, done with, a dead man as it were. Therefore in the dream he flings me to the dead teacher ("who is now dead—naturally "). I die a *natural* death. I have in fact given him a testimonial which has rendered possible his long stay in Vienna. Also I am his teacher. I have helped him to a new branch of knowledge : the recognition of the associations of his illness. There remains the analysis of the strange fact that the testimonial did not contain his name. And here it occurs to him that the testimonial contained another mysterious word. Weiser, his colleague, had in the school a nickname, because he had a sweetheart called Esther. On this account he was called " Estherlus." And in the testimonial there was written in large letters : *Carester*, a combination of Cara (dear) and —— again Esther, the queen of his heart, in other words : Regina Kaiser. The testimonial contained her name, but his name was lacking. This is connected with the hope I had expressed that the broken thread might be joined together and the friendship soon renewed. In this dream the hope of a new testimonial is expressed. Further, in connection with Jungmann, young men[3] and some homosexual memories of his childhood occur to him ; these show that this component by the transference of his feelings to my person has contributed to the success of the cure.

The end of the dream (Kainz-Tartuffe) reveals the resolve not to take his calling so seriously and to sham a little before the people without pangs of conscience. He will be a play-actor in life. His model will be Tartuffe. He comforts himself with the conscious-

---

[1] The reproach goes deeper. The teacher is identified with the father. Secretly he experiences a malicious joy in the fact that things are going badly with the teacher, and *will* do nothing to relieve him. The reproach therefore is for his heartlessness and his malice. In the masking memory also in fact he is " his father's assistant."

[2] [*Weise* = wise ; *Weiser* = teacher, guide. Trans.]

[3] [Young men = junge Männer. Trans.]

ness that he is no worse than other people, that his environment, his talents and his experiences have forced him into the track of the erotic ; he comforts himself further with the consciousness that in such a fine profession, by consolation, and by the edifying effect of his prayers he can restore to so many people the peace of mind which, through open conference with me, he has fully gained for himself.

At the close of the analysis I would draw attention to a few points. If we carefully read through the account of his illness given to me by the patient, we are specially struck by the secret sexual symbolism. I mention only certain expressions used in a double sense : " getting finished " ; further : " that it is only as good as I make it." etc. The whole prayer proceeds as symbols of eroticism. At one passage of his story of the disease the unconscious thoughts openly broke through. He uses, namely, the expression " Negligé—canal." He fears to fall into a negligé—canal. This finds its explanation in the fact that Regina Kaiser had repeatedly received him in a seductive negligé. Once she had sent for him in the greatest excitement. She had caught her husband being unfaithful to her and wished to get a divorce from him. In the excitement she forgot—or was it unconscious intention—that the negligé was unfastened in front. He saw her beautiful breasts. Shortly afterwards the breach occurred between the two women. Mrs. Kaiser had evidently expected a greater response from her friend. She wished to revenge herself. How happy many women are when they are so unhappy as to have to revenge themselves ! But he had neither the courage for a sin nor the strength to break with the beloved woman.

The violent accusations which the patient made against the prefects and against his wife were accusations against himself—projected outwardly.

We see how recent excitements make manifest the latent neurosis which had existed for years.

He goes home tranquil, cured.

After some weeks I received a letter from him in which he says that he functions without any feeling of anxiety even on week-days, and that he feels quite well. He once more thanks me cordially for completely curing him.

Truly, for six weeks—that was the duration of the treatment—a fine result of the psychanalytical method ![1]

[1] EPICRISIS :—After four years I received by chance news of the ex-patient. One day a lady suffering from agoraphobia came to consult me. She had heard that her priest had suffered from similar anxiety-conditions, and had been cured. Mr. J. B. gave her my address, and begged her to give his kind regards and to say he was perfectly well. Asked what the treatment was, the priest said : " Dr. S. will give you the drops which did me so much good." This with a peculiar smile. The lady, who had made a long journey to Vienna, now in all good faith asked for the wonderful drops, and was greatly disappointed when she heard that the treatment was only " psychic."

CHAPTER XXIII

FEAR OF BLUSHING (ERYTHROPHOBIA) AND FEAR OF SWEATING

FEAR of blushing is extraordinarily wide-spread. It is found in every stratum of society, among poor and rich, among solitaries and among persons who appear before the public. The stronger the fear, the stronger the obsession which causes the blushing as a psychic betrayal. *Every one who suffers from erythrophobia has a bad conscience.* As the blushing of the chaste maiden is really an unconscious confession of her sexuality, so the blushing of the adult neurotic represents fear of " being found out." Among these persons one finds the very gravest paraphilia, sadism, nekrophilism, anilingus, cannibalism, vampirism, inclination to lust-murder and rape. Of course harmless paraphilias such as homosexuality and exhibitionism may express themselves through blushing.

Men who suffer from blushing make clever attempts to hide the reddening. They get tanned in the sun, they grow a large beard ; they prefer to take their walks in the dark, are happy when it rains and they can carry a large umbrella that hides the face. They choose hats coming well down over the forehead. In speaking, they cannot look you in the eyes ; they are shy and embarrassed.

All these patients say that they have no other anxiety. I have seen officers blush on the occasion of an official appearance before their chief, when they feared appearing before him ; officers who had been several times decorated for extraordinary bravery, for whom the storming of a position was child's play.

Blushing affects not only the face. It may spread to the shoulders, the breast, the hands. Local blushing also occurs. There are erythrophobists who show only a red spot on a certain part of the face ; others two red spots like hectic cheeks. Others blush only with the ears.

Especially painful is this blushing of the neck and breast for ladies whose calling obliges them to appear *decolletés*. I knew one of the most famous singers of Europe who, in spite of rouge and powder, showed red spots on the breast at the moment of appearing. She strove in vain against it and finally had to abandon her profession. She could not bring herself to undergo analytical treatment. Another patient blushed at the neck when she looked at

anyone. I suggested that she might always wear high-cut blouses.
The patient replied :
" But I like wearing them open at the neck.   Pray, doctor, who
can wear high-necked blouses in summer ? "
It appears that this neurotic had "genitalised " the parts that
blushed—to use Freud's striking expression.   One blushes most
easily when the part of the skin concerned is an erogenous zone.
Many persons identify themselves with their genitals.   I know
men who identify themselves with the penis and compensate for
deficient erection by a forced stretching of the whole body.   Among
the impotent one can here and there observe this excessively stiff
bearing.   The erythrophobists have also genitalised the face.
Ferenczi says : " The identification of the whole ego with the face
is something common to human beings.   It seems to me probable
that the shifting of the libidinous emotions ' from below upwards '
(Freud) in the sublimation period causes (probably helped by the
lively vascular innervation) a secondary genitalisation of the
face, whose sexual rôle is at first only exhibitionist." (By " genitalisation " of a part of the body he understands with Freud
periodically increased hyperæmia, saturation with moisture, tur-
gescence, accompanied by corresponding nerve stimulations.)   But
this genitalisation of the face (which inevitably carries with it a
feeling of shame in respect of the face) is never the sole cause of the
erythrophobia.   There is always also bad conscience as a weighty
factor.
A similar phenomenon is sweating of the hands and of the face
which brings about a torturing fear of sweating and may make the
sufferer completely useless socially.   Fear of sweating often occurs
in conjunction with fear of blushing as the next case shows.

No. 115.—Mr. N. V., a thirty-six years old artillery captain, complains of
various nervous troubles.   The central point of his illness is his fear of attract-
ing attention and making himself ridiculous by blushing and sweating.   An
example will best explain how this fear acts.   If he has to go with his father
to a restaurant in the evening, he is occupied the whole day with the thought :
" Shall I be able to enter the place without blushing ? " ' This thought
torments him from morning till evening and hardly leaves room for any
other thought.   At length the dreaded hour arrives.   His father has gone
on before ; he is to follow.   That at once troubles him greatly.   How many
people will be there ? Will they stare and possibly laugh at him ? Even
before entering his heart beats as if it would burst.   He would much prefer
to turn back.   But he says to himself : " Come ! You must show that
you are a man.   You have gone through twenty battles.   You have six
decorations.   (In uniform it is never so bad.   Many men who dread open
spaces are fear-free when in uniform.   The uniform takes away self-con-
sciousness.)   So in you go ! "   He enters.   A hot feeling rises from his
stomach to his head ; his blood boils.   Sweat breaks out from every pore.
His head gets hot and red.   His hands sweat.   Lucky that he has his gloves
on in case he should have to shake hands with anyone.   At last he gets
through the torture of the entreé and the greetings, and seats himself at the
table.   He is bathed in sweat, his shirt wet.   The company notices this.
One asks why he is so exhausted.   He stammers out some excuse, stuttering
as he does so.   Finally the condition gradually passes, to be succeeded by
rage at his childish behaviour.

The root of this anxiety is his bad conscience. Even from childhood he has masturbated. When he was seven years old he began to play with his five years old sister. He kept up this play. At the age of fifteen he performed the first coitus with her. Before her wedding—she was nineteen years of age—he came once more to her in bed and took leave of her. Twice there was coitus.

Besides this he has various criminal acts—quite a number—on his conscience. He stole money from his mother's chest—he was then sixteen years old—which caused him an anxiety erection, and tremendous orgasm. (Apparently phantasy of incest with the mother.) Several times, too, he committed burglary without stealing anything, simply in order to bring about the longed-for orgasm of anxiety. The analysis shows that he plays with the fancy of a lust murder of little children and that these forbidden acts are substitution acts for the lust murder.

He has every reason to fear that he is seen through. He acts as if found out.

This case throws a bright light on the mechanism of anxiety emission. It is not true that the libido is transformed into anxiety without psychic help, as Freud has taught. Only the specific—in every case unconscious—phantasy brings about the orgasm. The scholar who does not finish his school-work and has an emission, had during the work some phantasy in which he was occupied with a definite sexual object which he wanted to attain.

To the neurotic everything becomes a play, a symbol.

Much simpler is the next case of erythrophobia :—

No. 116.—Mrs. I. L., thirty-two years old, no hereditary taint, has, so she says, never been nervous. She fell ill three years ago of blushing, and since the first time she blushes at every inopportune incident. Even the thought that she may blush, makes her blush. She is happily married to a much respected man, and states that in her marriage she finds mental and physical satisfaction. She decides on an analysis to be free from the terrible fate that embitters her life.

She is asked to report how the trouble first began. She reports as follows : She had two ladies visiting her. They were just having an exciting talk. One lady told her an indifferent incident and at that she blushed.

Will she give details ? What was the incident in question ?

" My husband is an advocate and had the representation of a high aristocrat, the richest man of our circle. The husband of this lady had taken the post away from him. And the lady was saying that as notary her husband was freed from military service. I thought of my poor husband who had just been called up, and was now on active service. I became blood-red. Really I did not want to let the ladies see that I was concerned about the loss of the post. I invited them and was very amiable with them. And I did not lose my composure at this report. I only became red."

Here we plainly see the connection between suppressed rage and blushing. Also shame at being defeated seems to have played a part ; also a third factor as I can readily show. She is a Jewess and lives in a Christian town where she mixes only with the Christian families. " One cannot associate with the Jews," she says. The two ladies were Christians.

The second case of blushing confirmed my supposition. She had a talk with a gentleman about Zionism, a talk that was very exciting, and suddenly she became blood-red. I explained to her that she had always been ashamed of herself in front of Zionists, because she had continually denied her Jewish descent.

She mixed only with Christian society and was privately very proud of this, looking down on her co-religionists with contempt.

" Evidently you were ashamed in the presence of the Zionist because you denied your Jewish origin. In both cases we have to do with the feeling of inferiority to the Christian which the Jew experiences. You are a very proud, self-conscious woman, and cannot endure this feeling."

She wishes to set me right and reports a case with which the Jewish question had nothing to do. She had to pay frequent visits to a highly placed lady, by birth a Frenchwoman. This happened several times a week. She always had to find something to talk about. So once she told about a case in which she had been struck by the elegant behaviour of a young man. She said : " The man must be from Paris, because he knows so well how to behave." He was very good-looking too. She found out that he had been brought up in Paris. As she related this, she blushed furiously.

I give her to understand that the youth had found favour with her, which she violently denies. No man can find favour with her at first sight. She must first know his soul and his mind.

We find out that she is very reserved and has greatly restrained her lively temperament at the wish of her husband. Her husband likes sedateness and refinement. She must accommodate herself to his tastes. I explain to her that all compulsion must finally manifest itself in some neurotic symptom.

The next day she comes to me in great excitement. She says she has not slept the whole night. I am on a false scent. I am imagining a vain thing. I think that the young man found favour with her. With her no man can possibly find favour on purely physical grounds. It was the feeling of shame in presence of the Frenchwoman, a feeling of the defeat and the triumph of the French. She is instructed that hurt pride very frequently manifests itself in blushing. She admits that she has always been very ambitious, and always wanted to be first.

Gradually the unhappiness of the marriage comes to light. Her husband loves her passionately, he is the best of husbands, her marriage is the happiest possible, but he will have his own way in everything. When she says anything, he says : " You are quite right, my child ! But ——" and then he proves just the opposite to her. In the education of the children and in the house, everything must be as he wishes. It is worst in company ; he pursues her with his glances and criticises her so that it is impossible for her to be at ease. As a girl she was self-possessed and everyone praised the calm of her deportment. Now she is always trembling as to whether she has done right, fearing the criticism of her husband, which she reads in his looks. She has found it very difficult to accommodate herself to the little ways of the country. She has been used to the great town and suffered under this. Only the children and the duties connected with them could partially fill the gap.

The analysis meets with great resistance. She comes too late. She has sick headache. She will not admit what is going on within her. The resentment under which she suffers constantly becomes more evident. She says she has passed many months in sanatoria. She suffered from heart neurosis, from attacks of anxiety and from stomach neurosis. Her husband was very kind and shrank from no sacrifice to make her well.

But she is unhappy in her marriage. He has destroyed her self-respect. He always insists that any little peculiarity of hers is Jewish. She has not forgotten these humiliations and would like to be revenged.

For some years she is anæsthetic. She thirsts for satisfaction. She is looking for another man. The war ought to have set her free from her husband. For that reason she was so strongly in favour of getting him exempted from service. She trembled at the thought that he might have to join the army. But it happened otherwise. The Christians were everywhere saying : " The Jews get out of it whenever they can." Then her husband joined up of his own accord. She could not hold him back then. His period of active service was terrible for her. Secretly she was longing to be set free by his death ; outwardly she was trembling for his life.

The Jew-complex then has been established in her in several ways. And, besides, there is the fact that she is much taken with a young man who is a Jew and who has lived in Paris. She wishes to keep this secret even from herself and betrays it to all the world. Her blushing confesses what her mouth represses.

Here she breaks off the analysis. Of her further experiences I have heard nothing. Probably her erythrophobia has a deeper origin. The analysis showed even at the beginning that it was a case of the stirrings of an evil conscience.

Fear of blushing and of sweating are among the most difficult and the most thankless tasks of the psycho-therapist. Hypnosis mostly fails completely ; analysis can boast of great triumphs. Yet I have seen patients who have vainly sought help. from several physicians, analysts of every school and from individual psychologists and have not found it. That shows us how deep the roots of the trouble may often go. If these patients are not cured, they shut themselves off from all the world. The dread of blushing makes them shy of meeting people. They become eccentrics, recluses, bury themselves in loneliness or shut themselves up in a room, and only at night slink through the streets like secret criminals. Many a mysterious suicide may be traced to dread of blushing. Only the mental physician knows the agonies which these patients suffer. That there is a little pleasure mingled with this agony I have already mentioned. This pleasure component is deeply hidden.

In rare cases the erythrophobia is converted into its opposite, into shamelessness. That is the strange method by which a lady of my acquaintance freed herself from this trouble. She became a celebrated demi-mondaine.

She once said to me, wittily enough : " The only thing I could blush for now is that I cannot blush for anything."

CHAPTER XXIV

DREAD OF THE RAILWAY, DREAD OF GETTING COLD, DREAD OF EXAMINATIONS, AND PSYCHIC IMPOTENCE

THE little everyday phobias also prove to be accessible by psychological analysis. The cases of dread of railway travelling which exhibit clearly relations with the sex-life are interesting in this respect. Freud remarks hereon in his [1]" Treatises on Sexual Theory " (Deuticke, 1906) :

" Rocking, as is well known, is constantly used for getting restless children to sleep. On older children the shaking of carriage journeys, and later of railway journeys, exerts such a fascination that all boys at least want at some time in their lives to be conductors and coachmen. They will take a mysterious interest of extraordinary intensity in the processes of the railway and at the age when fancy is active (shortly before puberty) they make them the kernel of an exquisite sexual symbolism. The compulsion for associating railway travelling with sexuality arises evidently from the pleasurable character of the sensations of motion. If now we have the repression which converts so many childish preferences into the opposite, the same persons when they are growing up or grown up will turn with disgust from rocking and shaking, will be frightfully exhausted by a railway journey, or inclined to anxiety attacks during the journey, and will protect themselves by dread of the railway from a repetition of the painful experience."

Every case of dread of the railway may be psychologically explained, *and sea sickness and railway sickness seem to me to be a special form of parapathia.*

No. 117.—I was treating a patient who was suffering from very grave anxiety hysteria. He feared he would suffer from disease of the spine, often thought he was so suffering, passed sleepless nights because he had such violent anxiety attacks that the physician was compelled to sit many hours by his couch to tranquillise him. Every week he suffered the horrors of death, took leave of his dear ones every time, and so on. Discretion forbids me to give further details of the history of his illness. Only one detail I will mention. The patient suffered from dread of tunnels. As he consulted many professors, and visited various institutions he had to travel a great deal. This travelling was for him a special torment because he had to get out before every tunnel. Thus, e.g., he could not travel to Baden by Vienna without interruption because there was a little tunnel to pass through. He got out at the station before, travelled over the distance in a carriage, and eventually rejoined the.railway.

[1] Abhandlungen zur Sexualtheorie.

The analysis showed the following relationship between this dread and his experiences. His father had died very early and his mother was still a young, jolly woman. While she did not trouble herself much about the bringing up of the other children, she showed for him an absolutely blind partiality. She took him with her everywhere, even on the journeys which she made with her lovers. The first of these journeys, immediately after the death of her husband, was over the Semmering, which, as is well-known, has a great many tunnels, into Italy. Now the boy, who was then four years old, noticed that in the tunnels—the compartment was darkened—something took place between his mother and the strange gentleman who called himself " Uncle." It may have been only caresses but the boy's fancy already rich and directed towards sex by several observations, invented something out of it. A propos of this I will again insist that *fancies may have the same harmful influence as experiences.* It is quite indifferent whether in the case of hysterical persons we have to do with a psychic trauma that they have really experienced, or with one that exists only in imagination, which they have built up on facts within their experience. (The material is genuine, the use of it a false one). The repressed idea acts as such in ruinous fashion. Thus, with our patient, the painful experiences of his childhood. His mother, whom he loved excessively, had in this case shown herself a prostitute. This brought upon him new and severe conflicts and ended in suicide. I could not complete the psychic treatment because I had to leave the neighbourhood fourteen days after beginning it.

I have mentioned the case only to explain the cure of the tunnel dread, which improved after the short analysis. Immediately thereafter the patient was able to pass through the same tunnels on the Semmering without any delay.

Other forms of the tunnel dread originate in birth-, womb- and coitus-fantasies. Religious motives too, play a part in the tunnel dread. In one of my neurotics I discovered the notion that he was travelling into the darkness of hell. The railway is often compared with the devil. The entrance into the tunnel symbolises the gate of hell. On account of his criminal phantasies the neurotic fears the judgment of God and everlasting damnation. The tunnel arouses the fear of hell which is ever latent within him and makes it manifest.

But the opposite of railway dread, the longing for journeys by rail, can also be easily explained by psycho-analysis. We have already considered in detail a case of this sort, that of the Rabbi (Chapter XXI.).

I have under close observation a lad of eighteen years, suffering from " dementia præcox," who is very remiss. What is specially striking about him is a passionate love for motion by cycle, carriage, rail and boat. His latest ideal is a motor cycle. Otherwise apathetic and torpid, he becomes lively if the talk turns on the motor cycle. In the train, too, he gets quite excited. His eyes flash, his halting speech becomes fluent. After a journey by motor cycle or by rail he becomes impotent for some hours. He suffers also from emissions. At these times he always dreams that he is travelling. Either he rises with an air-balloon, he flies with two wings, or he travels by motor. He has then a sensation of lust and wakes up with an emission. His mother had the habit when he was a child of tossing him into the air and catching him again, which gave him a wonderful feeling compounded of fear and libido. This was perhaps one of the sources of his railway neurosis.

Railway dread, sea sickness, dread of rocking, are often to be traced to experiences of childhood in which these actions were at first accompanied with pleasure, then caused pain, so that the idea opposed to pleasure, namely, disgust, or the repressed component of the libido, viz., fear, comes to the front. Another important source of the railway dread is the criminal source. These patients had all played with the fancy that the railway train will run over a hated rival, e.g., the brother, or the dreaded father. What they wished for others will befall themselves. They will certainly be run over. *Thus behind every phobia hides the old infantile criminal phantasy.* He who dreads the fire has at some time wished to play the arsonist. He who cannot bear the sight of blood, was once in his phantasies, a murderer.

Among other things there is combined with the railway dread *the dread of getting cold.* This neurosis is one of the gravest and most unpleasant because ultimately makes the person a prisoner in his dwelling. In the less serious forms of the disease the patients fear the rapid motion of the body or of a carriage because they may get heated and then cold. In the train they look anxiously to see if all the windows are closed. They fear the draught and cover themselves with thick outer clothing to escape the danger of draught. Even in summer they travel in a closed carriage and scarcely dare to open the window of a carriage. They are constantly haunted by the danger of first getting hot, and then on cooling, bringing on inflammation of the lungs.

It is a case of persons who dread their own passionate nature. They tremble at the thought of love. For they could not endure the loss of love. They are like people who will never keep a dog because they once suffered great grief through the loss of one.

Also the *dread of collisions and accidents* may be mingled with the ordinary railway dread. I know a lady who lives in constant fear of collisions. It is not difficult to guess what kind of collision she fears. In the street she suffers from the dread that she may collide with some unknown person. In spite of her fervent temperament and her immense wealth she lives the life of a nun. She cannot be induced to travel by rail and passes the summer in Vienna and close by. The danger of a collision haunts her early and late and persecutes her in her dreams, in which collisions alternate with erotic scenes. In life she poses as a free moralist, who would permit herself anything if the right man should come. Her dread of collisions shows that she is not rightly seeking the right man. The infantile source of railway dread, which *Freud* discovered, does not exhaust her whole being.

I can maintain the same thing of another phobia as of the railway dread. One very frequently encounters *the dread of examinations*, which is by many doctors taken to be only a symptom of increased general nervousness. Examination dread in its severe form, is a neurosis. There are students who are splendidly prepared, who have a complete command of their subject ; nevertheless they are not capable of taking their examination. They have the feeling that they are not yet ready, at the last moment they find a yawning gulf in their knowledge, they fear failure, and so year after year passes, they become " back numbers," and either give up studying altogether or finally, under specially powerful pressure of social circumstances, they take their examination. This neurosis also plainly shows relationship to a diseased *vita sexualis*. One of my patients confessed to me that every one of his examinations, even at the grammar school, was accompanied by emissions. The more violent were the emotions of fear the more pleasurable was the accompanying sexual condition. This patient was not capable of taking his examinations at the University, and abandoned his studies. As a substitute for the examination dread there began then an obstinate sleeplessness accompanied by fits of terror. He was attacked in bed by violent palpitation of the heart, had the feeling that something frightful must happen and in bed spent most of the time rolling sleeplessly from side to side. This dread was easy to cure. The patient lived with his sister ; they kept house together. Their rooms adjoined each other, their relations had always been very tender. As several dream analyses proved to me, the craving of this patient was directed towards his sister. This incest thought was entirely excluded from consciousness. In the evening when the craving awoke, there came with it the idea that something frightful must happen to him. This frightful thing was the incest which he desired just as much as, on ethical grounds, he abhorred it. The cure of this case was very easily brought about. The sister removed to an aunt (she too, suffered from similar symptoms) and the patient took another lodging where the environment was not linked by association with the exciting ideas. After some days the feelings of dread had vanished and the patient enjoyed an extraordinarily deep and sound sleep.[1]

I have frequently found that behind phobia may be detected suppressed paraphilia, old criminal phantasies, and especially repressed incest thoughts. Examination dread in particular is

[1] His emission in the examination showed that for him the examination signified " undressing."

always a transferred anxiety idea. In reality the anxiety refers to something other than the examination. But in accordance with the mechanism of the compulsory idea, it is transferred from an idea painful to the consciousness to a less painful idea and is now accompanied by that affect which should attend the painful idea. This may be noticed in normal persons also. It is well-known that the examination dream is one of the most frequent anxiety dreams of the normal person. He dreams that he has to undergo an examination and cannot pass it. Mostly one has such a dream when one has to make an important decision in life, but frequently also when libido and potency are evidently out of proportion to one another, when one fears a sexual failure.

The examination anxiety of the neurotic often reveals itself as sexual dread. Mostly these people are also impotent. Fear of the woman corresponds to their fear of the examiner. . . . . Another source is the secret religious feeling of these neurotics. Every test becomes a test before God, who will weigh them and find them too light. All these people are really very pious people who are apparently free-thinkers. In the intellect they have overcome their faith, but the affect holds fast the old faith of childhood.[1]

No. 119.—The following case was very exactly analysed by me. I begin with a description of the circumstances of his anxiety which I have already published in another place. This is also the case of a medical student who had prepared himself as much as fifteen years ago for his doctor-examination. The particulars are taken from his diaries which he keeps with painful precision.

Mr. Z. K., candidate in medicine, never passes his examinations. Not that he has been idle. He is the most industrious of all those who attend the lectures ; he is the first there ; he takes down in shorthand every lecture of his teacher.

But the date of the examination stands before him like a spectre and he is ever asking himself again if he knows everything exactly, if he has mastered the whole subject to the last dot of the i's. How if the examiner, just by chance, should put a question to him which he could not answer ?

At this thought he is bathed in a cold sweat. No ! he dares not expose himself to this danger. He must go into the examination with a feeling of absolute security. And he studies till far into the night, orders special works on the subject, because the text-books do not seem to him sufficiently detailed. For him there is no merriment, not a jovial hour, no night of revelry. He has but one wish, to have done with it quickly, that he may be able to throw off the terrible burden of it. Gradually there matures in

[1] Goethe, who was so great in his knowledge of the soul, says of the harp-player in "Wilhelm Meister" : "Reason had set our brother free, but his heart was soft ; the earlier impressions of religion became lively, and human doubts took possession of him. The liberated, free reason acquitted him ; his feelings, his religion, all customary ideas declared him to be a criminal."

him the feeling of certainty. Now he is absolutely sure ; he will take the examination. Something unexpected happens. He appears at the examinations of the others and places himself among the colleagues who are listening, among those poor wreckers whose whole hope is set thereon that they may be able to answer the weightiest questions posed by the strict professor through frequent hearing of the examinations.

Remarkable ! How little the students know ! What a lot he could have said in the place of these candidates. What a wealth of wisdom stands at his command. His resolve stands firm. On the morrow he will give in his name for examination.

But in the evening his confidence in victory begins already to give way to a slight distrust. Suppose it was after all a chance that he knew everything so well. Would it not be wise to go once more and once more to compare his knowledge with that of the other candidates ? So said, so done. He again enters the examination hall and seats himself in the background, in order not to attract attention. All lonely he sits there, hardly greeted by here and there an old acquaintance. Who should know him here ? His fellows have long since passed as doctors, and he has no relations with this young generation which fills the benches here. Only once in a way a face he knows appears. They are mostly fellow-students who have spent the years merrily in their clubs, drinkers, old fellows. Who would have dared to suggest to him that he, the best in his class, would be obliged to sit on the same bench with these " back numbers " for whom he had always had a compassionate contempt ?

Ah, if he might now sit there, if he had only had the courage to give in his name sooner ! How he would have been able to shine to-day. For again the examination shows him that he could far surpass in knowledge all the candidates who sit there.

Angry, out of humour and yet full of confidence, the candidate hurries home. To-morrow he will give in his name come what may. He takes a sacred vow to bind himself. This time he will not let himself be conquered by his anxiety feelings. This time he will not be the victim of his childish cowardice.

He carries out his resolve. He gives in his name. Three weeks stand between him and his examination. He sits increasingly over his books and rushes through the well-known pages. Here and there he notices a gap in his knowledge. Is he not deceiving himself ? Has not his memory played him false ? What would have happened if the professor had asked him this very question ? His disquiet increases. He becomes sleepless. The examination rises up before him like a frightful vision. He sees himself trembling and stammering before the examiner, unable to say a word. No, no ! in this condition he is not capable of passing an examination. He must have a rest first, tranquillise his nerves, tone himself up. As things are it is absolutely impossible.

In this mood he seeks me out and begs for a hypnosis. He remembers that Krafft-Ebing once freed a midwife who was suffering from examination dread by a successful hypnosis. She presented herself calmly at the examination and passed with distinction. Now it is only in the rarest cases that hypnosis succeeds with those phobias. The inhibitory ideas are stronger than the power of suggestion.

And in this case, too, the hypnosis failed. Psycho-therapy, on the other hand, was completely successful. It turned out that the man had formerly been relatively impotent. With every *puella publica* he was absolutely impotent and he had not trusted himself with other girls or women. At the same time he had every night strong erections, especially in the morning.

The further analysis showed that he lived on terms of violent strife with his father. As he said, on account of the examination. But closer investigation showed that even before his examination difficulties he could not get on with his father, so that in consequence he did not live at home. He had various strange tastes. He liked the company of elderly ladies best, and raked up old facts about the marriage of his parents.

He brought me several proofs that he was not the son of his parents. Thus in a way he made his mother a prostitute. He believed he had sure proofs that his father was impotent. He was not the least like his father, and so forth. Finally he confessed to me that as a child he had so loved his mother that even thus early he had been jealous of his father. Only within the last few days he had had a dream accompanied by an emission, which had so excited him that he had asked a parson who was a friend of his, whether it was a sin to commit incest in a dream.

In short behind his impotence there was hidden, repressed into the unconscious, a passion for his mother, an incest idea. Through the repression his love was anchored fast in the bottom of his soul. With the help of the analysis this repression was ended, and the patient was able to proceed calmly to his examination and without special nervousness or excitement to secure the longed-for doctor's degree.

Behind every examination dread we are able to look for grave repressions. The dread is transferred, it refers to a sinful sexual or criminal longing. Behind the examination before the teacher are hidden other, for the patient far more important, examinations. How will he stand before women ? ' And still more important : How will he stand before God ? Every neurotic is indeed a secret criminal. He has every reason to fear the examination before God. The examination dreams have a similar meaning, and these according to my experience of very frequent occurrence, especially with poets. Dread of mathematics or of Latin has a special symbolic meaning which I have discussed in detail in " Die Sprache des Traumes " (" The Language of the Dream.") The neurotics who suffer from examination dread are often erythrophobists, are shy before company and before people generally. In many cases we shall establish a relative impotence. There are several forms of impotence. Here we will speak only of that which is really only a dread of impotence. Many men experience at one time or another a sexual failure. Then the thought gets hold of them that they are impotent. This fear idea now dominates their whole thought, and hinders the automatic course of the sex act. When they approach the woman they are dominated by the single idea : Will it come off or not ? Then naturally it does not come off. Such patients have the most powerful erections at nights, mostly in the morning. For them Albert's wise saying holds good : " Where there is psychic impotence the diplomacy of a beautiful woman celebrates its greatest triumph." But miraculous cures may also be achieved by the energetic physician who is capable of inspiring confidence. An especially curative effect results from forbidding coitus. When one imposes on such a patient some months' abstinence, one may be sure that after some time he will come in triumph announcing his success. Especially if one has set his mind at ease, has promised the certain return of potency and has introduced some therapeutic agent that acts by suggestion (psychophorus, cold water bottles on the spine, electric treatment). These cases are all of the same type.

No. 120.—Mr. J. W., an otherwise very potent man, wishes on a journey to have intercourse with a chamber-maid. He is absolutely impotent. As we learn afterwards the chamber-maid had an eruption on the face and he had heard the day before that a friend had suddenly had to be sent to a lunatic asylum on account of syphilis in the brain. He now firmly believes he is impotent. He comes to me and asks me to help him. Otherwise he will shoot himself. When he was abroad (he says) he was already impotent. Then he came home from the journey and with his wife it was the same thing. I explain to him that the impotence came on acutely in consequence of a repressed idea of disgust and fear (lues), that his illness really represents only a fear of a fear. He must go home, in the evening drink a glass of old wine, take twenty drops of validol and read a chapter of a piquant book. The rest will follow in due course. The next day he presented himself healed.

Such cases are known to every practitioner. But on the other hand very obstinate ones which defy all therapy. According to my experience the most certain treatment is the analytical.

I will only add a few remarks. Many cases exhibit a sexual trauma in youth, in which a member of the family, the mother or the sister (indeed, in one of my cases, the grandmother) plays a part.

No. 121.—Dr. Ernst Bloch publishes a very instructive example showing how the carelessness of parents may destroy a man's life-happiness. (A contribution to Freud's Sexual-theory der Neurosen, Wiener Klin., Wochenschr., 1907, No. 52). A grave case of neurosis with psychic impotence. At the age of five years he was wakened by a noise which his parents made in coitus. He heard his mother's " groans," which produced in him a certain feeling of pleasure. He now tried to imitate this example. He aroused his four year old sister from her sleep and wanted to use force to her. She cried out, frightened, the parents were made aware of his design and the *father thrashed him soundly.* Later he entirely forgot the scene. After marriage it appeared that he was incapable of effecting a coitus. He has indeed plenty of erections. But when he gets into bed with his wife the erection ceases at once. He has been married eight years and lives aside not with his wife. Several times a week he has emissions after powerful erections. The scene overheard in his childhood is ever rising before his mind's eye. The image of his mother comes between his wife and him. This is a true *obsession* produced by repression. His sexuality is fixed to his mother. His consciousness of guilt comes from the same source.

The case is quite typical. I cannot here go into this subject more in detail. Most cases of anxiety hysteria and compulsion neurosis present a relative psychic impotence, which indeed is in part connected with a secret inclination to perversion.

A psychic impotence shows the following characteristics :

(1) An incest idea can often be detected.

(2) Consciousness of guilt has an inhibitory influence. This consciousness of guilt is remorse for masturbation, and bad conscience on account of the incest phantasies.

(3.) The memory of the first sexual aggression is often owing to various influences accompanied by displeasure. This is especially the case when, as above, blows followed the aggression.

(4.) An evident homosexual component and other unconscious perversions lessen the energy of the heterosexual instinct.

(5.) The impotence is partly a punishment and is voluntarily retained from unconscious motives of penance for the criminal phantasies.

(6.) The impotent finds in the pleasure of asceticism a substitute for the pleasure he has lost.

(7.) Impotence is used from unconscious motives of piety and from ethical principles to ensure purity (Disease as a refuge).

(8.) *Over-estimation of the sexual object, which hinders an intimate approach.* In these cases coitus is felt to be a lowering and a fouling of the object. Among these are the men who are very potent with a prostitute and helpless with a decent woman.[1]

Here I add a fragment of an analysis of psychic impotence which specially illustrates the principle of retribution.[2] In these cases the phantasy of castration plays a great part. The children, out of revenge because they have been threatened with castration for masturbation, are always full of criminal phantasies of castrating their father. When now the father dies, deep remorse follows

[1] Gerhart Hauptmann has brilliantly described this type in his most profound drama, " Griseldis." The Markgraf violates milkmaids and can do nothing with ladies of his own rank.

[2] Ferenczi, who confirms my results in his paper, " Analytical Interpretation and Treatment of Psycho-sexual impotence in the man," says very aptly : " Sexual inhibition is a veto of the unconscious."

and (as a consequence of self-punishment) impotence. Men always punish themselves by this, that they withdraw themselves from the dearest and best.

But asceticism itself may become pleasure if the masochistic component is strongly enough developed.

No. 122.—A twenty-four year old medical student comes to me in great excitement. Something horrible had happened to him. For some months he has loved a girl who returns his love. For months he has urged her to give herself to him entirely. The girl had angrily rejected all proposals and had broken off intercourse with him. Some days ago she wrote to him that at her parents' wish she must marry a man she does not love. But she wishes first to belong to him. Now he was in fearful excitement, tormented by permanent erections, until the hour of the rendezvous arrived. They went into the hotel. *Here he was so excited that he wept.* To his consternation no erection followed although until then he had always been able to take part in coitus without the least hindrance.

This is briefly the preliminary history. Now he is so excited that for weeks he has not been able to study. He has also the most remarkable dreams which he cannot explain. His father died years ago. He was a hard-hearted and strict father whom he positively hated. His mother had always been very kind and tender to him. Now he dreamed it was all the other way about. *In the dream he had a dear and very tender father, whereas the mother was a horrible Megaera. He attacked his mother, then, and strangled her. Then he appeared in the dock charged with matricide.*

Evidently he wishes to protect himself from the influence of the mother and to eradicate his hate against the father.

In another dream he went for a walk with two girls, daughters of a counsellor of a provincial Court, and again appeared suddenly before a court of justice.

From these dreams we observe that on the one hand a strong criminal complex must be present, on the other fear of the consequences of a crime which might bring him before a court of justice. This is confirmed by a stereotyped dream which is periodically repeated. After it he wakes in terror with palpitation of the heart. He stands in truth before an abyss. I propose an analysis to him with which he readily agrees.

The first dream he brings me is remarkable enough. It runs :—

" *I sat with a woman, of whom I only know that she was a woman, in the angle of a low-arched niche built into a deep wall. We both sat there a long time silent. Suddenly there bent round the corner a being whose face was lighted from within as by an electric lamp. It gazed at us for a long time with its glowing eyes, and said : O !* "

The solution of this dream is not difficult to the expert who knows the *religious symbolism of dreams.* The woman in the niche of the wall is the mother of God. He is the Christ-child (Christus-neurosis).[1] His second ego, as he believes the " moral " ego, but in reality the " lustful " ego stared with glowing eyes at the mother of God. The first conclusion is that an *inner* light illuminated him and that therefore he spared the maiden. Evidently moral inhibitory ideas had taken away his potency. The girl was to marry in two weeks. Had he any right to withhold her virginity from the legal husband ? Might not the husband notice that she was no longer a virgin and send her home with abuse and disgrace ?

The second meaning of the dream is traceable to a glowing love for the mother. He looks at this mother with glowing eyes. But what signifies the mysterious " O " ? No association connected with it occurs to the patient.

" Do you not know any poem in which the " O " plays a great part ? "

" Yes, there is some ballad or other which ends that way."

" What is it called and what is it about ? "

" I don't know."

[1] Compare " The Language of the Dream."

DREAD OF THE RAILWAY 251

"I will help you. It is called 'Edward.'"
"Right, Edward."
"What is it about?"
"About a knight who is slain and falls from his horse."
"No. It begins: 'Edward, how is thy sword so red, Edward?
'I have struck my hawk dead, mother, O mother, O!'"
"Right—now I know quite well."
"Do you know the end also?"
"No. I have quite forgotten the last verse."
"Edward has killed his father, he wishes to expiate this, and his foot shall never rest on earth, then he curses his mother and then finally comes the grand climax of the ballad : 'For you, it was you, who advised me! O!' It is just this 'O' which brings out the art of the reciter."
"I know, for a few days ago I recited the ballad aloud in my rooms."
I showed him how strong the repression of patricide-thought must be. In the first dream the converse of this thought appeared. He loved the father and killed the mother. In the second dream he adhered to the latent dream thoughts.[1]
"I had another interesting dream last night," says the patient and reads the next dream to me. As a dream picture it is a curiosity and really very interesting. There followed two other dreams which we will give immediately after the first one :—

I. :—"*I dreamed of an immeasurably high plane placed at an angle of about sixty or seventy degrees and having the appearance of a majolika ; the colour was yellowish, in many places resembling in colour the human skin. The beginning and the end of this plane were covered with masses of mist. Distributed over the whole flat surface in symmetrical order were raised portions in the form of a hexagon, one metre in diameter and raised about fifty cm. from the surface of the raised portion. On this surface moved about naked young men and naked girls, some alone some in close embrace. All had their feet in a peculiar position in that the upper and lower parts of the leg were exactly fitted to four sides of these raised hexagons. All these young people were moving downwards and disappeared gradually in the lower masses of mist. The motion was very peculiar. It was like the gliding of a leaf in slowly flowing water. The leaf as it swims remains attached to any obstacle, breaks away again and so repeats the same game. All these young people swam in the air to one of the raised hexagons, sat down on it, remained sitting some time, got up again, swam on further and so on . . . . And all with their feet in the peculiar position. I myself followed many of the others quite alone also in the same position. When I came to the raised portions where the others had just stayed, I noticed these to have a peculiar greasiness and sliminess. And I called out with an evident feeling of astonished incredulity : ' You are copulating ? ' A derisive laughter was the answer.*"

II. :—"*As a soldier in the manoeuvres I rested in a wooden hut which was as long as my body to the knees, and on the open side was closed by the heavy wing of the open door of a barn. The feet up to the knees—just above which was the under-edge of the barn-door were covered with straw which I saw through the door. Suddenly I heard some one call with a loud voice from a direction I could not determine ' Miloakaberg.'*"

III. :—"*My ego was divided into two parts. The one part was standing behind a table upon which, spread out flat, lay many large bright green apples. The other part was standing before the table among other people. The apples were in the horizontal plane of the eye, so that standing among the spectators one saw only the first row. The first part of my ego, which stood behind the table, said : ' I beg, Saturner.'*"

---

[1] Cf. A. J. Storfer, "On the Special Position of Patricide" (Writings on the Applied Science of the Soul. Leipzig and Vienna, Franz Deutiche, 1911).

The first dream is a rare type. It is a so-called Spermatozoan dream.[1] The patient's ideas confirm the interpretation. He is a student of medicine. I ask if he now works at histology?

" Of course, every day."

" What do the hexagons remind you of ? "

" They are bladder-epithelium cells."

Now the interpretation is plain. The sloping plane the colour of the skin is the penis. But why the number sixty to seventy ?

" How old was your father when he died ? "

" Sixty-five years ! "

" Between sixty and seventy, then ! "

In this dream he is a spermatozoon and according to the infantile sex theory swims about in the bladder till he comes to the mother. The obstacles are cells. Phagocytosis occurs to his mind. He comes through the air into the vagina (greasy, slimy !) and finds that it is a coitus.

The next dream is a womb-fancy.[2] He is in the womb. Straw, of course, easily catches fire. The puzzling word, " Miloakaberg " is explained as follows :

He dissects it into Mil—oaka—and—Berg.[3] As to " Mil " it occurs to him that his mother is called Mila. As to " oaka " he says, one may also divide into " Mi " and " loaka." Then I am under the necessity of putting in a *k*, i.e., " kloaka." But this is the cloaca, such as the duck-bills have, or the vagina of the mother. The word means then : the *mons Veneris* of the mother or the cloaca and the *mons* of Mila.

The last dream has religious symbolism. Apples, of course, are in the Bible the symbol for forbidden sin. The dream tells us of grave sins. But what is the meaning of the mysterious " I beg, *Saturner.*"

At first *satis* occurs to him. Beyond this he cannot go. I point out to him that *Saturner* contains the word *Saturn*. Did he know anything of Saturn and the Saturnalia ? They were Bacchanals with strong erotic tendencies. Slowly I bring him to the fact that Saturn was also called Chronos and was by Zeus—" cut to pieces," he puts in. " No, he was *castrated.*"

" Now you know why you were impotent. You had the phantasy of castrating your father. As a punishment you, according to the lex-talionis, became impotent. Did you weep when your father died ? "

" No, I could not shed a tear."

" You see. Before the girl, you made up for that. It was a sacrifice to appease the manes of the dead father so deeply wronged by you."

Now he mentions further ideas that have occurred to him. Lately he is constantly having to mention the word *Poison*. He says, too, that for some time he has suffered from dread of syphilis, and that in spite of the assurance of all the physicians he took a harmless balamitis for syphilis. Also he was afraid of having paranoia, tabes and paralysis. I point out to him that behind this causeless dread of syphilis lurks the suspicion of having inherited lues from his father.

We return to the word " Saturner." Does he know that lead poisoning is called Saturnism ?

" To be sure. Some years ago I went through an attack of lead-poisoning because I had used lead colours for painting. I would not believe the doctor and took the gingivitis for secondary hues."

Now we know the meaning of the word *Satis* also. He has piled up sins enough. His father cries *Satis* to him, that is also to cut short his satyriasis. He professes to be an atheist. But he reads the Bible for its interest and

[1] This is the first spermatozoa dream that I have found. This discovery was soon confirmed by Marcinowski (" Gezeichnete Traüme," Zentralbl. für Psychoanalyse, Bd. II.) and Silberer (" Spermatozoentraüme," Jahrbuch f. Psychoanalyse, Bd. IV., *pp.* 141 and 708).

[2] Cf. " The Language of the Dream," the chapter, " Womb-dreams."

[3] *Berg* is German for *Mountain*. Translator.

poetry. He visits the churches because it gives him tone and tranquility. O—he would like to believe if he could! He goes to the Court Chapel on Sundays only to hear the sacred music. He is a devotee who will not confess his devotion. He has a stereotyped dream :

" I am reading in a book that I like very much and that I have never read properly. I read aloud and wake up and then half-asleep go on reading. Then I wake up and still see the letters and cannot quote a word of what I have been reading.

This book is the Bible, the book of all books and the prayer book. He prays in dream and by day he is ashamed of his devotion.

We see that he is suffering from a heavy consciousness of guilt with regard to his father. He wished to kill his father! (Edward and Zeus). He himself will be a god (Christ!) He dreams of great medical discoveries which shall benefit mankind. It is a transformation of the religious ideas of redemption. And so concluded the first sitting.

I will not continue this analysis. It shows us the patient's evil ideas and his punishment. His dead father becomes his judge and calls to him a thundering " Satis."

Other cases of impotence depend on criminal phantasies. Unconscious sadists especially, who wish to murder or strangle the woman, easily become impotent. The impotence is then a safety-valve against the criminal impulses. The histories of patients belonging to this category are given in the fourth chapter of this work. There I have treated this subject exhaustively. Here I give only a few indications to illustrate the connection between fear and impotence.

Only two more brief examples of the crippling of aggression by trauma.

A twenty-eight year old medical student suffers from impotence. As a six-year old boy he got into bed with his brother and attempted a sexual act. His father happened to come into the room and thrashed the little one most pitiably. Every time when he wants to make a sexual aggression he experiences an inhibition. Like a warning from distant days, " It will again end in blows."

Another observation :—A thirty-four year old advocate suffers from psychic impotence. The analysis reveals that as a five year old boy he had a beating from his mother because in her bed he attempted indecent pinches.

Of course these infantile traumas do not explain the whole mechanism of a psychic impotence. They are only the nuclei of the crystallisation of the parapathia. And from my present experiences I should maintain that these traumatic cases are comparatively rare and that psychic impotence often represents a very complicated structure. Ethical and religious inhibitions, " fear of woman," and hidden paraphilia combine to produce the picture of an impotence. In the analysis the " cannot " of the impotent one reveals itself as a " will not." Again impotence is one of the man's weapons in the battle of the sexes and enables him to humiliate his partner and to evade crises (Adler). We must remember, too, that many endure similar traumatisms without

K*

injury. The recollection of a trauma signifies often only the repressed longing for its repetition. Besides we must admit that Adler is right when he maintains many a neurotic himself makes traumatisms into a real trauma.

Here let this suffice. One point of view results with absolute certainty from these examples. The only rational treatment for psychic impotence is the analytic method. I can declare with pride : I have succeeded almost always in curing by psycho-analysis alone grave cases of psychic impotence which had for years been treated in vain by the older methods. Psycho-analysis alone is capable of overcoming all inhibitions which prevent a powerful erection. These inhibitions are internal obstacles of which the patient is never fully conscious.

I have yet to mention the fear of infection, especially syphilo-phobia. One of my patients, a physician, could not free himself from this phobia in spite of minutely examining the sexual object every time. It is a precautionary measure to shield the purity of the patient in face of temptations. Syphilis becomes the symbol of the impure (and of incest). The patients tremble for their eternal salvation and in order to attain heaven they make them-selves a hell upon earth.

Syphilo-phobia is also found as a mask for homosexuality. Fear of infections is often only a kind of self-protection. Among im-potents one finds very many who give this fear as the root and cause of their impotence. In the analysis it reveals itself as a fear put forward to hide other deeper motives.

It is precisely psychic impotence which demands the greatest ingenuity, the keenest observation and the finest diplomatic art of the psycho-therapatist. But it has one great advantage : it proves the power of psycho-therapy by results which the patient does not attempt to deny (as happens in so many other cases).

In the female sex also occur all sorts of similar phenomena. " Dread of man " may assume pathological forms and leads to " Evasion of marriage." There are girls who break off every engagement, take their lives before the wedding, or run away on the bridal night from " fear of the pain of defloration."

Fear of pregnancy, too, plays a great part in modern mental life. Of course women also suffer from fear of sexual infections. (Several of these cases are to be found in Vol. III.).

Highly organised feminine minds fear " to lose their ego," to be merged in the man, which expresses itself among other things in a " fear of falling in love." Also dread of an unhappy marriage, dread of a cruel man stand in the way of a normal development especially when unhappy experiences from one's own childhood have made marriage appear as a fight between the sexes. In the psychogenesis of homosexuality such emotions of anxiety form the centre point of various forces which tend to draw the individual

away from the other sex and nearer to his own.   Both " homosexual neurosis " and various paraphilias are fundamentally
latent phobias.

CHAPTER XXV

THE PROFESSIONAL NEUROSIS OF A SINGER

ARTISTS very easily fall ill of conditions of nervous dread which have reference to their calling. Actors fear losing their memory. Singers tremble for their voices. Women pianists suffer from the dread that they may break down in a public performance. Violin players fear that their arms may be crippled, so as to hinder their playing. Such nosophobial conditions generally yield to the reassuring suggestion of the physician.

Much more difficult to cure are artists who have once suddenly broken down in public or who, in consequence of nervousness, no longer appear.

Such disorders are mostly very complicated, and only relieved by a thorough analysis. To throw some light on this obscure region I will publish, as a modest contribution, the complete analysis of an occupation neurosis of this sort in the case of a professional singer. This is at the same time a human document important for the history of modern culture. It reveals more of real life to us than we can get from newspapers, novels and dramas.

No. 123.—Miss N. R., let us call her by her first name, Nastasia —a concert-singer, thirty-two years of age, has been suffering for two years from dread of appearing in public. Even at home she is not capable of singing the smallest song. She is nervous before a number of people, especially before women. She never goes to a theatre or a concert ; she feels that the women are looking down on her with contempt. They criticise her and find her ridiculous. They laugh at her. She often weeps for many hours in the day. Her voice often becomes harsh, simply in speaking. In singing she cannot produce a note. Often she suffers from *taedium vitae*. She asks whether I am not of the opinion that a cancer is forming in her throat. But the objective investigation shows quite normal organs. I tell her that it is a mental trouble and propose a mental treatment, to which she joyfully assents.

I will now try to reproduce the facts in the order in which I had them from her. The anamnesis is incomplete. But we abide by the principle of letting the patient say what she likes in the first sittings without diverting her thoughts by intrusive questions.

Although the patient's history is expressed in an extremely incomplete and fragmentary way, we can yet see from its structure, about where the repressed complexes are to be sought. Even from the first narration one can see where the kernel of the neurosis lies.

She comes from a healthy family, has no hereditary taint; her father died from a cancer in the rectum.

As to the first years of her childhood she cannot communicate anything of importance. She grew up in Petersburg as daughter of a teacher, had no friends and play-fellows, which as she thinks has had an effect on her whole life. As a child she was very pious and occupied herself with religious questions. In spite of this she could not be induced to be confirmed at fourteen years of age, because she took everything literally and felt she had not the strength to undertake the full responsibility for a religious life. She would rack her brains for days over certain passages in the Bible and the prayer book. She was not confirmed until she was seventeen. But it was no light matter; she had to be forced to it by begging and threatening. She was dissatisfied with everybody. In her opinion people were not leading Christian lives. Indeed, she wished to become a preacher herself and to make known the word of God. But at her confirmation she did not take the Communion. She did not feel convinced that she would feel *pure* enough at the moment of the holy act. She had a beautiful voice, and at first wished to sing only in church in order to please God. Here her splendid voice attracted an organist who told her mother that he would teach her singing and develop her art. And she made rapid progress. Unfortunately the teacher fell so violently in love with his pupil that he made her an offer of marriage. She was indifferent to the man. Indeed, when they were together he repelled her. Only when she was alone she had a feeling for him which, however, she called not " love " but " motherly feeling." He soon saw how hopeless was his suit and sent her to another teacher. Here, too, she was dissatisfied, so that one day she resolved to set off quite alone to Berlin and there to perfect her singing.

The story of this journey sounds very romantic and gives glimpses of the fantastic nature of hysterical women. But as I convinced myself later, the patient is thoroughly truthful and has not embroidered this first story at all. In Warsaw there entered the train which was taking her from Petersberg to Berlin a strikingly handsome elegant looking man, a professor of Warsaw. They entered into conversation, and she had the feeling all the time that the man might offer violence to her. He behaved himself irreproachably, however, and promised to visit her the next day. He came as he had promised, addressed her at once by her Christian name, " Nastasia," and behaved with great familiarity. However, she followed him because she believed she could not do otherwise. He took her then in a carriage to his friends. The whole time she was thinking : " *Whatever will he do with you ?* "[1] And then they came to an elegant palace where he took her to a splendid apartment, and introduced her to an elderly American couple, who at once gave her a warm welcome. They were eccentrics who took a great liking to her. However, the professor had soon to go away before the two became very intimate. After some years he once attempted to play the lover, in order as he said, to repay himself, but she did not yield to his entreaties. She studied hard. After about a year the professor's brother came to Berlin, fell in love with her and made her a proposal of marriage. He was " fabulously " rich and begged her only not to say " No " to him or he must take his life. " You can think it over quietly," he said, " but you must not say ' No ' to me ; otherwise I shall take my life." She was not in a position to accept this man and one night she left Berlin to return to her parents in Petersburg. In the meantime her destiny had fulfilled itself. She had received a recommendation to a famous violinist. When she entered his room she experienced something like a complete involuntary subjugation. It was as if the man had hypnotized her. She knew at once, " You will belong to this man ; he can do what he likes with you." A telegram from her friends called her back from Petersburg. She may return to Berlin without fear. The rich suitor will no longer force himself upon her, he will wait until her stubborn will is softened. The poor young fellow died two years later of *cancer in the throat.* In the meantime her training was completed, everyone praised her splendid voice and her grasp of her work, and she went on a provincial stage to acquire routine. She had been there only a few days when the director invited her to an interview in his house, and gave her to understand that she pleased him very much and that he would do his utmost to assist her training if she would show herself not unfriendly to him. Then he tried to put his arm round her waist and to kiss her. She uttered some energetic words of refusal and the result was that during the whole season she was able to appear only once and then only as a substitute. So began her career ! With her second engagement she had no better fortune. There it was again the bandmaster who, after the study of a part, embraced her and wanted to kiss her, to which she responded with a blow in the face and " You are a shameless, insolent man ! " So here, too, began a real martyrdom. She received notice and waged war on the bandmaster by giving a concert which should demonstrate her gifts to the public. The concert was a splendid success, but her enjoyment of the stage was utterly destroyed, and she became a concert singer. She travelled—for she soon became famous—through the whole world ; earned a great deal and gave a great deal away. In the

---

[1] This question refers to the cure. So does the feeling *as if the man might offer violence to her.* In the first sitting thoughts about the mental physician who is conducting the cure, play a great part also in this narration.

meantime she had become the musician's mistress. Let us call him Pawlow. Her fame grew and her successes were very great. But only, as she states, " because she could throw into her singing all her misfortunes and disappointment." She maintains that she "masturbated" every time on the stage. That sent the people into transports. The last time she sang a cycle of Russian folk-songs in Petersburg. The success was extraordinary, but after the concert she felt so tired and exhausted that she thought : " I can sing no more." *She feared her own voice.* And since then she has not been able to sing a note.

Such the story of her life-career. I call her attention to some peculiarities of this record of her trouble, which passes over such important things in silence and gives prominence to such trifles. Especially to the confirmation. Here one must note plainly that she has greatly occupied herself with physical things because that was the way by which she came to be so pre-occupied with metaphysical things. She states—and this in convincing fashion— that she has never physically masturbated. Of sex matters she had no notion until long after the confirmation. How did it come that she would not take the communion ? That she explains, was only her exaltation of mind. As early as thirteen years old, it was her way to have such high-flown ideas. Thus, e.g., she had composed a fairly long essay on Platonic love. This ended the first sitting. It is noteworthy that she talked for an hour of the men she had refused. A certain regret for so much despised love, for the lost fortune of the first serious suitor, which now by inheritance would have been her own, was clearly evident beneath her indignation. For the rest, she presented herself to me with her wonderful successes, her original character and her prudery.

The next time, since nothing occurred to her spontaneously and she opposed a great resistance to the analysis, I tried to find out the circumstances under which she came to lose her voice. She states that it was not a cycle of Russian songs but of songs by a young poet ; the story was terribly sad and depicted the wandering of a forsaken mother with her child through Siberia. This had excited her fearfully. The public was so affected that several women fell in a swoon, and every one in the hall sobbed and shivered. It was difficult to find any connection between the subject of the song and the personal experiences of the singer. She ceased speaking. Nothing more occurred to her. She had already told me everything. So I try an association experiment and asked her to mention some words which may arbitrarily suggest themselves to her. She begins at once and names the series : Dog, Tree, Wood, Way, Flower, Spring, Forester, Hill, Sun, Deep shade, Wind, Stream. Before " Stream " there was rather a long pause. Then come the words Roe, Finger-post, Heather, Stone. Then I usually arrange to have one or two associated words mentioned for each of the words given. In this case the associations were : Dog—

faithful ; Tree—bush ; Wood—cool ; Way—broad ; Flower—red ; Spring—fresh ; Forester—healthy ; Hill—view ; Sun—warm ; Deep shade—rest ; Wind—strife ; Roe—beauty ; Finger-post—reach ; Stone—overcome. Now I get the explanation of these associations and behold ! it appears that these associations are the expression for certain repressed complexes. For three or four hours a word will appear mysterious, arbitrarily chosen, and then all of a sudden comes the explanation. The dog is faithful—she is now leading a dog's life. For she has not yet told me the most important thing. That P. is married and has a wife in Peters-burg. The wife will not get a divorce although he has never lived with her for ten years. It often seems to her as if she has lost her will. The dog is the symbol of fidelity. (A later explanation of the symbol " dog " comes in a dream afterwards). She, too, is faithful. But it hurts her that she cannot marry P. The better sort of houses are all closed to her, because she is not his legal wife ; so she never goes into society. Also she cannot live in the same house with P. " Tree, wood, way." Her favourite haunt is the woodland. When she walks with P. through the woods she is overcome by an " almost mad " love—She is always modest and reserved. But when he thus goes before her in the wood it comes over her that she must cry out to him : " Embrace me and take possession of me." She could—in this one situation in life—demand of him that he should caress her as he does at night. Why this happens in the wood she cannot conceive. But in walking through a wood she is liable to show a weakness for other men too. " Tree, wood and way " lead now direct to the sexual complex. " Flower —red " a world-old symbol. To pluck flowers (deflorer !) usual expression for seeking amatory indulgence. " Spring "—frequent symbol for bladder. Of course for picking flowers in the wood there must be a " healthy forester." " Hill " (*mons Veneris*), " Sun " (joy in life), " Deep shadows " (one gets round the eyes if one lives too fast), " Wind " (inexplicable for the moment—seems to be connected with an anal complex which will appear later) lead to " *Stream* (Fluss) although after a long pause (ten seconds !). Here it occurs to her that as a girl she has suffered from leucorrhœa (Fluss)[1] which made her feel very unclean. A lady used to come and syringe her daily. As a child washing was of all things her greatest passion. " I was insanely fond of washing," she says, " especially dolls' linen. I should have liked of all things to become a washerwoman." (The washings are symbolic. They are to serve instead of the purity that is lacking.) She still washes her hands several times a day, and her whole body twice a day. She always washes after stool, and after making water. She washes her nose and throat daily ; but she does not syringe the vagina,

[1] The word *Fluss* in the original means, *stream, river,* and also *flow, catarrh, leucorrhoea.*

because she does not now suffer from leucorrhœa.[1] That was only in her youth. Now the association " Roe—beauty " becomes comprehensible. She often said of herself that she was like a young roe. " Finger-post " expresses the longing to escape from the mental labyrinth ; " Heather," with the association, " melancholy," calls to mind a song of a poor forsaken maiden driven to wander through the world alone, over sharp stones with bare feet ; she is such a poor pilgrim who has to wander over sharp stones.

Now I myself say to her a number of arbitrarily chosen words, of which three become specially conspicuous through the delay in her reaction. These are : *man—egoist ; sofa—convenient ; passion—cruel.* We come to speak of P., who she considers is of a rather egoistic disposition. All men are egoists. For the moment these associations suggest nothing more to her. Later, however, we shall see that she has here betrayed important complexes, certainly the sadistic complex. The next day she begins her association series with : *stool—carpet—curtain.* Further, after a pause : *street, carriage, person, dog, tree, hotel, garden, railway, view, hill, valley, stream, wood, woodland way, bench, bird, spring, shade.* We shall soon learn that all these words are of great importance for her life, and that they occur to her only on account of their intimate connection with her repressed complexes.

For *stool* the association *green* occurs. At first she cannot explain this. She believes that her father had at home a convenient green stool before his writing table. Now, however, it suggests to her that as a ten year old child she suffered from a very strange obsession. She had the feeling that she must never leave anything behind in a strange house, especially never attend to a call of nature there. She did not spit, she could on no account be induced, by no matter what urgency, to relieve herself there. She always ran home. She believed in fact that something costly would be lost, that she would become unhappy, as if it was a part of her, of all of them. This attachment to her house and garden was so great that she thought, *if her father should come to die,* she would marry his successor just to be able to remain in the house. These obsessions she cannot explain. But as they occurred to her immediately after the associations " stool " and " green." I tell her that they must evidently have some relation with these. And then it occurs to her. She was a little girl, four years old, and sat on her father's lap. Then her father gave her a bright copper coin to play with, which she suddenly swallowed. The household became greatly excited ; they sent for a physician who thought it might be dangerous, because copper gets covered with verdigris. Now she became the object of the most anxious attention in the house. She had to use a little pot for stool, and father always came and

[1] The most frequent cause of leucorrhœa with little girls is, of course, masturbation. In a double sense they feel " unclean."

looked in to see if the coin was there yet. And lo! on the second day the coin was found, and it was quite green. (Hence the association : stool—green.) This scene had made a great impression on the child. At other times the father, whom she greatly honoured and loved, had not troubled much about her. Only then had he devoted all his attention and tenderness to her. This little experience influenced all the future ; the stool still plays to-day a great part in her life. The obsessive feeling that she cannot leave anything in a strange house has the same origin. For in those two critical days it was impressed on the child to take care and not go to stool outside the house, otherwise the coin would not be found. And so there remained with her as a substitute for the suppressed wish : " If only my father would occupy himself with me and my body ! "—the obsession that she must not leave anything behind anywhere. For in fact she wished every day that she had such a coin so that she looked on her stool like money, as a valuable property of the family. (These associations between stool and money are so widespread that one would be almost disposed to consider the incident as imaginary, but that the coin faithfully preserved by her, and also her mother's account confirm the reality of the experience.) Anal processes still play a great part in her life to-day. Also she has to-day a great feeling of pleasure in making a stool, she does it twice a day always with a certain erotic enjoyment, with a great apparatus of preparations. She finds great joy in sitting, in her room she must have great accommodation for sitting, quite a number of seats, arm-chairs, and settees. She must have plenty of cushions at hand if she is to feel comfortable. Psychologically, too, the " anal character "[1] as Freud has called it is expressed by three attributes. Those people with whom the anus represents an erogenic zone are according to the consequent sublimation of the analeroticism (1) pedantic and order loving ; (2) obstinate and (3) very covetous. These qualities she has, all of them, to a certain extent. With the discovery of this fact the second sitting ends.

The next day she remembers a dream of a type she often had as a girl. She sat on a horse and rode round an apple tree which was blossoming. She wanted to pluck a twig and did so. But the blossoms fell off like snow.

This dream, so beautiful and poetic, had a concealed connection with her reading. At that time she had been reading Emilia Galotti, which had made a great impression on her. The well-known saying : " A rose broken ere the storm stripped it bare," gave her food for much thought. She played tragic solo scenes in which at the close she took her life. The situation, sitting on and riding a horse. is typical and represents the reversed phantasy of a coitus. But in this case a coitus without consequences. She

---

[1] Charakter und Analerotik. Psychiatr.-neurolag. Wochenschrift. IX. year, No. 52. " Orderly, frugal and self-willed," Freud calls these analerotics.

broke the blossoms from the tree, without its coming to fruit. She remained pure as snow. Apple tree—a connection with the Bible which in her religious period she read with passionate devotion (tree of the knowledge of good and evil). To sit, to ride on the horse, the picture reminds her of the scenes in which she sat on her father's knee and rode hopp—hopp—hopp, which gave her a pleasant feeling. Breaking twigs, tearing one down for herself, souvenir of the infantile masturbation. In other words, this is one of those beautiful ideal dreams which so often pass through girls' minds and which are yet only the symbolic ideal incorporation of a sexual desire. In the association experiment of the last day there were still some words which were not completely explained. To-day they are taken up and yield quite interesting points of view. After "Wood—woodland way," there came once the association *noise*. It then occurs to her that even now she has one idiosyncracy. She hates noise in a wood. She cannot bear it if P. walks through a wood with her and treads on the dry leaves so that it makes a noticeable noise. That is intolerable for her. As a child she was never in the woods! Or—yes! It suddenly occurs to her that she was in the woods only once a year, and indeed with the whole school. And that was *hateful*. The noise was positively loathsome to her. Of course, behind this there is hidden jealousy of her father. She went to the woods with many children and, as teacher, the father had to busy himself with them a great deal, caressed some of them, and so on. Then she became frightfully jealous and hated these excursions. For she wanted to have her father all to herself. At such times she would have liked to have torn him from the children and to have kissed and embraced him a thousand times. Now two things are explained : first, why she gets sexually excited when she goes through the wood with her lover *alone ;* it is the memory of the infantile scene when out of jealousy she wanted so much to embrace her father ; secondly, it explains the dislike for any noise in the wood because with the association " Woodland way " is aroused her aversion for the noise of the excursions. Her love still belongs to her father. She fell in love with P. only because he reminded her of her father. Also he is twenty-two years older than she. He might quite well be her father. Also he is as strict and pedantic in his ways as her father. Her father had wonderfully beautiful hands. She fell in love with P.'s hands !

Another very interesting, constantly recurring fancy in earlier years was the feeling that she had *lived twice before : once as a young man who lived a very gay life and died young, and the second time as a priestess who danced religious dances.* I call her attention to the plain meaning that this is evidently the expression of the two tendencies that are warring in her breast. She must as a young girl have been very gay and full of high spirits, a state of feeling which, however, soon died away. And then, as we know, came the pious, religious period, when she wanted to be a preacher. She has lived through both these stages, but these memories are cloak-memories and conceal psychic processes of her childhood. At once she calls to mind a little experience which strikingly confirms this. Once she had drunk too much so that P. had to take her from the restaurant to a room in the hotel. Then she tore her blouse open and said : " If I were a young man I should have to have a fresh woman every night." But this is the reversal of the wish as a young girl to be possessed by a different man every day. On the other hand, there is manifest here an evident homosexual disposition. We shall see how far this is correct.

Two little dreams bring marked erotic relationships. One : *" I danced in a white dress with an umbrella, then changed into the black dress which I wear every day."* Umbrella = sex symbol for penis.[1] Dance = copulate. This is a coitus scene after which she dresses in black. But the addition " which I wear every day " " gives to think." It seems a confirmation but must in reality be a disguise. It was a dress that she did not wear every day, namely, a mourning dress. Since she woke up with a certain feeling of fear, it seems as if she was harbouring secret thoughts relating to P.'s death. She would like to have her freedom again. That is certainly confirmed later. All phobia patients show the same thing. In dreams and in their phantasies they all do away with those they love. Hence arises in part her deep consciousness of guilt. Next day she brings a stereotyped dream which often comes to her. She had a child, and the child was cold, and was forsaken and in need of protection. This is an evident exhibition dream (child meaning vagina). She can remember countless such children dreams. They also occur as waking dreams in the day-time. The child that needs protection expresses also her dissatis-faction with P. For the rest it was her most fervent wish to have a child by P.[2]

The next detailed dream leads us yet deeper into the problem of her illness.

" I was in a barn. Several artists were there, but all musicians. A couple came from behind, they were very hot and were wiping them-selves dry. They were a pianist and a violinist. They said it was unbearable there, it was too hot. Also I talked with a gentleman who is a great scoundrel. He said : ' I have discovered something new. Let us try it together. It will be grand. We will not speak of it to anyone.' Then somebody came and said : ' You, Miss N., you

---

[1] Very frequently, evidently because the umbrella is raised (representing an erection).

[2] We think of the occasion when the neurosis became manifest. She sang a song of a mother, who wandered freezing with a child through Siberia. That was her history. She froze in the company of her cold lover. She and her " child," which we must take symbolically. (Cf. " The Language of the Dream." *The role of relatives in the dream*).

cannot sing, your number must be left out.' I had the feeling that the circumstances were such that I could not appear. Then the gentleman wished to play something from Schumann as a substitute for my number. The little Mischa Elman was there too, but as a great artist. I sat on a long carriage and had many tarts. They were badly packed. I said : ' That is the bad " Vienna packing."' Then some one gave me a book with which one could make purchases, but I had a feeling of shame as if that was not quite honourable. And yet I had a desire to try it. The temptation was there. Whether anything happened then, I cannot remember."

Clearly it is an erotic dream, which conceals a number of men to whom she had taken a fancy and who were unattainable for her. These were mostly musicians and artists. She gave a long list of well-known names. One she reproached with having no heart, another she told he was not worth a woman's troubling about. To the third she said, after his performance : " If I were a young girl I would kiss you now." In short, they are all men who have not possessed her and who now move in her dreams in a way which indicates her " anal " character.[1] Further, the recollection takes her to a scoundrel, a man from whom she had expected special sensations in the region of erotics. (" I have discovered something new. Let us try it together.") Of importance is the sentence that she cannot sing, and that now her number is left out, because it perhaps explains to us why she cannot sing. A little contribution appears. Here the dream, the analysis of which was scarcely indicated here, manifests itself as a scoff at P., whose potency seems to have fallen short of her requirements. Her *number (!)* is omitted[2] and the circumstances are to blame for this. She asks P. for love and he plays classical compositions to her. See the sentence with the ironical expression, " The gentleman " : " *The gentleman wished to play something from Schumann as a substitute for my number which had been left out.*" Pawlow's favourite number on the violin is the " Reverie " of Schumann.

He gives huge sums for nice dress boots and has a charming small foot (Schumann). " The little Mischa Elman was there too, as a great artist," is the phantasy of a " little fellow " (penis) which can perform much. The bad packing of the tarts is a scoff at P. The sweets are not well packed, they fall out too soon. But then comes the plain phantasy that she is a prostitute. She has a book for buying, sets her snares and seeks out just as many men as she pleases. This interpretation of the dream makes her quite sad. She had never thought that she was such a wicked person. To comfort her I point out that really only over-moral women get ill because they have to repress so much of the natural instincts,

[1] (" A couple came from behind. They were very hot.")

[2] And also the wish : " Oh, may P. die, so that I may dispose of myself as I please."

whereas the so-called bad ones remain healthy because they can live out their instincts. That consoles her to some extent. At the following sitting she comes into the room and hands me a little present. It is a richly carved ruler from Petersburg. The words which occurred to her the day before are : *Sofa—writing-table —soft—warm—fire—bare foot—spirit—flame—cylinder—dog—stool book-case*—and then after a rather long pause—*instrument—flower— window, door—foot stool—singing waters.* The transference begins to come into play. She has handed me a ruler, therewith conferring on me to a certain extent the same rights as her father. But the ruler has also another meaning. For she tells me she must make a confession. In gross material intercourse she never finds satisfaction. But when she has stimulating conversation with men about art and science, then she has such a feeling of satisfaction and in such moments wishes to have a child. She often thinks why are things so horribly arranged ? Why can one not produce by speaking and kissing, a child that shall combine in itself all the properties of both the producers ? Now I point out to her that symbolically she has really done that. For she has given me a little stick, from which I conclude that she is erotically excited by our conversation, which she at once admits.[1] I point out to her that to-day she has ostentatiously laid her vanity-bag on the sofa, a symptomatic act which amounts to a challenge. And now we remark, to our amusement, that the word-series which she produced the day before contains the same train of thought. It begins with *sofa*, comes to the *writing-table*, where I sit, proceeds through *soft, warm* and *fire* to the *bare foot*, whereat it occurs to her that she likes very much to go about bare foot at home (cf. the first series—Stone—bare foot) and that she thinks a great deal of her beautiful foot. " Spirit-flame, cylinder, dog, stool," owe their significance to the erotic complex. The doubt whether I, as a savant who is occupied with books (book-case) will occupy myself with her is ended after a rather long pause with the association, *instrument*. That it is an instrument for opening that is meant is clear, and that this instrument then finds window and door open is easily understood. " Foot stool " refers to her joy in sitting (she would like to sit at my feet) while " Singing waters " symbolises a coitus scene.

I now point out to her that she is in the stage of *transference*, and that it is for this reason she occupies herself with my person. I do not omit to make it clear to her that the success of the cure is only possible if the danger of this transference is averted in good time, and that this is most easily effected by expressing oneself openly about it. In the next association experiment, in which I choose

---

[1] Compare the analysis of a case of obsession neurosis in a woman teacher : " Diagnostiche assoziation studien," No. 6 (1906). A girl sits on her teacher's lap. Then she says, laughing : " The teacher can never get away from his occupation. He even has a ruler in his trouser's pocket." (*Jung*.)

some words, there are some interesting points. To *backwards* comes after a rather long pause *dark* (anal complex). To *number* comes seven, which at first she cannot explain. The next day she brings the explanation. P. is the seventh child of his parents and was always called No. Seven at home. We now know also which number must be left out. To *tart* comes after a long pause, *not eatable*, which again expresses her aversion for P. His caresses are evidently insufficient. The bad Vienna packing so that the tarts fall out too soon ! (Ejaculatio præcox.)

I must refrain from going into other interesting associations, because we must consider a much more important dream, which makes her phobia psychologically comprehensible. Up till now it had always remained a mystery why she has ceased to sing. There came, to be sure, in the association experiments and the dream analyses, memories which explained a great deal. But not all. One of the memories plays an important part because she was proud of it. She said as early as the first sitting " that she had never been jealous, and had even brought a woman to P. herself." Yes, for in fact he was an artist and needed excitement. This was a dancer from the Petersburg *corps de ballet*, splendidly beautiful, and celebrated. P. loved her to distraction. Even then I suspected that this must be connected with her dread of appearing in public. And the dream brought me complete certainty. It ran thus :

" *I was in a great banking house which was very high, and all at once I could not resist : I sang, but not a song. It sounded tremendous. Then there came an official and said he must give notice because he could not endure it (because I made such a scene). I quieted him and said : ' I will not do it again.' Then I saw one of our actresses. She was quite naked, undressed like a prostitute. Then I was given something to count. But I could not get above twenty-two. There was always some confusion. It was cold and she begged me to give her one of the woollen cloths with which I had counted. All at once I was in an old-fashioned concert-costume. It was like a half crinoline. I untied the ribbons in order to be able to walk faster and to hold the dress up better. Then it began to rain. Sonja said I must call out for an umbrella, and P. said he was bringing one. He was dressed as for a great festival. She said : ' But for me too.' I thought : ' You don't know P. a bit. There I must go alone.' "*

The dream touches the deepest problems of her parapathy. We shall soon see how it lays bare the mystery, why she can no longer sing. Let us begin the analysis : " *She was in a great banking house.*" She loves a house with plenty of accommodation for sitting, many benches.[1] Then occurs to her the bank[1] from which P. always gets his money. Also her house in Potsdam, near Berlin,

---

[1] The word *Bank* in the original means *bench* and also *bank* or *banking house*.—Translator.

occurs to her (*Potz — Damm*).[1] "*It was very high*" refers to a sexual phantasy of the structure of her vagina. A physician told her her larynx was large and high-built. Evidently it is a phantasy of a great penis which occurs in all cases of anxiety hysteria. "*All at once I could not resist,*" it goes on. At that time she had in Potsdam, where she lived, an experience to be described later. It continues : "*I sang, but not a song.*" As a child she had a habit of going about and singing wild notes, composing something and at the close she would in her phantasy kill herself, and she fell dead on the ground. She remembers an attempt at suicide which she made in Potsdam. Really not an attempt, only a thought of suicide. At that time, she had, as she said, brought P. and the dancer together. In reality they had met at a seaside resort and had come to know and to love each other. It turns out that not only had she done nothing to bring the two together, but she suffered so much from jealousy that she brought about a separation between P. and his beloved. She had believed at the time that she had the magnanimity to look on while P. lived for a time with another. But that was beyond her power. She wrote to him once from Petersburg that he must choose between her and the dancer ; she could not share him. Then she came to Berlin and made a regular scene. (This made a great deal of noise.) P. now lay down on the sofa and fell asleep, but she opened a book that lay there which was a present from " her." It bore an inscription to P. of an extraordinary passionate nature : " I bind thee with a thousand chains which thou wilt never break ! " When she read that she stole from the room to commit suicide. She wanted to throw herself into the water. But P. seems to have noticed something or, unconsciously, she did not do it so quietly as she wished. In short, he hurried after her, caught her in time and brought her back by gentle force. He promised to make an end of the whole thing. Originally P. wanted to forsake her. To this refers : "*He gives notice to leave ; he wanted to leave her because he cannot endure it.*" But yet another experience occurs to her. She once had an interview with the ballet dancer in Petersburg. She was so shameless that she did not hesitate to seek her out in her Petersburg residence and to ask her for a recommendation to the Director of the Petersburg Opera with whom she was on very good terms. Of course the false woman did this only as a pretence in order to get to know her and perhaps to meet P. again and to get him again into her net. This excited her frightfully at the time. But what had excited her yet more was that she had found in one of the dancer's letters the sentence : " How can you think so much of a person like Nastasia. *She has certainly a shocking voice. I cannot conceive how you, as a musical man, can endure listening to her ugly voice.*" She had then under the impression of the visit temporarily lost her voice. She was hoarse and her voice failed. In the

[1] A German oath. *Potz* = *Gotts* or *Gottes* (God's).—Translator.

presence of this Sonja she could not produce a single clear note. This letter excited her tremendously. It brought things to a crisis and she demanded of P. that he should write the dancer a farewell letter. He wrote three letters. None of them would do, and finally she dictated one to him, and that he sent. At last she had vanquished the hated rival. But at what a cost! Relations with the seductive Circe were broken off. But all the same P. had not forgotten the beautiful dancer. He has a slow, sluggish mental digestion. From time to time he still speaks of her again. Therefore here in the dream she calls him the " *official.*" As *official*, too, there occurs to her a young fellow who is an admirer of P., and obtrudes himself upon him. *But he will not associate with him.* The continuation of the dream contains a fine revenge on the dancer who has caused her so much trouble. She sees her naked as a prostitute. " *She gives her something to count. But she cannot get above twenty-two.*" P. is twenty-two years older than she. She was twenty-two years old when she became acquainted with P. The dancer is twenty-two years old. Above this number she cannot get. Now it occurs to her that in the dream she always counted eight, ten, twenty-two. Ten years she has lived with P., eight years she had lived with him when it nearly came to a breach on account of the dancer. Now she avenges herself on her for robbing her of two years of her life. She dresses very simply. She knew that the dancer wore fine *silk* underclothing. In the dream Sonja is naked and she covers her with two *woollen* cloths. The continuation of the dream refers to a memory in which an actress named Kurt played a part. The connection is prostitute, courtesan, Kurt. Once when it rained, she had lent her a reform-dress. Mrs. Kurt had also a husband who made hot love to her. But she repulsed him, she behaved very differently from the dancer. She did not mix in other people's affairs. She did not take other women's husbands away from them. And yet—did she not? She had taken the husband away from P.'s wife. But he was already separated from his wife and lived apart from her. The end of the dream is the phantasy that she marries P. " *She goes to fetch her umbrella.*" Naturally the dancer demands one, too (" *for me, too.*") She answers, however, smartly : " *Here I must go myself.*" This is indeed her present resolve : she would like to go to Petersburg for a time to recover her tranquillity.

This dream then again reveals a solution of the mystery, why she cannot sing. Firstly, she does not want to earn anything, so that P. must provide for her as for his wife. Secondly, she cannot hear her voice because involuntarily she remembers the saying of the dancer. It is also as if she wished to punish P. because his beloved found her voice ugly. For this reason P. shall never hear her voice again. She repeats that at the last concert she sang so despairingly that everyone was struck by it, and the people were quite staggered. She sang a ballad in which an unhappy woman was hunted like a wild beast. A gentleman of her acquaintance (then an *official*) said to her : " That was rather a cry than singing." The next day she comes in ill-humour. She is tired as if she had been beaten. " As if I had," she says, smiling, " given her a thrashing with the ruler." The dream which she brings is rather important. " *A strange woman has hidden her child. I must not see it. At this I scolded and cried terribly. Then I see P. with another lady like a shadow, as if he were in a salt mine or in a pit.*" The strange woman about whom she makes such a fuss is my wife (the transference continues). But it is also Frau P., who will not do her the favour to die. Whenever she takes up a Russian newspaper she always expects to see this woman's death announced. It occurs to her also that in the electric railway she has an obsession. She was present once when a woman was run over. Since then she cannot help thinking of this in the electric train without having some fear for herself. She has the feeling that *another woman will be run over*. And now it occurs to her that Mrs. P. was once run over by a train, and remained alive in spite of it. Her obsession in the electric train springs from the repressed thought : " Oh, if Mrs. P. would die ! Oh, if she had only died when she was run over."[1] Her child signifies the genitals to which she alone is entitled. A member (" the little one ") belonging to her has been hidden. *Then she saw P. like a shadow in the grave.* The story of the salt-mine was as follows. She was once with P. in a salt mine. She liked it exceedingly and felt quite well there. But he could not bear the heavy air, it seemed to stifle him. In the dream she avenges herself for his unfaithfulness with the dancer and causes him to die in the pit. P. and " another lady " are in the kingdom of shadows, they lie in the grave. I point out to her that parallel with her love for P., there is another tendency, hate for the man who has robbed her of ten years of her life and has torn her away from her career. Then a number of things occur to her with which she has to reproach P. He is too soft. He gives words only, never deeds. He would never stand up brutally to his wife and force the divorce upon her. She has the longing of the outcast for respectability. He has already had opportunities when that would have been possible. Then she considers that he did not restrain her with sufficient energy when she told him that she was going home to Petersburg. He took that simply as a matter of fact.

The next day still stands under the sign of the transference. Little occurs to her. The association experiment (free association words to which the reaction words are afterwards added) gives a series of words which refer to me. *Child*—beautiful; *books*—many; *pocket*—black; *hair*—black; *feather*[2]—broad; *lamp*—

---

[1] She wished to make another woman dumb, and became dumb herself. (Lex talionis).

[2] The day before she had brought me a case filled with broad feathers as a present for my writing table.

bright ; *tea*—delicious.; *writing-table*—large ; *book-case*—much ; *bird*—yellow ; *piano*—small ; *carriage*—convenient ; *pictures*— gay coloured ; *bust*—sleeping ; *wife*—poured ; *portieres*—brown ; *letter holder*—red ; *carpet*—soft ; *stove*—white ; *glasses*—green. *Child* again occurs as a phallus symbol. *Books* is known to us from the dream where she is a prostitute. *Pocket* and *hairs* both black (female genital organ) through *feather*—broad (male) and *lamp*—bright (female) to *tea* with the association delicious. Yesterday she wanted to have a cup of tea when she got home and P. did not wish it. That she cannot pardon him that she must always be his slave. This reproach is necessary so that she may excuse her love-thoughts for me. For immediately after *tea* comes the association *writing-table*—large and *book-case*—much. Book-case puzzled me for a long time. I wanted to interpret it as *savant*, but the patient did not agree with this explanation ; then it occurred to me that, after all, the case serves to hold the books, that she requires many testimonies of love, so that *book*-case[1] represents the symbol for a very potent man. Then follows *bird*—yellow (flesh colour) ; *piano*—play (frequent symbol for copulate). She is proud of her little piano. She is a convenient *carriage*. Then follow *pictures* (she brought me pictures to-day in which she is photographed half-naked in the sea and her attractive bust is very evident). After a short pause follows *wife*, the great obstacle that stands in the way, *partieres* (which keep the light off) are brown, while the *pocket* is black. *Letter case*, by which she means an under-blanket, which is red. *Soft carpet* which has the same meaning as the convenient carriage, leads to *stove*, one of the most frequent symbols for women who are passionate. *Glasses* is at first not quite clear, and refers to the fact that her lover received eighteen glasses from her mother. (A contribution to the meaning of the dream before the last : eight plus ten).

At the following sitting there occurs to her a recollection which is the typical recollection of a woman who suffers from hysteria. We shall seldom find a case of anxiety hysteria in which the phantasy of a gigantic penis does not play a great part. With our patient it has already been indicated ; witness the ruler and the beginning of the dream of the banking house, where it goes up very high. The recollection refers to the period between the twelfth and thirteenth years of her life. She came out of school with her friend. Behind a tree stood a man who suddenly exposed himself. He had trousers which flap down in front like the peasants' and there she saw something enormous surrounded with bushy hair. She ran home crying ; her father asked her what had happened, and she said she could only tell it to her mother. This was a gentleman she knew, a little, weak man who was married and had six children. She knows for certain that in her phantasy the penis

---

[1] Every book represents a " number." In large libraries the books are labelled with numbers.

had magnified itself considerably because she did not expect anything so gigantic to belong to such a weak man. It was no phantasy but a real experience. The man was not prosecuted.
The next day she experienced a great joy. *She sang again for
the first time for two years, two songs and a dramatic scene, continuing
for an hour without getting tired. Her voice sounded splendid! She
and P. wept for joy.*
The next day she had to tell me something painful. She had
received a letter from Petersburg in which she was informed that
her brother's wife was very seriously ill. For a second the thought
thrilled through her, if this woman should die she would go to
Petersburg and keep house for her brother, then she would really
be provided for. The brother is younger than she and is strikingly
like her father. When she saw him last she was amazed that in
speech, in gait, and in bearing, he so entirely resembled her father.
She knows that her brother has a rare admiration for her so that
his wife was jealous for a time. The original thought must have
run otherwise. She wanted to take her mother's place. There
was one person too many. If the mother dies I shall be her
successor. We remember that she had an obsession, if the father
dies, she will marry his successor. This obsession was only the
masking of a more painful thought. Because she identified the
brother with the father she must now identify the seriously ill wife
of the brother with her mother and hence the death thought. Then
she wrote her brother a letter in which she inquired with exaggerated
tenderness as to the state of his wife.
She brings me another dream : *She is with me in the room, and
sings the part of Gretchen in " Faust." She begs to have the little
table pushed on one side, she would like to stand there. Then she sang.
It was not the right place. She was not standing as she wished.*
She groaned so that she wakened P. from his sleep. We remember
that in one of her last dreams she quarrelled with a woman and
then awoke weeping. This was my wife. In this case too, we
have to do with the results of the transference. The little table
that she wants out of the way, stands to the left of the piano.
The reason why she wishes to stand there is interesting. Close to
the little table hangs a large pastel of my wife which she always
looks at while she has to wait till it is her turn. She wants to place
herself near my wife. We understand then why *she was not standing
as she wished.* In passing, it may be mentioned that the dream
has also another meaning, that *to sing* means for her also *to copulate,*
that P.'s deficient potency is scoffed at. Now it occurs to her that
she has another obsession. She dreads counting. That we saw

---

¹ These thoughts of death reveal the strongly *sadistic* side of her character.
Once more she wished to make a human being dumb. The dead can no
longer speak and sing. She punished herself with the suffering which best
symbolised this infliction of dumbness. As a singer she was dead after
losing her voice.

in the dream where she could not get above twenty-two. On the other hand she loves the number three. She always feels tranquil when she finds a trio. She was third in the relation between papa and mamma, she is the third in the relation with P., and the recollection came to her now simply because she wanted to be the third in any case. She does not wish to turn my wife out, she does not wish to stand in the right place, she only wishes to be at the left hand, the third. Here dawns something of her oppressive consciousness of guilt, always present in neurosis.

In the next sitting there is another dream : "*I was on a great heath. There was nothing but clouds, but suddenly out of the mist there grew clear, and moved, a form like the hull of a ship which could hover in the air. It was perpendicular and had suddenly stood upright. Then I jumped about and several dogs also, but the dogs were quicker than I.*" She takes the dream to be symbolic. Her fate, her future, were hitherto wrapped in clouds. Now it seems as if her ship of life would find a goal. The piece cut out of the mist she describes as like the bulwarks of a ship. There occurs to her an experience of her life when she was twelve years old. (We see the hysterical amnesia beginning gradually to yield). She was visiting a school-friend and came to a smooth place (it was winter) she was afraid to cross it, she might fall. Then a gentleman came up to her, took her by the hand and told her not to be afraid. He asked her if her parents were kind to her, whether she had plenty of fun, and she was a honey-sweet, dear girl. Could she not go with him ? When she said she was going to mother, he said she should say she was going to a friend, and he would take her to the theatre. He held her by the hand so hard that it hurt her and wanted to kiss and embrace her ; and then she felt a hard object like a ruler. But she promised to come back and ran away quickly. At home she told the incident at once and the whole family started on the track of the evil-doer. But he was nowhere to be found. This too, was no hysterical fancy but an experience. She smelt very strong of patchouli and her clothes smelt so nice for some days afterwards that all the household noticed it. In this embrace by the man who rose up out of the mist, the erected penis which projected like a piece cut out of the mist, must have greatly excited her. And now the affair with the three dogs becomes clearer. As a supplement there occurs to her : *There was a little water there, too, and she was afraid of getting dirty. But the three little dogs— there was a yellow one, a white one, and a black one—all jumped over it beautifully at once.* The water with which one fears to get dirty is the bladder ; the association—bladder, urinate, penis leads naturally to the dogs, which, as well by their peculiar way of urinating as by their copulating, early excited the girl's attention and therefore play a great part as a sexual symbol in the dream. The yellow dog is P. (he has flax-coloured hair), the black one is myself, and the white one her father. It is a sex dream in which three men are at her disposal, all of whom perform the jump over the water beautifully and gracefully. The conclusion ("the dogs were quicker than I") is explained by the fact that at that time she ran away from the men, which she evidently regretted. Now she was not so nimble and was overtaken.

This dream betrays the fact, of which we had an inkling already in her first narrative, that she keenly regretted having so often in life played the virtuous one, and that P. had not been worth the great sacrifice of her chastity.

In the days that follow she is greatly excited ; she can indeed sing, but her voice becomes unaccountably hoarse. She complains of all sorts of inexplicable feelings of fear. There are almost insurmountable obstacles. But some days later again she is in a pleasanter humour and brings the following dream : "*I dreamt that I had been dizzy and fell down several times. My family did not understand this, except my cousin who always helps me. All at once I fell over a four-cornered wooden chest and bruised my arm. Then in the distance, I see a little child, which is standing in a very dangerous position. I become giddy and fall.*" From this dream I learn that she had suffered from fits in which she fell down and lost consciousness. The first time she felt dizzy was when she looked down into the bear's pit. Then it was repeated at the steep places of a mountain, especially when P., who went first, complained of giddiness. The *cousin* is a girl by whom she is greatly admired, an ugly, thin girl (four cornered chest, homosexual thought) ; the chest reminds her of a coffin. When she sees a coffin exhibited she thinks involuntarily : " Is it meant for Mrs. P. ? " There suddenly occurs to her an incident which was of great importance in her life. Her father once admired another woman and lived on very bad terms with her mother. Once there was a violent quarrel between the parents. The father uttered an offensive word to the mother. She got into a passion and called her father to task. " I will not have anyone speak to my mother like that." The father banged the door so violently that he hurt her arm badly. She ran to her room crying, packed her things, and would not remain another moment in the house. Then her father came up and sobbed, and begged her to forgive him, and embraced her fervently and kissed her. She felt at the time that this was too humiliating for her father. The continuation of the dream is a little child *standing in a channel between black and white marble.* This is a penis which rises from an alabaster skin, is surrounded by black hairs and stands dangerously. (The reminiscence from her childhood). The transference is not yet at an end. In the dream she falls with me, after her arm is injured, i.e., after P. is buried and lies in the wooden chest. She hopes too, that, like the father, I will embrace her if she threatens to go away. I expect, therefore, that in a few days she will express a wish to break off the cure. This she punctually does. When I tell her that she has identified me with her father, and now hopes that I will beg of her to remain with me, that I will fall at her feet and kiss her, she smilingly confesses to such a thought. I point out to her also that it was jealousy which made her attack her father, not only love for her mother.

The dream speaks of sudden crashes and falls. Here we may throw a penetrating glance into the genesis of various hysterical attacks of dizziness and swooning. I request her to inform me of her recollections of this sort of thing. She knows nothing at all. Not till the next day has another bit of the amnesia vanished.

The patient now remembers her various swooning fits. She suffered the first swoon when she was seventeen or eighteen years old. Mamma angrily told her about her uncle's housekeeper that he was going to marry her. Then she had a feeling of *disgust* and fell in a faint. She seems to have looked frightful. She knows that the lady in question has also suffered from hysterical cramps. Evidently Nastasia had suppressed the wish to become housekeeper to her father. The swoon was a sort of cataleptic rigidity, *but then came fits introduced by a splendid feeling of delight.*[1] Such a fit ran its course as follows : From the back there came a sensation as if she had lost all feeling, as though all physical sensations would vanish. Only her hand seemed to her as large as if it were made of marble.[2] Her head became clear as if she could grasp and comprehend everything. Then for the space of a second came a feeling as if she was oppressed by the might of a strong foreign force. A letting herself go, a surrender, so that she could give up everything. These attacks are easier to understand because they always took place at a time of sexual abstinence. She remembers many attacks before she had the connection with P. ; then came a great interval, and later the attacks began again when P was ill and she again lived in abstinence. The last attack took place during her critical experience with the dancer. It occurs to her further that she had a similar slight attack when she was a child only four or five years old. Her mother was then pregnant and big-bellied, and she went for a walk with her. And she suddenly said : " I am so weak, I cannot walk, I feel I am going to faint. You must carry me." She was jealous of the coming baby. Even to this day she often has such " slight attacks," as she calls them. A *pleasant* feeling as though she had no inside. As if she was getting giddy. As though a post was being turned round inside her. As if the post could expand her inside. During the slight attack she turns first pale, then red. It is evidently a process similar to orgasm, in which the sensation of a gigantic penis (post) is produced. And now it occurs to her all at once that as a child she did masturbate and indeed after a peculiar manner. In the school there was a balustrade down which the school boys used to

[1] Cf. the sweet fainting fits of Mrs. M. B. P. 100.
[2] Phantasy of a great stone-hard penis.

slide. She too, liked sliding down the balustrade and in doing so she experienced a pleasant feeling made up of fear and pleasure. It is due to this mode of masturbating that later on the patient could not bear any kind of swinging. Jolting made her sick and on board ship also she very easily became sea-sick. Now we know what the dizziness meant. On the other hand this reminiscence has cleared up a mysterious part of the mist dream. The memory of balustrade and ship come from childhood, from the time when the first sexual sensations were started by a balustrade. On the other hand on board ship she had to fight to repress these ideas.

She remembers too, that she once fell in a swoon in church. This was when sins and their punishment were being discussed. She considered herself to be a real sinner, and escaped from this painful consciousness by a prompt faint. At the next sitting she complains of pains in the coccyx, a coccygodynia. The first time, she had this pain on the high seas when she was seriously ill. There she saw a man who strongly reminded her of her father. The father was then suffering from cancer of the rectum. Immediately after his death she suffered from these pains in the rectum. In general she has the faculty of being able to suffer in sympathy with others. If her mother had neuralgia it could easily happen that she felt the same pains. If any one talks of toothache, then she also feels toothache. If anyone tells a horrible story of the tortures which someone has endured, she feels a violent pain in the upper thighs which radiates as far as the sex organs. She is an extremely sympathetic person, as in general sympathy is to be attributed to a masochistic excitement tinged with pleasure. Masochism and sadism are plainly stamped in her nature. We shall soon see that the next following sittings will confirm this.

For the sake of completeness, as in this case I have given all the dreams, I will now briefly mention the following. It runs : " *I was with two cousins and was about to spread my bread with butter and there was also a smoked herring from the isle of Rugen. It was so fat, and white, and beautiful. The bones came out easily. Not separate but like a skeleton. One cousin, the younger, said : ' Nastasia will eat the flesh of a herring on her bread and butter.' But the elder said : ' I don't believe it ; a singer who plays " Margaret " will not put so much on a piece of bread and butter.' *"

With the two cousins distinctly homosexual memories set in. One of her cousins is her greatest admirer. She has already been mentioned in one dream and is quite jealous when she forms a friendship with another girl. Thus she once said : " Now Nastasia is going to Paris with Vera, and when she comes back she belongs to me alone." Eating bread-and-butter, frequent symbol for coitus, as also is eating sweets. The smoked herring is P., who smokes excessively the whole day long. *He is fat, white and beautiful*, refers to her liking for his skin. *The bones came out easily* has more than one meaning. Since her star-part was " Margaret," that refers to her parting from P. She leaves P. light-heartedly. Not indeed completely separated, but the love is dead (but like a skeleton). The other meaning is the wish that P. may die. Finally there is concealed behind this dream a new paraphilia, fellatio. She narrates several reminiscences referring to this and referring mostly to what I had heard already.

The next dream makes us fully acquainted with her sadistic tendencies. *Thy sky was vividly illuminated. Countless flying machines filled the air. All were occupied with people who looked like silhouettes. The flying machines swing their legs as if they could walk in the air, all with a turning motion. Some fell down into the water but they rose again into the air. Others landed in green meadows. All the people were clothed in white and they sat on the green grass engaged in conversation. There was a ladies club there, too, and when I looked in they all had little spots of blood on their faces. The ladies were half naked, clothed only to the waistband. The legs too, had red spots on them.*"

Like all her dreams this dream too, is almost undisguisedly erotic. " *The sky was vividly illuminated.*" As a girl she had made herself a sky-bed which she lighted in wonderful fashion with a red hanging lamp. What visions appeared to her in this bed, we learn from the next sentence : " *Countless flying machines filled the air.*" A flying machine is like an umbrella, the symbol for a penis. " *All were occupied with people who looked like silhouettes.*" This refers to her sadistic wishes that persons whom she loves may die. They become shadows. She is like a vampire ; in dreams she causes the death of every one she kisses. " *The flying machines swung their legs* " is easily comprehensible. The turning motion is known to us from the fainting fits. The " *fall into the water* " (bladder) has already often been noted. " *They rise again into the air* " (another erection). " *But without danger* "—she wished for a fall into sin that would not endanger her. The most frequent phantasy of young girls who fear the consequences of erotic pleasures. " *Others landed in green meadows* " leads to a quite new complex. We know already that talking in a sitting position means for her the highest sexual enjoyment. " *Clothed in white* "—in night-dresses. To this refers " *All the people were clothed in white, and they sat on the green grass engaged in conversation.*" There was a ladies' club there too—here homosexual and sadistic tendencies evidently set in. A number of memories come back to her connected with this. She was once sea-sick and vomited so often that she got red and blue spots in the face (Echymoses). As a ten years old child she saw a trick-rider in a circus who fell from her horse, and was carried along for some distance. She sprang on to the horse again, tried to smile, but the tears ran down her cheeks. She was hurt in the side. First a few drops of blood oozed through her tights, then blood came very rapidly. This rider had thrown her into raptures, the whole incident had made a great impression on her. A comrade

L

expressed the wish to run away and also to become trick-riders. That she enjoys seeing naked women is shown by her strong exhibitionist and homosexual tendency. She likes to walk about naked in her room and as a girl played being a naked nymph here and there in her garden, and was once unpleasantly surprised at this.[1]

A number of occasions occur to her, when she has treated men with blows. In her first engagement when she was sitting on the stage, highly excited as " Ortrud " before the church, " Telramund" thrust his hand through a slit in her costume into the neighbourhood of her sex organs. She hissed : " Stop it, you impudent man ! " But this did not help her at all. After the act she gave him two boxes on the ear so that he tumbled backwards. She reproduces also a scene in the railway carriage when an officer of the Guards attempted an assault on her, which also ended in her giving the assailant a blow in the face. All the misery of the women artists exposed to any attack comes to light in these confessions. Another gentleman, who warmly protected her, and who was the most decent of all, once embraced her violently and she felt that he masturbated. She also remembers with fright an attempt at rape by a well-known author who attempted to make her his own in a carriage. For three weeks she had blue spots on her arms and could not appear.

This is only a small selection of the sadistic-masochistic thoughts which rise up from the amnesia. The green meadow of the dream comes from a well-known picture which she has often seen offered for sale in Berlin. Naked persons sit in green meadows, also little children sitting on green pots are depicted there. " Ladies' club " suggests a number of ladies whom she has really loved ; among others one, Rose, who for a time was her companion, plays a great part.

Let us not spend any more time over these small matters, but proceed to the next dream. " *I find myself between working women who have been making white embroideries. Then I am with my grandmother at the house of an ambassador. She shows me that the left side of my blouse is torn. I was much ashamed. I had no stockings on. When I wanted to draw them on they fell apart. Pawlow secretly gave me a pair of black silk ones which were lined with dark red silk.*"

" The working women "—they are hand-workers—refer to masturbation. Various ladies occur to her, among them my maid, who have specially taken her fancy. The hand-work had the form of a lozenge. She remembers that as a girl she once embroidered such a lozenge on a purse and wrote in it her initial " N." When her mother saw that she was quite angry, she only

[1] Other interpretations connect the dream with the religious life. She is in heaven among angels and indeed among fallen angels only, who cannot rise again. Also criminality plays a part, as well as a phantasy of pregnancy.

learned later that this was something highly indecent. It was the symbol for the feminine sex organ, and prostitutes of her neighbourhood have this put on their things. In the dream, the grandmother has the following meaning. Pawlow had discovered that she was no woman, there was something lacking, she had no nipples. Her mother too, had no nipples and therefore did not nurse her children. On the other hand her grandmother had brought eight children into the world and had nursed them all herself. In the dream her left blouse is torn because she had such a large nipple that it tore the blouse. For as a supplement it occurred to her : " *Under the blouse there was a hard, pointed object, which had torn the blouse.*" " Ambassador " produces some reminiscences which in part refer to the homosexual region.

The stocking story, however, is entirely made up of homosexual memories. She is much interested in ladies' stockings, and it occurs to her that a niece of Pawlow's once gave her six stockings lined with red and said to her : " If some time you leave Pawlow, then you must become my wife. Then we will never part." In this dream she to a certain extent dismisses the man, and turns to that form of sexual satisfaction which she can attain even with women (hand-work !).

Now, again, it becomes clear to us why she is afraid of women. *Her fear of women is repressed love.* Her homosexual tendency is perhaps stronger than the heterosexual. She reports too, that she has oscillated in her love for her mother and for her father. She has often called Pawlow, " Mother."

In the next dream she makes me also into a woman. *She sees me in an apron and with a knife as if I were a surgeon.* The analysis is compared with an operation. Further explanation is superfluous. Also she admits that she feels better and gains weight daily, which is evidently not pleasant for Pawlow, for he prefers to see her thin and suffering. A thin and suffering woman is his ideal. Again, she reveals a part of her thoughts of illness. *She was ill the better to please Pawlow, in other words to make herself interesting.*

In the last sitting but one we arrive at the complete solution of this psychic drama. There the psychic probe goes down to the bottom and finds the sensitive point. She begins by saying that she cannot conceive why she hates Sonja and it turns out that she has identified herself with the dancer and loved her. When she was alone she did all sorts of dance exercises, would also open the piano at the top with her naked foot, copied famous dancers, and so forth. That is, she behaved as if she were not the singer Nastasia but the dancer Sonja, and as dancer of course she needs no voice.

Why did she do this ? Because she felt a deep consciousness of guilt. That which Sonja brought her was surely only her just punishment. She had wanted to intrude as the third in the relation between her father and mother. She had intruded between Pawlow and his wife. Was it not the retribution of fate that Sonja should intrude between her and Pawlow. And suddenly it occurs to her why, when Sonja visited her in Petersburg, she lost her voice. When Sonja had the audacity to appear before her, her first impulse was : "Now hurl yourself upon her and throttle her." This impulse she suppressed, and immediately she felt her throat clutched as it were with a grip of iron. She wished to kill Sonja, i.e., to possess her. She envied Pawlow that he was a man and could possess the beautiful Sonja. She was more jealous of Sonja than of Pawlow.

On the next day she took leave of me after she had sung to me for an hour quite unembarrassed and with full command of her artistic capabilities. She reported to me one more little dream. *She had seen on my writing table an open lamp, which she had extinguished and taken with her.* The transference is at an end ; she was the open lamp, which had burnt as long as the cure lasted. I was a little light that had lighted her in the darkness and shown her the way.

The phenomenon, why she had lost her voice, is settled in many ways. She sang no more because she wanted to work no more, because she wanted to compel Pawlow to provide for her as for a wife. Also the inducement of illness as a refuge came into consideration, because she was tired of the many attacks to which a woman artist is exposed. Further, she sang no more so that Sonja should not hear her ugly voice. She sang no more because she wanted to be ill, so that as an invalid she would please Pawlow better. And she sang no more because she wanted to be to Pawlow what Sonja had been : a woman loved for the sake of her beauty, a dancer who could indeed dance, but could not sing. She became dumb because she wanted to make others dumb. She wanted to throttle Sonja and throttled her throat. She was a criminal and homosexual. Her fear of people and especially of women is to be traced to the repression of all these unconscious tendencies.

Only he who has experienced how even in the middle of the cure the hitherto mute songstress under the stress of the loosened inhibitions, positively shouted out Schubert's song : "Nun muss sich alles, alles wenden "—can form a conception of the immense power of the analytical methods. The patient has left Pawlow, he has found in the dancer full compensation for her. She is devoting herself again to her artistic career. Only the future can tell us more. The last news is very good. She has repeatedly sung in public.

CHAPTER XXVI

GIDDINESS AND FEAR OF MOUNTAINS
THE FEAR OF FALLING

A KNOWLEDGE of neurotic giddiness may spare the physician many unpleasant mistakes. I have already pointed out elsewhere that neurotic giddiness is mostly directed to the left. To be sure there are exceptions. Often organic trouble alternates with neurosis. Here a decision can be arrived at only by a thorough investigation and the discovery of any psychic causes that may be operating.

No. 124.—How important is the psycho-analysis of every feeling of giddiness we see by the following case :—Herr M. G., police official, comes to me one day complaining that he is " carrying about with him " some sort of serious illness. He feels as if all his strength was gone, and believes it must be some secret disease which he doesn't know, that is preying upon him. At times he feels a pressure in the head and his feet shamble and tremble as if they would not carry him. All day long he is faint and weary ; in the evening he feels a little better. His hands are weak and hang nerveless at his side. *Yesterday in the cafe he had a feeling as if he must hold on to his seat with all his strength or he would fall. It was as if he were giddy. It regularly dragged him to the left.* He is forty years of age, free from hereditary taint, organically perfectly sound ; appetite pretty good, stool regular, sleep unperturbed. Asked if he suffers from feelings of fear, he says that fourteen days ago he had a violent attack of fear. Suddenly in his office he felt very bad. He kept saying to himself : " *You're going downhill. You will die before your time.*" The attack was so violent that he got the police surgeon, who happened to be present, to examine him. The doctor told him he was quite sound, it was only a nervous spasm of the heart. Two days later he found himself suffering for want of breath. He kept drawing deep breaths and struggling for air and could not go to sleep because he believed his heart was diseased.[1] He would have liked to cry if as a man and an officer he had not been ashamed to. Now he seems disgusted with everything ; he has no real initiative. The week before he ought to have started on an official journey in order to discover a criminal, and he did not go for fear something might happen to him. Yesterday he forced himself to go out for a walk, but after a few steps he became so tired that he had to rest on a seat, and there he remained for hours sitting and staring straight in front of him.

His relations, struck by his way of going on, had forced him to consult a professor who pronounced him to be " neurasthenic," and ordered him to seek distraction.

The patient, big and thin, and rather pale, brought out these statements in jerks, with suppressed excitement. He is no stranger to me. I treated him some years ago for " acute parapathia " in consequence of a psychic conflict and I know that his marriage is unhappy : that his wife, jealous, and mentally his superior, is constantly nagging him and makes his home a hell. I ask what sort of a life he now leads sexually and find that for three

[1] An attack of ærophagia.

months he has practised complete abstinence. The present illness with its grave symptoms began a fortnight ago with the first attack of fear. Here again, as so often before, it was a dream that put me on the right track. I ask if the patient has vivid dreams, and he admits this.

" Only to-day I had a dream from which I woke up in a fright. I had an encounter with a gendarme and I had to make a note of it so that he should not take my name." And he added, " Too silly, to dream such nonsense ! "

" Is the dream connected with anything that happened yesterday ? "

" No, I don't know of anything."

" Has nothing of the sort ever happened to you ? "

" No. Yes, though ! Right ! Once when I was cycling I ran into a gendarme, and had to apologise to him so that he shouldn't report me at the police station. But that was many years ago. I had long forgotten that."

To accept this explanation as satisfactory and to explain this as simply a reminiscent dream would be to declare oneself a bungler in the difficult art of dream interpretation. The gendarme and the watchman are frequently in dreams a symbol for the wife who keeps watch less the husband prove unfaithful. (The same symbol stands vice versa for the husband). Accordingly I asked :

" Did you have a quarrel with your wife yesterday ? "

" Yes," he answered, " a very violent one."

Hence the explanation of the statement : " I had an encounter with a gendarme." His wife is a huge woman and behaves exactly like a gendarme to him. These questions having as I think settled the sources of the dream I now get the patient to tell me himself what occurs to him. So I say : " Pray shut your eyes a moment and tell me what else occurs to you with regard to the dream."

" Nothing at all," said the patient.

In such a case one must wait quietly till the resistance is overcome. For some minutes I quietly wait for further answers. Again the patient says " Nothing at all." Then he goes on, " Or something which really has nothing whatever to do with it."

" And that is ? "

" A Mrs. Degen. That must be connected with gendarme," he says, smiling, " because the gendarme carries a sword." (*Degen.*)

" Has this lady any relations with your wife ? "

" No, she doesn't even know her."

It was a slow and faltering " No," so that I said to myself, " The key to the mystery is hidden here." The dream about the gendarme, too, seemed to me in so far suspicious as it pointed to some fear of a lawsuit (cf. the case of the barrister, *p.* 164, No. 103).

" In what relation do you stand to this woman ? " I ask.

" I will tell you the truth, doctor ; for six months I have had no intercourse with my wife. And I had a connection with this Mrs. Degen which she broke off three months ago. Since then I have been living in complete abstinence."

" And did you accept this rupture with complete indifference ? "

" On the contrary ! I was frightfully upset about it. You see, doctor, I couldn't make out why she broke it off so suddenly."

" And have you seen her or written to her since then ? "

" A fortnight ago (that is on the day of the attack of fear) I saw her at a tramcar waiting-room. It gave me a shock and I made as if I didn't see her. By the way, in the last few days I've often suffered from shakings-up of that sort. Yesterday afternoon I lay down to sleep and felt such a violent shock that I woke up with palpitation of the heart."

" Why did you not speak to the lady ? "

" My pride forbids," he cried out excitedly. " Never, never will I do that. Besides I despise her. She was so well dressed that I believe she is kept by someone. She has left her husband, too."

" When did you hear of that, then ? "

" I read in the newspaper that her husband had gone bankrupt, and that his wife had left the house with her child."

Now I began to understand the gendarme. " Were you not afraid that if the matter came into court you might be drawn in ? "

" To be sure," said he, " to be sure, I was afraid. The hearing comes on in a few days. And I've been thinking all the time, what shall I do if the wife says that she had a connection with me ? "

" Why should she say that ? Did you part in anger ? "

" Oh, nothing of the sort ! But to make it easier for the husband."

" How would that make it easier for the husband ? "

" Because for more than a year I kept her. I gave her so much every month because I knew they were hard up at home. But she didn't do it for the sake of the money. I can't tell you how fond we were of each other."

" If this woman was so fond of you, why did she leave you then ? "

" Probably I gave her too little. Evidently she needs ' money.' "

" Were you the only favoured one ? "

" At that time, yes ; she gave me her oath it was so. But before me she had already had another lover : Privy Councillor X, between ourselves."

" Do you think she has gone back to him ? "

" Possibly, but not likely. He will take care of that. His experiences have been too unpleasant already with this woman. The husband knew what their relations were, favoured them in fact, and one day threatened a divorce suit and got a big sum out of the Privy Councillor."

" Ah," said I, " now I see. You are afraid of getting yourself involved in a troublesome lawsuit. You are afraid that the woman has told her husband the truth, and that in his need the man will try to blackmail you. You are afraid that it will come to the ears of your wife."

" Yes, I thought of that the day before yesterday. What shall I do if the lady demands money from me, and then if I don't give it her, goes to my wife and tells everything."

" So that the dream about the gendarme has a deeper meaning. You have already planned out what you shall say to your wife in case your fears are realised. You live in constant dread that this affair may involve you in serious consequences. But in your anxiety one thing has escaped you. You saw the woman a fortnight ago. Her dress was of striking elegance. That means that she has found a richer lover than you. I think she won't want to spoil this new love affair with lawsuits, and that she will be glad if you leave her alone."

I discuss the subject again several times with the patient. The cure was so amazingly rapid that his friends could not contain their astonishment. A weighty additional factor was that the sudden rupture of the liaison meant a decided abatement of the vanity which was a marked characteristic in him. Besides—he still loved this woman and could not forget her. He would have liked best to have avenged himself on the faithless one. If we take into account further that a lawsuit might have cost him his position, and that he feared an irreparable conflict with his wife, we shall form some idea of the burden of this secret. It is an interesting fact that the patient did not know that his physical condition had anything to do with this incident. He had so far succeeded in repressing all thoughts about it that they only flashed out occasionally for a few minutes a few times a day. Only the successful analysis made thoroughly plain to him the origin of the symptoms, and explained to him also how it was that the dream, which he has described as " too silly," could throw him into such a state of excitement.

The dizziness has here a special significance. It corresponds to the fear of falling from a secure social position, and has certainly arisen through conversion, so that it is really a *hysterical* symptom ! Moreover, the well-known way in which anxiety neurotics suddenly start at night has ultimately the same psychic origin. The patients fall from their ethical heights into the abyss.   Below them, in fact, is hell and above is heaven.   Every fall therefore is a fall from heaven into hell.   (A fall into sin).   Frequently dizziness is only a symptom of intoxication.   But almost every one of these organic symptoms has ultimately a psychic origin, as we have here shown by numerous examples.

Feuchtersleben, the great physician and thinker, knew precisely the nature of this dizziness.   In his book—still readable at the present day—" Textbook of Medical Psychology " (Vienna, 1845) in speaking of conditions of monomania, he observes that it is important to watch the transition stages since the anomalies are certainly no lyric leaps in the epic course of life.   " Who is there," he says, " who has not had at some moment the feeling, however transitory, that he must leap from a height into the depths ?   Did not the poets base on this feeling their tales of the water-nymphs, the Lorelei, etc., with their allurements ?   Is the height-dizziness anything else than the loss of perceptive power produced by the conflict with such feelings ?   So the threads of the psychic and the physical life are mutually interwoven."

Here Feuchtersleben associates himself with the theory set up by Hess in 1791, that dizziness results when the mental pictures succeed each other too quickly.   With the aid of some examples we have become more intimately acquainted with the genesis of dizziness. We learned that, in neurotics, dizziness may represent a symptom of intoxication but we cannot help believing that at any rate ultimately its cause is psychic.   I will mention only the case of the cashier who was overtaken by giddiness as he was crossing a public place.   Here the cause was undoubtedly the suppressed plan to abscond.   We have also " falling " in the symbolic sense as when we speak of a girl who succumbs to temptation as a " fallen woman."   If the dizziness was only an intoxication-dizziness it should occur on various occasions.   By our analyses, however, it has always been possible to demonstrate the psychic connection. How plain is the genesis of the dizziness in the case of the singer, N. W. !   Her dreams showed us that as a child she experienced dizziness and lust when sliding down the balustrade.   And so to the present day a violent libido expresses itself in her as dizziness. Of course, only a libido which seems to her a sin, a falling into sin.

I call to mind the case of the sixty-four-year old man (P., No. 46) who for some months suffered so severely from dizziness that he reeled in the street.   Yet he could stand on one leg with his eyes shut.   The dizziness was always towards the left.   In the course of the very interesting investigation I found that, twenty years before, he had a liaison with two women, each of whom was to remain in ignorance of the other.   He repeatedly said to himself : " You are an infamous swindler."[1]   He was more drawn to his mistress—to the left—than to his wife.   The dizziness served also

[1]*Schwindler.* [*Schwindel* means giddiness and also swindle.—Tr.]

to protect his virtue. It prevented him from visiting his mistress daily. He visited her only on " good " days.

From this point of view we shall more readily understand many cases of height-dizziness and height-fear. Height-dizziness is always a fear of the abyss, a fear that " something frightful " may happen. It overtakes people even in places where there is no cause for a moment's fear. To the psychologist every case of dizziness sets the problem : " What is behind this ? " Similarly mountain-fear is a phobia of which the psychic mechanism is revealed only in psycho-analysis.

I have at my disposal some observations which render comprehensible the psychological components of height-dizziness.

No. 125.—One of my patients, Mr. A. Z., was always passionately fond of mountaineering. Let us bear in mind that it is not love of nature alone that drives men to the mountains. It is exuberant energy, the tameness of existence, the longing for physical activity, an obscure sexual impulse, but it is also a way of escape from oneself ; it is eroticism with its values changed, sublimated love of conquest, and in many cases direct longing for death. So that only a small proportion of the accidents in the mountains are really accidents. Mostly they are cases of suicide completed as it were automatically (cf. Freud, " Psychopathology of Everyday Life "). Now our tourist, A. Z., was once suddenly overtaken by dizziness after he had been struggling for some months against *taedium vitae*. All of a sudden on a plateau of the Rax, the idea flashed upon him : " Now you can put a speedy end to your weary life." And half an hour later, before a steep path, he came to a standstill and could go no further. He became violently dizzy. It was as though his consciousness had been divided into A and B. A said : " Throw yourself down." B feared the fall and produced the dizziness.

In most cases there is, behind the phobia, fear of retribution, the old childish fear of the punishment of God. Such patients wanted to throw some particular person over a precipice (active criminal fantasies !).

Many persons who suffer from dizziness have as children evoked sexual sensations by dizziness (swinging). Mountain sickness is analogous to sea and railway sickness. Another form includes patients in whom the dizziness developed only in later life. These have already had to struggle with the temptation to throw themselves out of windows or the like.

In the " Archives de Psychologie " Flournoy has published a remarkable case—that of a young man who had repeatedly consulted the professor concerning a torturing fear. This young man lived in constant fear that he would fall down a precipice and so perish. Although both logic and the physician assured him that he had only not to climb a mountain and he could not fall down, this phobia was of extraordinary strength and made him wretched. And sure enough one day this ill-fated man really did throw himself down from a declivity that was not at all dangerous in itself and came to an untimely end. Who in this case would believe that his feeling was prophetic ? No—the youth evidently went voluntarily to his death. His fear corresponded only to a repressed

I.*

wish. As the song says : "Half was he drawn, half sank he of himself." (*Goethe:* "Der Fischer.")

He had sat down and gone to sleep by the slope. Then out of the unconscious arose the desire stronger than his will to live. In his dream he made an awkward movement and found peace for ever.

A great proportion of the mountain accidents are suicides. The false step is often to be traced to the influence of the unconscious which suddenly assumes command of the motor apparatus.

Exact analyses of height-dizziness always show the longing for death. In most cases, besides the criminal fantasies already known to us, one will come upon pleasurable memories of swinging in childhood. These then, becoming painful, were repressed, and as a reaction from them there set in vomiting and disgust, dizziness, etc.

An excellent example is the case of the singer which I published in the previous chapter. She will often climb the steepest mountains without dizziness. On days when life seems joyless she is attacked by violent dizziness. *After* the analysis she suffered neither from sea-sickness nor from mountain-fear.

I once observed in the mountains a married couple who were suddenly overtaken by giddiness, both at once. The man had just passed the place where Tourville hurled his wife down the precipice. He said to his wife—as if in jest : " How would it be now, if I were to throw you down ? " She laughed and was overcome by violent dizziness, and he also.

Here, too, a repressed criminal thought was playing a part. Such little observations render comprehensible the phobias in which this fear has become a pathological fixture.

CHAPTER XXVII

FEAR OF GHOSTS AND OF THE DEAD
SPIRITUALISM AND SPIRIT-WRITING

FEAR of the dead is one of the most frequent cases of fear. There is always something uncanny about a dead body. There are many persons, otherwise of good courage, who cannot sleep in a room where there is a dead body. With a neurotic this fear may rise to the point of obsession. There are people so nervous that they cannot enter a house where there is a dead body ; they cannot even speak of a dead man.

If we analyse this feeling we always come upon the idea that the dead awake and may turn upon the living. The mere idea of the dead rising, without any idea of their making an attack, causes even courageous persons to tremble. It is especially the feeling of the uncanny which comes upon us if we overstep the bounds of the known. A world in which we lose our sense of direction strikes us as uncanny.

The idea of a life after death is not only comforting and elevating to us, it is also uncanny, so long as we have no certain tidings from that world.

As a preliminary stage to fear of the dead, the fear of being buried alive is very wide-spread. In many wills one finds directions for a stab in the heart as a precaution against being buried alive. Among these neurotics one finds a great many who suffer from womb-fantasies. And in fact every human being was once buried alive, when he lived in his mother's womb. In the neurotic repression of this ridiculous incest-phantasy, the monstrous nature of which does not prevent its being relatively frequent, the desire for a fœtal existence expresses itself as fear of being buried alive.

All these people collect as proof a great record of cases supposed to have happened, which, however, cannot stand further investigation. Most of these tales belong to the region of fable.

Dread of the dead is always connected with a bad conscience as is also dread of ghosts, i.e., a fear that the dead will punish one, resulting from one's own evil thoughts. The following case is of great psychological interest.

No. 126.—Mr. J. B., sixty-one years of age, has been for twenty years suffering under the obsession that he cannot live in a house in which anyone has died. Otherwise a quite normal human being, he suffers agonies of fear if there is a corpse in the same house. He at once rushes from the house. But this phobia extends to houses in which at any time someone has died.

Therefore he lives in new houses only, leaving directly if a death happens there. It is remarkable that he has not built a house for himself, although his means would allow it. But, again, he cannot live alone in a house. He must have plenty of people about him or he is attacked with torments of restlessness and uncertainty.

The basis of this phobia was found to be a pronounced necrophilia. He is always thinking of corpses—in the negative form also as a defence. His horizon is filled with corpses. For fear of a necrophilic act he avoids houses where people are dying. That he avoids houses in which people died many years before is due to the fact that the thought excites him sexually. Again in self-defence against his necrophilic and other sexual tendencies he needs the presence of many people. In a small house he might easily yield to temptation. Rapid cure after psycho-analytical explanation.

Oddly enough, dread of ghosts and of the dead is often transformed into the opposite—into spiritualism. Patients attempt in this way to overcome their fear by associating with ghosts.

Without attempting to answer the question whether spiritualism is justified or not, I must, from the humane standpoint admit the great consoling power of this doctrine. Spiritualism is a religion of substitution and completion. There is in men an infinite longing for the supersensuous, for something beyond, for the marvellous. They seize with eagerness any cup that may quench this thirst for the mystical.

For the psychological comprehension of converse with spirits it is necessary to have an exact knowledge of the mechanism of outward projection of internal processes. *Every spirit, like every hallucination, is a projection of that within us, or more plainly, of our " unconsciousness."* The paranoic who is pursued by enemies is pursued by his own thoughts ; the hysteric who hears offensive cries is abusing himself. It is the voice of the judge within that he hears. The spirit quoted by the spiritualists is their " own " (unconscious) spirit. Everything that the spirit writes is dictated by one's own ego. But how comes it about that this embodiment of that within them appears to the patients and to spiritualists so foreign and so hostile ? How comes it that thoughts arise which are foreign to consciousness, knowledge comes into consciousness which was before a sealed book, qualities appear which contradict the nature of the person suffering from the hallucination ?

In these cases we have always to do with persons divided in two, in each breast two tendencies striving for mastery. This " dissociation " renders possible a separation into an observing, critical, meditative person and a person projected outwards, uncritical, fantastic. In grave cases of dissociation there may even be three personalities. Neurosis results from the conflict between the inner and the outer being. Psychosis represents the overpowering of the outer by the inner being. Before the critical intellect is overpowered there comes a transition stage which we may describe as conflict between intellect and emotion. The stronger emotionality of the one personality, the inner or the outer, decides the victory.

The illusions of the mentally afflicted were often supersensuously influenced. If in early times it was the voice of God or of the saints that the patients heard, if mostly it was the tendency to religious hallucinations, visions, whispering voices, appearances in dream that manifested itself, so to-day besides the religious factors which will never lose their importance, it is telepathic influence and spirits in the spiritualistic sense that play a great part. But it would be reversing things altogether to attack religion or spiritualism, and to maintain that they had caused the disease. They are only the occasion, though we must add that there are brains which cannot bear the strain of metaphysical questions. They remain healthy so long as no great demands are made on them. For health they demand a simple scheme of things. If they are suddenly overburdened and come into contact with the terror of the supernatural they become disordered. Every normal person knows that there are questions about which one cannot think, indeed must not think. I have often heard very wise and critical people say that they dare not meditate on the question of " infinity," or on " time and space," otherwise something in the head threatened to go wrong. It would be to drive them out of their senses.

Therefore all neurotics and all enthusiasts likely to be carried away by idle fancies, all who are by heredity disposed to psychosis (e.g., slight periodics, zyclothymen, pronounced hysterics, psychopathic inferiorities) must be restrained from meddling with spiritualism and especially with spirit-writing.

That many people thus occupied keep very well, and indeed in especially high spirits, I have repeatedly noticed. For many it is a joke, others find consolation in it, to a third section it gives a heightened realisation of their own personality which they have hitherto lacked. They feel themselves exalted by association with eminent spirits. They have the advantage of other mortals (what all men long for—and especially neurotics).

A man in the fifties tells me in my consultation hour his experiences with the spirits he had called up. Owing to the barrenness of his occupation he had long lost all joy in life. For three years he had gone in for spiritualism. He is now in rapport with the greatest spirits. His spirit circle is frequented only by the most important spirits of all time. Yesterday Goethe dictated a new poem to them. Also they had already spoken with Kant, and Spinoza. " Look here," cried the patient, " life is a joy to me now ! What company had I before ? Grumbling State officials, a tedious sit at meals at the restaurant, and some old friends of my youth. Now I talk with Goethe, with Napoleon, with Schiller, with Bismarck, and discuss with them all the questions of the day."[1]

If we test the mental condition of these people we find them mostly quite normal except for this spiritualistic delusion. Once I ventured to ask this gentleman whether it was then his belief that Goethe condescended so readily to everyone. I said I had already heard from other spiritualists that it was especially Goethe that they liked to converse with. What would happen then if

[1] I have described this phenomenon in detail according to her report in my book, " Die Träume der Dichter." Published by J. F. Bergmann, *p.* 137.

two or more wanted a chat with Goethe at the same time ? Thereupon he gave a superior smile and said they had often been told
"I am busy just now," or, "To-day I can't speak." The spirits
were all very kind and accessible. A very fine poetess once
informed me that the spirits had dictated a whole book to her.
This was Clara Blüthgen, whose " Sounds from the Beyond " came
by spirit-writing. Also a little volume of aphorisms (quite excellent
ones, by the way), called " Drops of Ink," owes its origin to the
spirits. The poetess had not suffered at all by this experience,
she remains mentally fresh and was able to bear the severe reverses
of the war and to find consolation in new creative work.

Other examples have shown me that there are minds which cannot
bear spirit-writing. It is therefore a very venturesome thing unless
one's inner being is established with absolute firmness to plunge
deeply into spiritualism. Especially people who suffer from grave
psychic conflicts, who are divided within, should be restrained from
this dangerous sport.

Even to engage in waking suggestions and in hypnoses may
cause very grave conditions from neuroses to psychoses. With
hysterical persons there may arise after hypnoses transitory symptoms of hysterical lunacy.

No. 127.—A girl, hitherto quite normal, is hypnotised by a professional
hypnotiser in the hospital where she is engaged as sister. She is very easy
to hypnotise and carries out all sorts of post-hypnotic orders over which the
patients make very merry. All the next day she is lost in reverie, stares
straight in front of her, cannot be employed for any work. Sleepless night.
Hallucinations. Hears voices and sees the hypnotiser with the face of a
devil. He is Mephisto who will take her to hell. Hears him declaim : " Thou
dear child, come, go with me, right lovely games I'll play with thee." The
next day confused, speech wandering, refuses food, thinks herself sinful.
After two pantopon tablets (0.01) partial calm. Light sleep. On the third
day no hallucinations but deep depression. Cannot cease thinking of the
hypnotiser, afraid of being in his power. He could do what he liked with
her. At the request of her sister she is hypnotised by me. Receives the
assurance that the spell is broken and that no hypnotiser can do anything
to her. Also she receives the suggestion never to let herself be hypnotised
again and to forget the whole hypnosis. After this, her last hypnosis, she
will completely forget the first one. She will laugh at the hypnotiser. And
she is to have no fear of me. She is now secure against any hypnosis and
any sudden attack. The success was amazing, hysteria being characterised
by sudden changes of outlook and of mood. The temporary hysterical
psychosis, caused by sexual excitement and sexual fear arising during the
hypnosis, was cured. I had an opportunity of observing her months later.
She was again, as before the hypnosis, the happy healthy sister.

The hypnosis had brought to light her latent hysteria. The
psychogenesis of this psychosis was not difficult to recognise. She
was suffering from abstinence, she was virgin ; having to do with
many men, some of whom she had to see naked, had increased
her libido. So it came about that she took the hypnosis as a sexual
act, was fascinated by the hypnotiser, and fell in love with him,
and desired a rape during the hypnosis according to the principle
of all neurotics (discovered by me), " Pleasure without Guilt."

But we see how dangerous it may be to play with hypnosis, what power it gives to the hypnotiser and how the question, " injurious or harmless ? " can be answered only for each individual. (A lawsuit which took place in Vienna in 1919 raises a similar question. A girl maintains that through the suggestion of a well-known suggestor who gave exhibitions before the public, she was seduced and demands marriage or damages.[1])

I have also seen some cases of injuries through suggestion. Girls who always see the eyes of the experimenter before them and have more or less lost their balance.

No. 128.—After a sitting with a suggestor, Miss M. K. loses her sleep and falls ill with " maddening pains in the head," which compel the doctor to give several morphia injections daily. She roars with pain. It is as if a knife was being bored into both her eyes. She is brought to me in a carriage with head bound up. Cure in three days by psychotherapy (without hypnosis) simple talking to and explanation.

No. 129.—Sister B. attends in the hospital the demonstrations of an amateur waking suggestor. Since that day she has lost her balance. She cannot stop thinking of the eyes of Dr. S.—that was the suggestor's name. She believes that he follows her home and influences her thoughts. She gets herself transferred to the front where passionate feelings hitherto unknown to her awake. Firmly believes that Dr. S. influences her at a distance, and excites her. Writes him letters full of reproaches. Travels to Vienna and visits him in his lodgings, begs him to free her from his influence and not to persecute her any more. A systematic persecution-delusion grows up, in which S. plays the chief part. Reads allusions in the newspapers, notices that he has smuggled certain items of news into the advertisements, finds that he has sent the house-porter to watch her. Her mother's house-porter takes his mistress into her room. This is, of course, the devilish work of Dr. S., to excite her fancy and make her tractable. Again sends S. letters to the effect that she sees through his machinations. In four weeks with intense psychotherapeutic treatment this paranoic disease passes away. Diagnosis : Verisimile : hysterical lunacy or hysteria paranoides, unless one prefers, according to the proposal of Henneberg and Zichen to call these ideas " eknoia."

If for predisposed persons hypnosis and waking suggestion are a dangerous game which may do much harm, it seems to me that spiritualism, and especially spirit-writing, are in certain circumstances very mischievous. The next case gives a clear picture of a spirit-writing psychosis.

No. 130.—Miss N. M., thirty-two years old, from a neuropathic family, said to have been always nervous, weak constitution, anæmic, undernourished, was told by a friend of the exciting occupation, talking with spirits. She very quickly learns spirit-writing. She gets the spirits to dictate to her several poetical works. Also several spirits are called up, among others Mozart and a man whom she says she has never seen. Finally she decides

[1] Unfortunately almost all the hypnotisers and suggestors who practice in public have also a private practice in telepathy and even in graphology. A well-known telepathist, Mr. H., has in fact a medical man of straw behind whom he operates, and who has opened a " psychic clinic." Mr. H. is the assistant at the clinic of Dr. O. Only the psychotherapist who later has to do with the victims can estimate the harm done here. Of course there are also cures. These cures then serve as an advertisement and bring many new patients to the clinic.

to get into touch with Schiller. Schiller comes at once and is very nice to her. She is quite proud of her intimacy with Schiller. About three weeks after she has taken up spiritualism Schiller signifies that she should leave this world and go with him. But at this moment comes on the scene his wife, Lotte, who is very jealous of her, and threatens a fearful vengeance. One day in the café she cries out with the madness of hallucination : " She will throttle me ! She will take vengeance ! Help ! Help ! " She saw Charlotte Schiller and feared her vengeance for her intimacy with Schiller. She was taken from the café in an ambulance to the friend who had introduced her to spiritualism (but had herself remained quite healthy). There I find her in the greatest excitement, with every sign of an anxiety attack. Objective symptoms : maximal dilatation of pupils ; diminished corneal reflex ; throat reflex lacking ; tendon reflexes very lively ; indication of patellar clonus. She declines to speak of her experiences with the spirits. If she did the spirits would come back. It would be frightful. Lotte is a fearfully severe woman and has sworn vengeance upon her. Gradually she allows herself to be pacified and tells me of her hallucinations.

Under opium she rapidly becomes tranquil. Two days after leaving off the opium a severe attack of anxiety without hallucinations. She had a "terrible weakness of the heart " and a feeling that she must die. A physician quickly summoned gives her a caffein injection, simply to quiet her, as he said : " really not necessary." A typical attack of anxiety. Two weeks later feels comparatively well. Admits her delusions and promises to have nothing more to do with spiritualism.

The psychogenesis of this case is interesting. The patient had for years had a liaison with a married author, and evidently reproached herself violently for this. She suffered from a feeling of guilt that she would not admit to herself, and which therefore manifested itself in a disguised form. She transferred the conflict with her lover and his wife to Schiller and Lotte. So if we put in the place of Lotte the wife whom she had robbed of her husband the picture becomes very clear. She feared this woman's vengeance, she trembled before the punishment of the Heavenly Judge. The business with the spirits revived the faith of her infancy, which she imagined she had overcome. The punishment for her sins was inevitable, all the more that she was not faithful even to her lover and had fallen in love with a band-master who in her hallucinations turned up again as Mozart, disguised to be sure as quite another kind of band-master. The fear had plainly a religious origin.

We see from this case that the profound conflict from which the patient suffered would probably have led even without spiritualism to a neurosis or perhaps to transitory psychosis. The business with the spirits had accelerated the outbreak of the suffering.

On the other hand we may set the rapid passing away of the psychosis to the account of psychotherapy. I did not content myself with describing the hallucinations and with the assurance that there were no spirits, that all these were born of her own imagination. I tried to get to the kernel of her psychic conflict.

At first striving against it, then with more compliance and finally confidentially, freely, the patient entrusted me with the story of her life. I heard about the great love for the author, now overcome ; of the new love for a musician (band-master) in the hallucination. The patient soon understood that she had put Schiller in the place of the poet and Lotte in his wife's. The dénouement was surprising. The wife of her former lover came to her and spoke out her mind freely. She said that she had long forgiven her and had no thought of vengeance. She was not the only one or the first one with whom her husband had been unfaithful. She went even further and placed her house at her disposal. She and her daughter outdid each other in kindness to the patient. The whole affair was settled in the most beautiful way and soon belonged to the past. The illness lasted two weeks, whereas usually such psychoses last for months.

It would lead us away from our subject if I were to speak here of the importance of psychotherapy for the treatment of the psychoses. I would only say that it is the duty of the psychian to seek out mental causes and motives and to attempt a psychological analysis. In those who practise spirit-writing the psychic conflict manifests itself in such a way that the spirit is the dissentient voice and to a certain extent represents an objectivising of the conscience. *Spiritualist diseases are conscience diseases.* People rush into spiritualism who have a bad conscience trying in this way to find distraction and relief. In this sense spirit-writing is an attempt at cure, a sort of " reaction by distraction," at any rate an attempt at healing which often achieves the opposite.

CHAPTER XXVIII

ZOOPHOBIAS

ANIMAL phobiæ are extremely common. In fact one finds them in most people who have otherwise no neurotic characteristics whatever. One fears mice, another snakes, a third dogs (cynophobia), a fourth horses, a fifth insects (bees !), a sixth fleas. Every phobia is usually rationalised. The dog may be mad, the snake is perhaps venomous, infection may result from a bee-sting, flies convey infectious diseases, mice and rats are disgusting because they come in contact with dirt, toads are disgusting because they are damp, slippery, plump and ugly. The pathological nature of the fear of animals can be understood only if one sees that the emotion renders logical consideration impossible and that we have to do with a parapashia. The illogical nature of such a case is evident if we can estimate how far the phobia is removed from reality. When a lady suffering from fear of horses trembles for fear the horses might walk up the staircase to the third floor and bite her or trample on her, then the pathological character of that fear becomes evident even to the superficial observer.

A detailed description of the animal phobiæ would require a whole book. For most cases it is characteristic that the phobia begins in infancy. Almost all children have a great interest in animals. They identify themselves with animals or in a puzzling way begin to fear them. Freud in the " Analysis of the Phobia of a Five-year old Boy " has explained the fear of a horse as the fear of the father. In a later work he maintained that the animals symbolise the parents. That is true for many cases—as we shall see later—but it is not true for all, and does not exhaust the psychic structure of an animal phobia. Other factors are concerned which I will present in detail. To the phobist the animal always represents a special part of his own soul. Further the animal plays a great part as " the organ for executing criminal wishes." Through consciousness of sin (lex talionis) arises fear of the punishment of God. Precisely that animal will bite and kill us which we wanted to remove a hated rival from our path. Besides animals may represent all possible housemates or become representatives of a definite parapathia (Fellatio, cunnilingus, necrophilia, vampirism, sadism, mysophilia, etc.). All these components may unite to produce a phobia. We must never forget that the neuroses are built up in several dimensions and that several forces combine to express themselves in a certain symptom.

Let us begin with the analysis of a simple case before proceeding to more complicated ones :—

No. 131.—Mrs. N. C., thirty-two years old, separated from her husband, comes to be treated by me for fear of snakes. This fear has existed since childhood and has grown enormously in recent years. She would write beforehand to find out if there were snakes in a place. She asks the hotel-keeper if there are snakes in the garden. She rents a room on the fourth floor and is very anxious because there is a roof gutter near her window. The snake might crawl through the roof gutter into her room.

She grew up with three brothers and sisters in a rich gentleman's house. The father was extremely strict. Everyone in the house trembled before him. But he was a man of rare beauty with a wonderful voice. (She thinks a great deal of the voice.) Never in her life has she since met such a " wonderful man." At twenty she married for love and had ill luck. Her husband was a frivolous good-for-nothing who infected her with lues and gonorrhœa, and squandered a part of her large fortune, so that after four years she had to get a divorce from him. She describes her feelings with regard to wedded life as at first normal ; later, she had for this man nothing but disgust and loathing.

She avows a healthy natural sensuality. If she loved a man she would give herself to him. Even if it was a serving-man. If he only took her fancy. . . . But in reality she is religious and shuns all sin. At the moment she is in love and proof against any attack. And on whom has her choice fallen ? On an artist, sixty-five years old, a reproduction of her father. She is angry with him because he did not accept her. She says she offered herself to him plainly enough. She never doubted his potency. (" He is splendidly preserved.") Of course, she had chosen an object so little dangerous to protect her virtue and to avoid all temptations. She has no lack of suitors. But she rejects all suggestion of casual love-making. For she is in love with the artist and may not betray him.

She is much interested in the phallus. As a child she repeatedly saw her father's great phallus. She is not repelled by a male organ. A physician had told her that her aversion to snakes and her fear of them corresponded to her aversion to the phallus. She says that cannot be so ; that she has no such aversion ; that she had repeatedly taken her husband's phallus in her hand without any aversion or fear.

The analysis shows a strong homosexual disposition towards her sister and a friend. Small homosexual experiences in childhood were brought to light. But this was only one component of her phobia. I was able to demonstrate the following causes :—

(1) Fear of another sexual infection.[1]
(2) Fear of sin. (The snake in the Bible a symbol of sin).
(3) Fear of homosexuality.
(4) Warding off a fellatio-phantasy.
(5) Identification with the snake. (She is a false person, who has desired her mother's death).
(6) Relations to the poison complex. (She wished to poison her husband).
We see the fear of snakes is the fear of her own bad thoughts. After the analysis complete cure. After two years marriage for love.

The relation of the animal phobiæ to sexuality are mostly very transparent. In the simplest cases it is the normal sexuality which is condemned as " animal " by the prude and is symbolised

[1] Goethe in his " Venetian Epigrams " makes the snake the symbol of sex-infection.

in fear of animals. Hysterical girls who rave about purity show a pathological fear of bulls. Bulls might thrust their horns into their stomachs. The animal dreams of these patients betray them at once. They are persecuted by bulls or wild horses. It is their own passions from which they are trying to escape.

Infinitely more frequent is the fear of homosexuality, which expresses itself as fear of animals. In such men we find fear of snakes, rats and worms, also of bulls and stallions.

In women, defence against homosexuality may express itself as fear of mice and fear of toads. There are whole families whose female members suffer from fear of mice ; this fear is handed on from generation to generation apparently through the influence of the environment. The pathological character of this fear of mice appears from the following observation.

No. 132.—Mrs. H. K., thirty-nine years old, suffers from sleeplessness, extreme excitability, convulsions with temporary loss of consciousness. She has suffered since her youth from a terrible fear of mice, against which her mother and grandmother also had to struggle. She will have no hidden corners in her house, always has the garden searched, keeps several cats as a protection against mice. Her present attack dates from the visit of a relative who showed her a dear little mouse of old silver, which she had received as a present. She did not know that one must not utter the word mouse before the patient. At sight of the charming nicknack the lady gave a loud shriek and fell senseless to the ground.

The homosexual basis of this fear appears from the fact that all these patients fear the mouse may get under their clothes. Similarly a woman who suffers from fear of toads declares : " I cannot bear the thought that the toad might get between my legs. I have an inexpressible disgust for this creature. Why—if my gardener had already killed the toad, I cannot get rid of the thought that never-theless this toad might get under my clothes."[1]

The fear of dogs (cynophobia) which may grow into fear of mad dogs (rabiophobia) has various roots. Here I mention only cunni-lingus, fellatio, vampirism, mysophilia. Usually it is the fear of the wild beast within one's own breast.

Somewhat more rare is insect phobia, often symbolising the pricks of conscience, but sometimes a sex symbol. A study of the " analysis of a bird-phobia " in the next chapter will give an idea of the complicated nature of these problems.

I maintain that there is no animal which in certain circumstances may not become the object of a serious phobia. Obsessions too, show relations to zoophobia. The discussion of them is reserved for a later volume.

I now give the account of her dread of cats contributed by a very intelligent lady now forty-eight years of age. I will say at the outset that this is not a report of an analytical investigation. The report speaks for itself. I will here confine myself to a few remarks

[1] In legend the toad is always a sexual symbol. It usually changes on being kissed into a prince or a princess.

ZOOPHOBIAS 297

and refer the reader to the history of the patient which contains the analysis of a bird-phobia.

No. 133.—" When I first began to suffer from fear of cats I am not certain, but I suppose that the fear or rather the invincible horror which I feel at the sight or even in the proximity of a cat which I cannot see, goes much further back than I know. I was, as I have been told, a strong child well developed mentally and physically, without a specially nervous disposition. I was extremely fond of dogs, but appear to have had no liking for cats, for otherwise I could not understand even less than now, why my nurse should have told me a tale about a cat, warning me of their love of vengeance ; that this (although she meant it kindly) achieved just the opposite was certainly not her intention ; it simply showed lack of understanding of the child-mind.

" The story which made so deep and terrible an impression on me, was as follows :—

" ' A clergyman had a cat of which he was very fond ; the cat even had all its meals at his table. One day the bishop came to dinner, and the cat was banished to an outer room ; in the night the cat sneaked into the room, lay down on the breast of the sleeping clergyman and put its tail into his open mouth. In the morning the clergyman was found dead in his bed.'

" That telling of a cat's vengeance could not contribute to endear this animal to a child already timid is certain, but even pedagogues of the better class could not have expected the fearful effect which this story had on me. It is my misfortune that I was brought up, not in the age of the child, but in the seventies at a time when it was still believed that nervous disturbances could be suppressed with energy and by slight punishments. The first shock of which I was conscious happened in my ninth or tenth year. I had a little niece whom I dearly loved and whom, so far as I could, I mothered. It was summer ; the child lay, as I thought, in the perambulator, in the garden ; I wanted to look at the child or to take it out, threw back the curtains and saw, not the little one, but the black house cat, which was as frightened as I was, and jumped off over my head without touching me or injuring me. My first thought was : " The child is suffocated." There was no second thought because I lost consciousness. I believed that would have been the time to dissipate my fear of cats, by cautiously accustoming me to them, by systematic well thought out stories of the kindness and attachment of cats ; but unfortunately nothing was done in this direction ; they thought my fear would wear off if no notice was taken of it. To this day I recall with horror the unspeakable torture which the lessons in the garden caused me, when I ought to have been thinking of learning and all I could think of was whether the white and yellow tom-cat would come into the shrubbery. It is forty years since then and yet to-day as I write these lines the constant dread of my childhood grips me. From the day when I swooned the dread of cats runs like a black thread through my whole life. I, who loved living in the country, saw with fear the coming of summer, because I had to move from the safe first-floor flat in the town, into a summer residence situated if possible in a garden. Willingly as I made and make excursions the thought of entering a country inn is very painful to me because I am always afraid of meeting a cat there, so that I would always rather give up the excursion than experience on the way the fear of ' the fear.' The change of residence, the compulsory staying in the open air, and the constant fear when on an excursion of having to go into some house affected me physically. The family physician said I could not stand the heat. I believed him then, too ; now I know that only the strain on my nerves was responsible. Day and night I had not a minute in peace because I had constantly to be on the watch lest I should be surprised by a cat. I knew exactly whereabouts in the neighbourhood there were cats, whether they stayed in the garden and what they looked like. For a quite quiet cat to pass near me was a torture and I never again went alone to the place where I had met her. I was a grown-up girl and can vividly recollect how I once woke up in the night (I did not sleep alone) and found a cat on the foot of my bed. The uproar I made was so fearful that the whole family came running in for they believed that burglars were in the house. When in the following year the house really was broken into, I was not nearly so much afraid as in that night. What is so horrible in my condition is that cats are not so rare as crocodiles and if I don't want to be boxed up in my four walls I am exposed every moment to an encounter with a cat.

" In places where no one sees a cat and where I have often been without seeing one, I am suddenly overtaken with an unspeakable dread, I cease speaking, I change colour, feel bad inside, and feel the proximity of a cat as yet unseen. In a short time the cat appears ; I cannot tell whether through my constant watching I saw it before the others ; or whether I looked for it because I noticed the smell ; I only know that a place where I have had such an experience remains always connected with the thought of a cat and is avoided by me as far as possible. I believe that unconsciously I know the smell of the animal. We live in a house with a closed court-yard ; the porter has a dog, and there never was a cat in the whole house. One evening I come home after the gate is closed, stop at the staircase and declare I can go no further, for there is a cat in the house. Of course they laugh at me. After a long search they find a very little kitten which had gone astray. The animal was separated from me by about twelve steps and a screen. Often I should like to go into a shop, but I cannot because I have the feeling that there's a cat there ; and if in spite of this I have forced myself to enter, there always was a cat there. This not being able to forget the torture which I have felt at the sight of a cat or the unpleasant ideas which many words call forth in me, is a great burden in my life. If I call my travels to mind the first pictures which rise to memory are those places where I have seen a cat (e.g., Hotel St. Gotthard, white Angora cat, and so on) and only then come the pleasant impressions. It is very unpleasant to have such ideas connected with the St. Gotthard, but the case is much worse if these feelings of fear and misery are connected with places which absolutely must be visited. Words, too, arouse the cat-fear in me, e.g., clergymen, vicar, and more such. Unfortunately, my dread of cats was not improved by my marriage ; and it became much worse when I was expecting my baby. Much as I rejoiced over the child, I was in frightful anxiety the whole time lest I should meet a cat, because I was convinced that the child would be injured thereby. In places where otherwise I felt quite safe (theatres, concerts) a great fear would suddenly seize me that a cat might suddenly spring at my face and of course all artistic pleasure was over. During the whole time of my pregnancy I never went out alone for fear of meeting a cat. I was not to escape my fate. In the seventh month of my pregnancy I was terrified by a cat in the street and some days later I bore a dead child.

" I have often tried myself to get rid of the cat-fear. Once I so far succeeded in getting used to a white cat that I was able without special excitement to share a garden with her. To be sure this cat was a special cat ; she wore a little bell and was so gentle that she shared her bed with a bitch. When cat and bitch had young ones they took it in turns to look after them. I believe it was mostly due to the bell that I had less fear of this cat. I have very keen hearing rendered keener by fear, and as I could hear the animal I was secure against seeing it suddenly and also from the fear that it might get at me from behind. Once I tried by watching a cat in a cage for a long time to accustom myself to the sight of it, but alas ! with no success. Lately I was compelled with many other people to share a room with a cat for about half an hour. This time also I was—to my shame—the vanquished and had to atone for my ' heroic deed ' with a sleepless night interrupted by intestinal disorders.

" I could write for another hour but it would still be the same story ; in my life the cat has always proved the stronger ; yet I must say that I am not one of the weakest. Of late years it seems to me that I am more tranquil whether it is age or simply a false conclusion, for since the war we cannot travel, make few excursions and so avoid the chief causes for excitement. It may be interesting to know *that as a child until my sixteenth year I had a great dislike for furs, and a quite special fear of my father's great travelling fur which seemed to me to be made out of a number of cats. This condition has entirely abated."*

As a supplement to this account by the patient I would mention the following facts. She loved her father intensely, and was otherwise never afraid of him. She had the association *father—cat* only when he put on the great fur for travelling. Originally other furs also were revolting to her. Only of later years out of vanity she became accustomed to furs and tolerated also her husband's fur.

She tells me that her whole life has been spoilt by the fear of cats. It is always the vision of the "tail in the mouth" (her original expression) which has dominated her. Even the word "cat" could not be uttered without making her feel sick. Often she suffered for weeks from sickness and stomach trouble. At seventeen years of age she had a long stomach disease which the doctor declared to be ulcus ventriculi and which later revealed itself as stomach neurosis.

When her husband proposed to her she confessed her fear of cats to him and warned him not to bind himself to her. He treated the matter lightly, and as a physician hoped to rid her of the phobia. On the wedding night he had remarkable experiences. His young wife was quite unenlightened. Her experience consisted in a kiss which the "best man" at a wedding had given her. She was then so naïve that she believed that through the kiss she would become pregnant and bring a child into the world. On the wedding journey when her husband consummated the union in the railway carriage she thought him mad and dared not speak a word for fear she had to do with a lunatic. Only gradually she allowed him to enlighten her. Previous attempts at enlightenment by women friends were rejected. She laughed and refused to listen because she did not believe in such nonsense. (So great was the power of her hysterical repression.)

On the fourth day of her wedding trip she entered a restaurant where a cat ran past her. With a loud cry she fell in a swoon. She had to be taken to the hotel in a carriage. For two weeks from this day she suffered from vomiting and stomach trouble while continuing the journey.

She says that later she always had orgasm, remembers no abnormal sexual phantasies. Her marriage is extremely happy, although her cat phobia gave her husband a great deal of trouble and limited his life to certain "cat-free" places.

She does not remember any dream. She never dreams. Only in childhood there was a dream which constantly returns. She fell slowly to bottomless depths.

She was the youngest child and was spoilt beyond measure by her father whom she loved more than her mother. She was difficult to bring up, refractory, self-willed, dogmatic, and very jealous of her brothers and sisters. She had a sister five years older than herself who was greatly pampered by her brothers, which she never could bear.

Her whole condition has greatly improved because she has very intense scientific occupation. She has now risen superior to the affair, she can talk about cats, she can study her phobia scientifically. She tried to get accustomed to cats in the Zoological Gardens. Great cats (lions and tigers) do not affect her. But the sight of a wild cat made a shudder run through her and filled her with nameless disgust. Dogs she is passionately fond of. But all animals that remind her of cats are hateful to her. She has also a pronounced aversion to birds that flutter about the room, while a captive canary bird is indifferent to her.

A noted psycho-analyst traced her phobia to a passion for the governess which she could not understand and denied. The analytic treatment like all previous treatments, no success.

In order thoroughly to understand this cat-phobia one must know that persons who dread animals in this pathological fashion have identified themselves with the object of the dread. *The patient sees in the cat the mirrored image of herself.*

She is the false cat that with boundless jealousy envied her brothers and sisters the parents' love. She saw incorporated in the cat the criminal ideas of her childhood. Her wild impulses very early manifested themselves, but soon there developed a sensitive conscience which suppressed everything bad and projected it outwards into the cat. She suppressed, too, all sexual emotions and sex-knowledge so she was able to enter unenlightened into marriage and to believe in conceiving through a kiss.

One can plainly see the connection between the cat and the father. The father's fur was made entirely of cats' skin. Her aversion to all furs is the negative expression of a suppressed paraphilia, which has preserved itself in the expression, " tail in the mouth."

The analysis was evidently frustrated by her resistances. She had the gift of those who are dissociated of " hearing past " the words of the physician. She consists of two persons. One of them is determined not to know what the cat means. So all teaching remains barren. It runs off her like water from a duck's back.

It is very characteristic that she cannot remember any dream. She says she never dreams. That is not true. Everyone dreams constantly from the moment of falling asleep till he wakes up. But she must not know her dreams. She must not know what goes on within her. She leads a double life. She lives in a second world of dreams from which no bridge leads to the real world. The phobia alone represents her passions, her cravings, her battles and her victories in the second world.

But this phobia has determined her whole life. *The leitmotif of her existence is the dread of cats.* The cat is the tyrant of her existence, the representative of the false. The dog the symbol of the true is her friend. In her soul dog and cat wage an embittered strife. She could bear the sight of but one single cat. That was the kitten with the bell which lived happily with the dog. This cat's bell may have reminded her of her conscience, which continually sounds the bell, "*Be on guard against yourself!*"

CHAPTER XXIX

ANALYSIS OF A BIRD-PHOBIA

MOST animal phobiæ are shown by analysis to be a pathological fixation of infantile tendencies, a psychosexual
infantilism. But the matter is not so simple, and one
must not consider the analysis completed with the interpretation of the sex symbol. Otherwise one experiences the
humiliation of finding that in spite of all analyses and explanations
the phobia persists and is unaffected by all therapeutic measures ;
a fact which doubtless moved Freud to declare the phobiæ to be
" psychically unassailable," i.e., not of psychogenic origin.
In the following analysis it will be shown how dangerous it is
to conduct and interpret such an analysis on purely sex lines.
Most phobiæ are built up in a way much more complicated than the
beginner in analysis imagines. A symptom is determined in several
ways ; like the whole neurosis it is built up in several dimensions.
The following analysis of a bird-phobia will illustrate this.
No. 134.—Mr. J. K., a forty-one years old factory owner, has
suffered since childhood from various fear-conditions, the centre
point being an almost invincible fear of open spaces and a *fear of
birds*. The roots of the agora-phobia are connected with those
of the bird-phobia, so that for the present we may confine ourselves to the latter. From his childhood our patient fears all
birds. Even a bird in a cage which he encounters in someone's
house is unpleasant to him. It pains him, too, if he meets any kind
of bird (hen, goose, duck, etc.) in the open air ; these animals
seem sinister to him. This feeling of anticipation increases to
horror if he sees a bird flying about the room. Birds in the
air too, are a constant object of anxiety to him. The sight
of birds flapping their wings is intolerable to him. The idea that
a bird might flutter round him flapping its wings causes the strongest
feelings of terror. Equally great is the fear that the bird might
settle on his shoulder.
The physician who was treating him, a very able and experienced
therapeutist, considered the sexual significance of this phobia.
The German expression *vögeln* (Vogel = a bird) for a cohabitation
set him thinking of sexual defensive ideas especially of defence
against a fellatio phantasy (penis in ore). This solution was not
directly rejected by the patient but also not accepted, and brought

no alleviation of the painful condition.[1] As to the origin of the phobia the patient contributes some important recollections. He remembers *a parrot* which lived in his parents' house and was then given to an aunt. He had forgotten this parrot when on a visit to the aunt he suddenly saw the bird flutter into the room. Filled with terror he begged that the creature should be removed. He remembers also two " *inseparables* " which were kept in his parents' house. He believes one *inseparable* died, and the other also. Finally it occurs to him that an aunt was photographed with a pigeon in her hand.

More important appears the report of a very recent and remarkable impression which was several times repeated. From his residence to the office the shortest way was through the Zoological Gardens for which he had a permanent admission ticket. Like all phobists, he strove against his fear and tried to overcome it by the force of custom. A mysterious power drew him to the birds which he so dreaded. So every morning he went by the birds, always gripped by fear and horror. Then one morning he discovered a parrot which by its peculiar expression and its form reminded him of an old man. The bowed attitude, the troubled face, the glance of the dull eyes . . . this was no bird, this was a man in bird-form. It was especially horrible for him to look at this bird and yet he could not help looking at it again and again. . . .

Before we proceed to the explanation of this strange phenomenon we must speak of two other phobic phenomena. The first is his *fear of falling in love*. He fears that he may meet a woman with whom he must fall in love. This dread dates back some twenty years. At that time in a sanatorium he made the acquaintance of a girl who was greatly tormented and persecuted by her mother. Immediately he pitied her, and at once fell in love with her while he was comforting her. But at the same time he said something to the girl's companion which was intended to render impossible all thought of a marriage. He would always remain a bachelor, he would never marry, his circumstances did not permit him to marry. Nevertheless, he thought that through his sympathetic attitude he had made the impression of a suitor. He withdrew to his room and was seized with a violent attack of fear, so that the physician declared him to be a " hysteric." A few days later he left the sanatorium and went home. He had to meet the girl a few times more. He always took care to guard against any ideas of courtship. He sent congratulations only in conjunction with his brother, sent flowers with his brother's card as well as his own, never paid a visit alone. But from that time dates the fear of falling in love and of

[1] Freud, in his study, " A Childhood Memory of Leonardo da Vinci " (*pp.* 25 and 26) has set forth in detail the memory of this fantasy in connection with the pleasurable recollection of sucking. As to the bird as sex symbol see the paper by Friedrich S. Krauss, " Der Vogel." Int. Ztschrft f. ärtze. Psychoanalyse, Vol. I., 1913, *p.* 288.

an impression that might lay hold of him. He does not dare to look a woman in the eyes, and to speak a few words with her. The woman-conductor, the masseuse, the typist are just as much objects of this dread as the servant-girl, the cook, the housekeeper. Therefore he confines his walks to certain roads and even these he can only use in the company of his servant or his physician. His mistress also accompanies him on certain roads.

He likes this mistress very well because he is certain of not falling in love with her. He always keeps her at a due distance. He did not even choose her himself. His brother found her for him. He has never passed a night with her. He always comes only on a visit to her and copulates with his clothes on. They exchange no confidences, they do not say " thou " to one another. Nevertheless he plays with the thought of marrying the mistress, for he considers her a very reasonable, refined person and the fact that he is not in love with her seems to him a great advantage. Certainly she will never " get a hold of him."

He is quite potent with her and feels a strong orgasm in coitus. But besides this coitus with the mistress which is performed twice a week as "necessary hygienic measure " (doctors' orders) there is also a second mode of satisfying himself which shows a pronounced infantile character.

There lives in his house an old housekeeper whom he likes to have caress him. She pities his sufferings and when he is sleepless strokes him like a little child till he falls asleep. This often causes an emission. This form of gratification reminds him of the sport of a governess in his youth (eight to thirteen) who evidently contributed a great deal to originating his fear. She used to play with his penis. With the housekeeper he experiences a revival of this experience.

There is another circumstance which gives his case a peculiar stamp. He tends to connect every accident with his own guilt. If an acquaintance falls ill, e.g., with inflammation of the lungs, he feels absolutely compelled to rummage through his whole past to convince himself that he has no responsibility for this illness. Alas, if he has advised the patient to go up the Semmering and he had cooled down on that occasion ! Or if he had recommended a journey or a doctor that had turned out badly. Therefore he does not make known who are his physicians and cannot recommend them to anyone. If his advice is asked on a medical question he is silent. If it should turn out badly he might hold himself responsible.

Suppose that Mr. X, a neighbour, who was indifferent to him, had died of the influenza. At once the torment begins. He rummages and considers : When did he last see Mr. X ? What did he say to him ? If he himself had no relations with X, a third person might have acted as intermediary. There is no peace for him. For if he excludes all possibilities there remains a bitter residue, something uncertain, inexplicable, which accuses him and burdens him. He must be somehow guilty of the misfortune.

This peculiarity is connected with another. He has a secret belief that a business will go badly if he prophecies it : e.g., a new branch-depot of his firm is established. He opposes this and is out-voted. Then the conviction is borne in on him that it cannot prosper *and in every case it has gone badly.*

He confesses that he then really *wishes* that it *may go badly*, and that these wishes of his are always *fulfilled.* His prophecies are the desires of a malicious, vengeful, envious, supersensitive, ambitious man, who will not confess these hateful feelings to himself and who by good works and acts of charity is always proving to himself that he has " a good heart." His hypertrophied ambition is compensated and spurred on by an oppressive self-depreciation. He blames his illness for the self-depreciation, because it cripples him and makes him only half a man. What would he not achieve if he were well ! But the illness exempts him from the responsibility of achieving these mighty works, and of justifying his faith in his own " great historic mission." But he follows with envious eye the successes of others and especially of his brothers, whose vitality, energy and good health oppress him when he compares himself, the picture of misery, with them. One of these brothers, too, treats him badly and does not believe in his illness, says it is imagination.

His illness is sacred to him and any doubt of his suffering seems to him a grave crime. His whole life is a fight for his suffering.

But he knows that no one can offend him or humiliate him with importunity. Such acts always end in an illness or some severe reverse for the offender. His very thought, " something may go wrong "—and how often his resentment gives birth to such thoughts leads to its really going wrong.

He has a secret faith in the omnipotence of thought. Within he is vengeful, egoistic and never forgets an injury. As already mentioned he has boundless ambition and feels himself always put in the background. (He says his father treats him like a boy, his brothers laugh at him, his sisters heed him not at all.) But he wants to be the first in the family. He demands recognition and love, and especially from his father, who uses him as whipping-boy and visits every unpleasantness on him. He can say to him (the forty-one years old man !) " You are still a snivelling brat ! You understand nothing at all ! "

But he does not dare to oppose his father and to answer with something that might provoke the old man. For if the father should get a stroke he would never cease to reproach himself. Then he would be guilty of his father's death.

It is plain to every analyst that his attitude to his father is bipolar. He loves his father and hates him ; trembles for his life and wishes for his death, if only to get the management of the business into his own hands. And withal he finds that the father is not kind enough, and urges all his physicians to tell the father that he, the son, is severely ill, and is not equal to any excitement. In grotesque fashion he extorts the old man's pity. He moans and complains without ceasing. In his whole life he has never known a minute's comfort. He is always ill, always suffering, he does not know what happiness is. God only knows how he suffers. This attitude to his father has its special relations to his phobia. He cannot live without a motor-car. He is uneasy if the car is not standing at the door. If his father does not come to the business he is unhappy, and his fear increases. His father has got a chill somewhere. He cannot bear that. If his father is at the business he can send the car away. Often, however, the fear grows, and the father has to hold both his hands. All his thoughts centre round the car. Is the car at the door ? Has it plenty of spirit ? Has not the chaffeur gone home ?

This compulsion is explained from his fear of losing his old father. If the father is not at the business he wants the car. But not because the father protects and helps him against the fear, but because he lives in a definite fantasy and expectation. This expectation seems to have existed since childhood. *He wants the car when his father is not at the business because every second he expects the news that the old man is seriously ill, that he has had a stroke or some other accident.* Then he would have to go to him at once in the car, and to see that a doctor was brought. He would be able to attend to everything at once, without having to reproach himself.

His tormenting consciousness of guilt arises from the wishes for his father's death. His neurosis is a form of self-punishment for these wishes. For in spite of his wealth he is like a prisoner in a golden cage.

We learn, too, that from his childhood his father has treated him badly, while his mother was very kind and tender with him. That at least is his recollection.

And now we come to the explanation of the bird-phobia. One detail, the fear of the fluttering birds, is easily explained in the analysis, when he brings me a recollection from his earliest childhood. Among the Jews there exists the religious custom of " beating the sacrifice to death." Before the day of atonement a (black) hen is swung with full force round the head. This is the sacrificial hen, the expiatory sacrifice to the wrathful God. At the same time a prayer is pronounced and the cry is uttered : " Life to me, death to thee ! " For every person such a hen is sacrificed, for the adults a large, for the children a small black hen. (The bird of death !) This scene made a great impression on him as a child. At that time the wish must have arisen in him : " *May my father or my brother die !* " Every other dead person is for our patient a sacrifice, a substitute. If someone dies, a stranger or an acquaintance, he thinks : " Good that I am not the one ! " Also he directly desires death for his enemies and for those he envies ; he is filled with malicious joy. The fluttering wings of the birds arouse in him the association with the substitute-fowls and with his first criminal, egoistic malicious desires.

Now, too, we can understand the recollection of the " inseparables." He heard then that these creatures love each other so much that if one dies the other perishes for sorrow. And it seems to have been so in this case. At least he has an obscure memory of it. He loved his mother and hated his father. His first recollection shows this attitude. As is well-known, the first recollections—as covering recollections in the sense of Freud—refer to the most important scene of the child-life, the first attitude, its relation to the world and to its immediate surroundings. This recollection was as follows :

" I am standing before a jeweller's shop and am admiring a pair of ear-rings with large red stones. I think to myself : I will buy these ear-rings for my mother when I have the money. "

His second recollection also refers to the mother :—

" I see a great house, and say : ' I will buy that for my mother ! ' My brother finds the house too dirty and says he will buy mother a much more beautiful one."

These two recollections show at once that he would like to lay all the treasures of the world at his mother's feet. His father and mother were very fond of each other. He remembers only one conflict which happened when he was older, and his father would not recognise his illness while his mother said something must be done for the child, he must go into a sanatorium. He was always a sickly child and was therefore greatly spoilt by his mother. . . . His parents were the " inseparables." A happier marriage he had never seen. The idea of getting rid of the father, must have reminded him of the " inseparables " and have brought before him the terrible thought that his mother might at once follow his father to death. Such a love seemed to the child something terrible. A dread of every love must necessarily develop.

Now the connection with the parrot becomes clear. The parrot (papa-gei) is his papa.[1] To my question : " To what age can a parrot live ? " he answers promptly : " Oh, very old, sixty to seventy years ! "

The parrot reminds him of his old father, and wakens the voice of his conscience. His horror is the dread of his own evil thoughts. His phobia is punishment for and protection against the evil thoughts. For he is taken up with his dread that he can think of nothing else.

He consumes himself in longing for love. It is the dream of his life to be able to love and to be loved. The dread of this love dominates him in bipolar fashion. (To have to die if the beloved one dies !) His polygamic ideas also (he is a collector and a Don Juan in phantasy) resist such a tie. If one loves one woman one

[1] [The German for parrot is Papagei.—Tr.]

is lost to all others. But in his youth he already had two women : the governess and the mother. By a skilful management of existing circumstances his mistress takes the place of the mother and his housekeeper of the governess. He again has his two women who look after him and are fond of him, but he has so chosen them that his heart is not bound and that he need not be afraid of love. If his mistress dies he can get his brother to find another ; the house-keeper, too, can be replaced. They are not irreplaceable. He need not die when they do. He is not bound but open to all possibilities. But in the bird-phobia his evil conscience relieves itself. Like a perpetual warning the substitute-bird stands before his eyes, reminds him of his own wickedness and bids him fear the punishment of God. His fear of death is fear of the reckoning after death. God knows all and sees all. God knows also his evil thoughts.

The patient says he is not religious and does not trouble about God and religion. Driven into a corner he has to admit that he repeats to himself the fragments he remembers of a Hebrew prayer, and also that he murmurs children's prayers before falling asleep. He keeps up the memory of the day of atonement by his own pennance and fast-days. He has noticed that the attacks of fear are connected with the stomach. He cannot bear eating. Fasting alleviates the condition. Often he can only get rid of the fear by three or four fast-days. These fast-days too, have a religious significance and are substitutes for the fast-days which he does not observe, like the day of atonement. All his suffering has one final importance. He is working for the great scene of justification on the last day. What has his whole life been ? Trouble, fear, pain and suffering ! So that one can understand his saying that he has never had a happy moment in his life. His life is nothing but eternal suffering. It is his punishment for his thoughts of death. And only God knows how he suffers, because he ascribes all his suffering to the honour of God. He plays before God the role of the perpetual invalid, the Lazarus, the Job.

It is noteworthy that by drawing in air he himself produces his attacks, which may be of rare severity, presenting the picture of a sick man, deadly pale, struggling for breath and covered with sweat. He makes the deep sighing and inspirations of the æro-phagic neurotic, and is also able to pump air into the stomach by reflex swallowing and chewing motions. When the diaphragm is high there results then the feeling of tension in the abdomen and in the neighbourhood of the heart. He has to undo his trousers and his waistcoat buttons.

All the symptomatic acts and speeches show a strong homosexual component, which also explains his bipolar attitude to his father. What he with child-like confidence expects from his father are caresses such as he receives from the housekeeper. From the physicians, too, he always expects attention, and remarks with pride that all his physicians are his friends. He gives himself endless trouble to describe and explain his illness, and is always seeking for appreciation. Really he does everything possible to conceal the true motives of the neurosis and hide them by twisting them into the opposite. He shuns the truth and shows that secret pride in his illness which is manifested by all rich and original neurotics whom countless celebrated physicians have failed to help. He tells none of his physicians of his secret faith in the omnipotence of his thoughts. He is himself a bird of death. He is an unlucky wretch that brings every one ill luck. In the bird he fears and hates his inner ego, the cruel, malicious, envious ego, the croaking raven that always prophecies evil because he wishes evil to everyone.

Doubtless the strong impression of " striking the sacrifice " has determined the structure of his neurosis. He has shown anxiety-conditions from childhood. The child-phobiæ which are so very frequent but which have escaped the notice of most children's physicians are the forerunners of the phobiæ of adults. Their study would facilitate the understanding of all phobiæ. I refer to the short paper by Abraham " Zur Psychogenese der Strassenangst im Kindesalter " (Int. Ztschrift für ärzt Psycho-analyse, Vol. I, 1913, *p.* 256).

A five-year old boy shows both forms of the fear from which our patient suffered even in childhood. He cannot remain alone in the house and cannot go out without his mother. He cannot even go to his relatives who live over the way. And he cannot go out with the nurse-girl, for he says, " I won't be a walking boy, I will be mother's boy." His father goes on a journey and he is allowed to sleep with his mother. On the day his father is to come home, he says to his mother : " *It would be ever so much better if papa never came back from the journey !* "

Such observations show us *in nuce* how thoughts of the father's death originate. From the above discussion we may assume that similar desires have existed in the breast of our patient. The way in which he behaves to the father confirms this assumption and gives it a high degree of probability. The bird-phobia whose homosexual determination I will certainly not dispute, shows us his " *idée fixe* " in Janet's sense. About his father's head flutters incessantly the black bird of death, and that bird reminds him of the frailty and mortality of his progenitor, for whose life he trembles —trembles as violently as he longs for his money and the inheritance of his power.

The case explains also the psychic mechanism of fearful expectation. The phobists expect a misfortune, long for it and dread it. They tremble for the consummation and yet long for it. From this conflict they take refuge in the grievous prison of their suffering.[1]

---

[1] The case has great similarity with the bell-phobia of Morton Prince (Int. Z. f. P.A. Vol. I.). A forty year old woman dreads all church towers. In hypnosis it comes to light that during an operation on her mother the

M

CHAPTER XXX

STUTTERING. STAGE-FRIGHT. GENERAL VIEW OF THE PHOBIAS

ONE of the most frequent forms of fear hysteria is stuttering, the dread of speaking. Originally it is only the fear of betraying some secret by speaking. Then the fear is transferred to the speaking itself. The people then fear not being able to speak quietly without interruption. I have studied several examples of these neuroses and have always come to one conclusion : Stuttering is a psychic betrayal like slips of the tongue or of the pen. An unconscious complex interposes itself between the syllables and words. It is internal resistances which check the free flow of the speech, not false articulation, lack of breath, indistinct vocalisation, etc.

The neurosis always begins in childhood, mostly as pure anxiety neurosis. The child has something to hide (See the Chapter : "Anxiety neurosis of Children." If stuttering occurs in adults, it is always a case of repressed ideas. (Cf. the case of the Rabbi and of the Priest.)

The entourage creates out of stuttering in consequence of unconscious resistances the conscious fear of stuttering.

The beginning of stuttering is very aptly described by J. Barth (following Liebmann), (New Views on Stuttering, Stammering, Blustering and Deaf- and Dumbness. Wiener Klinische Rundschau, 1904). The child begins, on some occasion or other, to stutter a little. (Mostly—we may add—if it has come into contact with the sex-problem.) Others then begin to ridicule the child : "it is blamed and laughed at, it is scolded and threatened, it is beaten and the most dismal prospect for the future is held up before it. Through this behaviour of his environment the stutterer gets the greatest fear of speaking, the involuntarily unco-ordinated motions, at first weak, are considerably strengthened by the fear ; the breathing, too, becomes frequent and irregular through fear. Speech becomes worse and worse ; usually the parents start exercises. Stuttered words must be repeated, people seek out difficult

bells rang. She prayed fervently and hated the bells that made such a noise. Her bipolar attitude towards her mother manifested itself in a consciousness of guilt, which occurred also with regard to other people, so that she seemed hateful and worthless to herself. These bells are also a perpetual warning awakening the recollection of her hateful thoughts during her mother's operation. Evidently also a secret belief in the omnipotence of thought. (Cf. the case of the Rabbi and of the Priest).

sounds, draw the stutterer's attention to these, and make him constantly practise them. *And so the stutterer is artificially inoculated with fear of certain sounds.* Previously all abnormal breathing and speech motions were quite involuntary, now voluntary ones also begin."

The centre-point of stuttering *is fear of speaking.* The case is like that of psychic impotence where fear as an inhibitory idea checks the automatic course of the function.

We have analysed in detail two great examples of occupation stutterers (the rabbi and the priest). We have some other analyses, small and large, which prove that in future only psycho-analysis can be the therapy for stuttering.

No. 135.—A twelve year old boy suddenly began to stutter. After some days the troubled mother put him under my care. It appeared that the boy had been shown by an elder boy how to masturbate. Till then he had had no secret from his mother. When he came before her and wanted to say something, it occurred to him that the mother must notice something about him, and speech forsook him. According to our view we may say : The complex forced itself upon his speech, and disturbed the normal course of that function.

I quieted the boy and told him his mother would not punish him ; that he has only to tell the truth, and leave off masturbating ; that he is still a child and at that age such excitements may be injurious. The boy confessed to his mother and at once ceased to stutter.

Had I not been able to interfere so energetically the boy might have become a confirmed stutterer.

In connection with this case I would point out that I am by no means alone in taking this view. Whereas for a long time physical causes were conjectured for the diseases we call stuttering and even operations were suggested, of late the voices which declare stuttering to be a pure neurosis are on the increase.

I would only refer here to the book by Denhard, jun. (Das Stottern eine Psychose).

It is significant that stutterers only stutter when they have to speak before strangers. If they are alone they speak or read almost or quite as fast as any other person. Dr. E. Trömer (Wiener Klin. therap. Wochenschrift, 1905, No. 8) takes stuttering to be a neurosis, not quite in Denhard's sense (an anxiety neurosis) but an obsession neurosis. He does not deal with their psycho-analysis, but gives a number of cases in which without any practising he has effected a cure by hypnosis. He maintains that there are many stutterers whose stuttering the practise treatment rather aggravates, while in all cases hypnosis is helpful, and is sometimes the only remedy.

It is true that he himself admits that by his method relapses are very frequent ; this may result from the nature of the obsession not being exactly explained, since hypnosis has not the value of a successful psycho-analysis. One must remove those unconscious ideas which make the stuttering an obsession. Gutzmann also (" Zur Behandlung des Stotterns. Therapeutische Monatsh., 1909, October) ; and especially " Ueber die Behandlung d. Neurosen

der Stimme und Sprache," Med. Klinik, 1909, No. 20) who takes
stuttering to be a neurosis, is like Forel against hypnosis and refers
to Ziechen's statement: " I consider the hypnotic treatment in
youthful stuttering in view of the disadvantages connected with it
as simply mischievous." Gutzmann advocates a persuasion cure
in the sense of Dubois and Dejérine. Besides this he recommends
treatment of any digestive disturbances. As early as 1851 Romberg
had described a case of stuttering which was cured by purgatives
and strict diet. In such case the suggestion of the physician is
the strongest remedy. Such cures give no security against relapses.
Only psycho-analysis goes to the cause of the trouble. I have
already several such cases which were completely cured by a
psycho-analytical treatment. I said to myself : if I want to explain
stuttering psychologically I will consider those cases in which normal
persons stutter in ordinary life. And what are these cases ? If
any one is not sincere, if he is embarrassed, he stutters. The
accused stutters if he has to defend himself and he lacks the confidence of innocence. The lover stutters when he proposes and is
not certain that he will be listened to. Freud says quite correctly
that when there is embarrassed stammering and stuttering an
internal conflict is betrayed by the impediment in the speech.

No. 136.—In a second case of occasional stuttering and blushing in a ten
year old boy I again believed the reason to be that the boy was masturbating
and feared that this vice could be seen in his eyes. This I knew from the
fact that as soon as he thought himself unobserved he often looked in the
mirror and gazed at his eyes for a long time, and that he once asked me a
disguised question about it. So I casually bring the talk round to masturbation and say what a good thing it would be if the physician had any means
of recognising it. Then he could often give the children good advice. Unfortunately there was no such means, for the idea that blue rings round the eyes
betray sexual activity was mistaken, as there were many illnesses where the
same rings occur. How correctly I had guessed the cause of the illness—
whether through the diagnostician's instinct or by a happy chance—was
proved by the fact that from the next day onwards the boy stuttered no more.
The fear that one could see the masturbation in his eyes had caused an embarrassment which expressed itself in the stutter.

In the same way are explained the cases of which Denhard tells,
e.g., of a merchant who could not pronounce the word " petroleum "
although he dealt in it. An analysis of the word " petroleum "
would, as with our rabbi, yield a number of repressed thoughts
which are associatively linked with it, and are the cause of the
obsession.

No. 137.—The third case which I had the opportunity of treating concerned
a gentleman who could not pronounce words with A, especially where two
A's occurred. To pronounce a word like *cataract* cost him a great effort and
it was very painful to him to use any of these words in his speech. Once it
happened to him in company that instead of *papa* he said *popo*. Since then
he altogether avoids words in which A occurs. Psychanalysis showed
that the slip—*popo* for *papa*—was a very significant one because in the word
papa the two A's (in the child's meaning A—a is in Vienna equivalent to
excreta) had unconsciously forced themselves upon him. The man suffers
from sexual perversity, he is coprophilic and all his libido is intimately linked

with scatological fantasies. That is the reason why he could not pronounce *cataract.*

When I told him the cause of his stuttering, the obsession vanished at once, and on the next day he was able to use any A—a words freely and fluently.

In recent cases I consider an officious therapy of stuttering with the help of practice to be superfluous, and even harmful, because it directs the attention of the patient even more upon the stuttering ; but I do not think one can succeed with hypnosis alone. *The only right way is that which I have taken in every parapathy : a thorough psycho-analysis, with which in slight cases one often attains the goal in a surprisingly short time.*

In cases of long-standing the psycho-therapy must be combined with the usual practice-methods.[1]

I am unfortunately unable to publish a complete analysis of a stutterer in this place. It requires a book to itself, as does psychic impotence. I will only extract a short example from an analysis.

No. 138.—Mr. B. Z., a forty-two year old engineer, suffers from severe anxiety-hysteria with hallucinations and various obsessions. His greatest trouble is, however, that on various important occasions he begins to stutter. Already as a boy in his fifth year he began to stutter. At times there is an improvement. Great excitement brings on the stuttering again. Latterly he stutters on every occasion. When he is alone he speaks quite freely and fluently without ever coming to a standstill. He began to stutter as a boy after he had spied on the cook during a coitus.

The course of the psycho-analysis was fairly free. I note only the words in connection with which, or in which, he remained "stuck." Then with such a word I get an association series. Let us take a simple example—the word Slavonians. The words run : Slavonians—Satan—Marybridge—Durchmann—Satin—Madrigal—Silurian formation—Salt Mine—Slatina—Salve—Elias—Slavinsky—Bird Slamek—Veronal—Lamiæ—Securus.

All these words have an intimate significance for his repressed complexes. Satan = he has been led astray by the evil one. Marybridge = he has a mistress called Mary and through her he has had a great deal of suffering. Durchmann = a man who has ruined himself in building a railway (his case). Satin = he bought Mary petticoats of satin, now she demands silk ones. Madrigal = he went with her to see the " Mikado," where a madrigal was sung. The Slav names, Slamek and Slavinsky, are evil reminiscences of a law-suit which made him so neurotic that now he has to take veronal. Lamiæ are spirits who suck the blood of their victim. In this case, Mary. The other words have intimate relations which I cannot here detail. In short, the man had good reason to stumble over the word Slavonia. This word was so closely associated with the most unpleasant complexes that there necessarily resulted a resistance to speaking it.

The word Marybridge points to the religious complex ; on this bridge there is a Madonna with whom fallen girls find refuge. (He has brought many innocent girls to ruin). Lamiæ points to his criminal and sadistic complex (Vampirism !) He struggles with repressed bloodthirsty thoughts. Finally, there is a clear indication of masturbation, in whose fantasies all forbidden emotions mingle.[2] Similarly all the other stuttered words could be explained

---

[1] On the basis of these statements Alfred Appell (" Stammering and its Permanent Cure "—A Treatise on Psycho-Analytical Lines. London : Methuen & Co., 1911) tried the psycho-analytical method in severe cases of stuttering and achieved fine results.

[2] In the " Language of the Dream " I have pointed out that all syllables " on," " ona," and the like, can be referred to the onanism complex.

by the method of free associations. It was always internal resistances, repressed complexes over which the man stumbled. The stuttering in youth had also the same cause. The unconscious, repressed ideas were brought to light in a comparatively short time (eight weeks). The patient ceased to stutter. For reasons of medical discretion the detail of this highly interesting case cannot be published. Here I can unfortunately only give indications. But these indications may suffice to show roughly the method by which one can discover the internal resistances which oppose the free course of speech. It is not only sexual conflicts which cause stuttering. They certainly play the chief rôle, for one finds with all stutterers that their mouth represents an erogenic zone, that they are suckers, gourmets, kiss-fanatics. (They have eroticised speech and genitalised the mouth.) But criminal complexes also cause stuttering so that we come to the view that *the cause of stuttering is a bad conscience. Always in the centre of the disease stands the fear of a mental betrayal. Often several motives combine to produce the diseases, as the following case shows :—*

No. 140.—Mr. T. W., a twenty-nine year old official of the Ministry, has a remarkable form of stuttering. He stutters only with men, while with women whom it is his speciality to captivate, he can develop a great persuasive power, without the least impediment in his speech. For two years he was treated by Prof. W., and for a long time by the speech-physician, Dr. F. There was practically no result. The analysis shows a strong homo-sexual tendency, which expresses itself with every man as embarrassed stuttering. Moreover, he was in every respect perverted. In his fifteenth year he had sexual intercourse with his sister, and gave it up only because she refused to continue it. But his thoughts circle round her still. He is fearfully jealous and often quarrels with her because she comes home late or coquets with his friends. He candidly admits having incestual thoughts about his mother and says cynically that in animals such intercourse is not considered unnatural. He calls himself a freethinker but as the analysis shows is really orthodox. Moreover, there is an inclination to cleptomania. Little thefts are committed in a dream-like state with erection. Quick and complete cure after a three months' analysis. He marries, comes out of the House. The cure is maintained for six years without a single relapse.

Laubi, of Zürich advocates very warmly the analytic treatment of stuttering. ("Ueber den Wert der Psychoanalyse für Ætologie und Therapie des Stotterns und verwandter Sprachstörungen." Centralbl. f. Psychoanalyse, Vol. IV.) He considers it as a preparation for suggestive methods and therapeutic practice.[1]

Fröschels, too, the noted Vienna speech specialist, in his works stands for the psychic genesis and treatment of stuttering. ("Ueber die Behandlung des Stotterns." Centralbl. f. Psychoanalyse, Vol.

[1] Laubi's assertion that Frank was the first to submit stutterers to " psychocatharsis " is incorrect. The detailed representation of stuttering as anxiety neurosis with my analytical successes appears in my first edition of the Anxiety Conditions (1910). Interesting contributions are to be found in the works :—Eder, London : Stuttering a psycho-neurosis (Int. Z. f. ärzth. P. A.) Vol. I., C. H. Bluemel ; the psychology of stammering (New York, 1914), A. Liebmann ; " Die psychische Behandlung der Sprachstörungen " (O. Coblentz, Berlin, 1914) recommends suggestion, elocution and exercises. V. O. Mabel (Lancet No. 5008) advocates the same combination. Titius : " Ein Beitrag zur Kasuistik des Stotterns " (Allg. Ztschr. f. Psychiatr.) saw stuttering disappear in the case of persons mentally affected in the emotions.

III.) Unfortunately he is not master of the modern analytic technique and in his diagnoses never gets beyond the beginning. Hopfner, according to a personal communication, attaches importance to the discovery of criminal complexes.

I consider any other method than the analytic to be superfluous. The therapy of stuttering will soon be an exclusively analytic one.

From the analysis of the next case I publish only a fragment which contains an interesting obsessive practice :—

No. 141.—A stuttering boy whom I treated during the last year told me that he did not stutter when he laid his hand on his nose. He presses the right index-finger on the bridge of the nose, and at once he can speak fluently and clearly. This boy was an inveterate onanist. His secret fear was that one might perhaps get out of him, or perhaps perceive, that he masturbated. His father had once told him always to keep his hands outside the bed. So his father seemed to fear masturbation. Now what did he express by this symbolic act ? If he had his hand in his pocket he could masturbate. By laying his hand on his nose he made a demonstration to all the world : Now, look here, I am not masturbating, my hand is not even in my pocket, it is on my nose. Thus his nose was the symbol of the penis and to the expert he made known by this obsessive act just as much of his secret as he wished to hide. The same boy suffered for some time from a lying obsession. One day he told me a long story which I saw at once was a fabrication. I at once ask why he has lied to me. He defends himself, saying he couldn't help ; " it suddenly came over me and then I had to lie." Yesterday he lied to his father without any necessity. The teacher fell ill and they got off school. When he came home he told his father that they had a holiday because the roof of the school had to be mended. Asked whether he was glad to have a holiday : " Yes, I was very happy."

" So that really you were glad that the teacher had fallen ill, instead of being sorry for him, like a good pupil ? "

This he admits ; he had often wished that the teacher might get ill, and he did not like to make known this unworthy wish to his father. But he had wished also, as the analysis brought out, that his father might fall ill. This goes deeper than the previous conflicts, and I must be excused from giving the motives for this wish. But that was only one motive for this lie. The other was that he wished to test his father. He wanted to know whether his father really knew everything, in particular, whether his father could tell that he masturbated and that he was hiding within him very " bad thoughts."

This boy had had an unpleasant experience. He was being treated for stuttering by a specialist who had read in my book that stuttering is connected with masturbation and repressed sexual desires. After the boy had been handed over to him for treatment and he was alone with him, he tested his reflexes, and looking him searchingly in the face, said : " You masturbate ! " That was, of course, the worst thing he could have done. For this boy was in fact suffering from the fear that everyone could notice that he was masturbating. Precisely because of this fear he was embarrassed and stuttered in company, before his mother, before his father—in short, before everybody, whereas when he was alone he could, like all stutterers, speak quite fluently. Now by the specialist he was confirmed in the opinion that one could recognise his secret " vice " at the first glance. He showed everybody then by the obsessive act (the hand on the nose) that he was not masturbating. All this I learned from him. Now why had he lied to me ? As with a lie he had sought to frustrate his father's omniscience, so he lied to me also to " test " me and to find out whether I really could find out everything, because I had told him so many things about his mental life, which before me none had guessed in him. This lying took place from unconscious " repressed " motives and was therefore of obsessive character.

One can scarcely conceive the immense variety of criminal thoughts which raged in this intelligent boy. He was under the fascinating influence of his father, whom he at once feared, loved and hated. He was full of erotic fancies. Thus he confessed to me he would certainly become a woman-doctor because he would then have an opportunity to see all women naked—an interesting contribution to the chpater, " Choice of Occupation and Neurosis." He had countless incest-dreams in which his mother and his three sisters played a great part. He played with criminal fantasies of killing a younger brother.

At the same time he was religious and full of consciousness of guilt. Just in this year he took refuge in incredulity and asked himself repeatedly whether there was a God. He slandered Him to test Him. He made a false confession and lied to God as to me and to his father. And his bad conscience betrayed itself in the stuttering which occurred especially with the teachers, the father and the catechist.

Success was not immediate, as is seen so often in psycho-analytical cures. It occurred some months after an analysis of a few months and has now held good for twenty years.

Among officials one very frequently finds a peculiar form of parapathia. They cannot bear anyone to look over them as they write. Whereas usually they write faultlessly, the hand begins to tremble if someone looks on. They get red and greatly excited. The writing becomes trembling, characterless, indistinct. Slips of the pen occur. In all these cases there exists in high degree dissociation of the personality, there have been grave repressions. The fact that graphologists tell character and much more by the writing is the basis of their fear of betraying themselves by their writing.

If this trembling occurs only with a certain person one may deduce an erotic attitude to that person.

No. 143.—A nineteen year old girl cannot bear the head of the firm to look over her as she writes. She shows all the above-mentioned symptoms. The analysis shows that, without wishing to confess it to herself, she is in love with the head of the firm.

No. 144.—A thirty-four year old government official cannot bear his colleague in the office to look at what he is writing. Especially if he leans on him and lightly touches him, he begins to tremble all over, gets red and giddy, and cold sweat breaks out on his forehead. The analysis shows a strong homosexual inclination towards this colleague.

As with stuttering so it is with stage-fright. The physician has the difficult task of sharply distinguishing in such cases of general nervousness between the natural tendency of his character and neurosis ; and this is only possible through a psycho-analytical study of each case. I have seen the worst cases of stage-fright in masturbators who even in childhood suffer from a certain fear of publicity. For they fear people may detect the "vice" in them, avoid publicity and readily blush when they meet company. Many people who suffer from fear of blushing are masturbators.[1] Just as frequently anxiety neurotics suffer from stage-fright. I have already repeatedly drawn attention to the criminal disposition of all excessively shy persons.

[1] Cf. Bernhardt : " Beiträge zur Lehre von der Errötungsfurcht." Berl. Klin. Wochenschr., 1914.

It is incredible that even old experienced artists regularly suffer an attack of fright before a public performance. With most it is a matter of a moment only—until they feel themselves in touch with the public. But that numerous amateurs are in this way grievously injured, i.e., permanently injured, neither parents nor educators seem to know. And even physicians devote far too little attention to these conditions. Little has hitherto been published as to the organic accompaniments of the anxiety-affects. I have sometimes observed dilation of the heart and a small pulse accelerated to 160 beats (acute dilatation !) Other physicians have made similar observations, especially in students who fight duels. *It seems to me certain that through repetition of such anxiety conditions organic injury of the heart results.*[1] A single acute dilatation may perhaps be borne without injury. If they are repeated several times alterations certainly occur in the walls and valves of the heart. Physicians must therefore see to it that parents prevent nervous children from performing in public. The notorious compulsion to perform in public has already had many a victim. And it is reserved for later pedagogical reformers to do away altogether with the senseless system of examinations and to set up in its place the simple impression of the teacher.

We come to the end of our wanderings through the vast kingdom of the phobiæ. (At some stations it is true we have been able to pay only a flying visit). It remains to review briefly the various phobiæ and to attempt in few words to characterise them.

Naturally there has been no lack of attempts to classify the phobiæ. That I consider an idle task. If one knows exactly the mechanism of *one* phobia, one will be able to recognise the various kinds of phobia as variations of one and the same disease. *Janet* distinguishes :—

(1) *Les phobies des fonctions et les phobies des actions.* To these belong the fear of certain motions which may cause pain, e.g., the well known " akinesia algera " of Möbius : fear of moving, walking, running, jumping, fear of sitting (akathisia) of which Janet relates a delightful case.[2]

(2) *Les phobies des objects.* Fear of knives, forks, pointed articles, cheques, jewels, dust, bacteria, poisonous objects, verdigris, syphilis. A great part of these phobias will only be treated in the last volume of this work in connection with the description of compulsion neurosis.

(3) *Les phobies des situations,* with their important representative, the fear of open spaces. As a group belonging to these the *les phobies des situayions sociales,* as erythrophobia, fear of assemblies, theatres, attestations, examinations, etc.

[1] Dr. L. R. Müllie has called attention to the important fact that melancholy may cause degeneration of the heart-muscles. " Ueber die Beziehungen von seelischen Empfindungen zum Herzmuskel." Münchener med. Wochenschr., 1906.

[2] A very interesting case of akathisia is given in the fourth volume of this work, in the chapter : " Technique of Psychanalysis."

M*

We will not let this classification detain us, and proceed without constraint to discuss some of the most important phobiæ.

I will only mention that there is no object, no feeling, no situation which cannot in certain circumstances be the object of a phobia and a nervous obsession. The most interesting cases of fear we shall discuss in connection with compulsion neurosis. I mention as peculiarities : the fear of getting wet in the rain ; fear of school and of all objects connected with school ; fear of the barometer ; fear of the physician ; fear of watchmen ; fear of children ; fear of being forced to something against one's will in hypnosis ; fear of betraying oneself in sleep and talking nonsense ; fear of one's own thoughts ; fear of old books ; fear of new clothes and new shoes ; fear of losing something ; fear of unjust accusations ; fear of extortion ; fear of rubber tyres ; fear of automobiles ; fear of spreading a bad smell ; fear of emitting a flatus ; fear of having swallowed animals. These are only some examples from my experience just as they occur to me.

The most frequent phobia is *agoraphobia*, the fear of open spaces. We have analysed some examples of this phobia in detail. The bank official who wished to abscond, the woman who feared falling into sin, have probably impressed themselves on my readers' memories. All topophobic women fear their own weakness. The converse, the fear of closed spaces (claustro phobia) corresponds to an infantile fear of being shut up, also to the fear of remaining alone with another person.[1] People with a bad conscience, persons with a sensitive bladder who want to run outside every moment will suffer from this form of phobia. Cases of fear of sudden need (of diarrhœa and urine urgency) form transitions. I know neurotics who can make the longest journey without objection, because in the through carriage there is a closet, but who anxiously avoid the local railway because in case of need they are helpless. Fear of being alone (mono phobia) was shown by the lady whose husband was so impotent that she feared she would have to be faithless to him. People who cannot be alone need a watchman to guard them against their own bad thoughts. Night-fear (nyctophobia) is comprehensible because these patients (they are mostly women) fear also snakes, toads, or mice ; also burglars, thieves who hide under the bed. A man may be lying in wait for them, and so on. After what has been said, it should be clear to everyone that it is a case of fixed infantile fear, of repressed sexual wishes converted into fear. Night is the domain of the erotic and of crime. The fear of drunken persons, mentioned by Beard, is according to my experience to be traced to infantile trauma by a drunken man. A second factor : the drunken man knows no inhibitions.

Fear of heights with the painful idea of falling has been discussed

---

[1] Besides the criminal basis, a great part in the fear of confined spaces, closet, railway carriage, lift, is played by the so-called womb-fantasy which again is overdetermined by fear of death (coffin)—[mother and mother earth].

in the cases of the singer and the police official. It appeared that we had to do with a defensive neurosis to suppress the sexual excitement, once experienced with pleasure, in swinging, sliding, pushing, climbing. Also fear of a fall into sin, into the depths of crime, must be considered. In no phobia may we forget the never-failing criminal basis.

The fear of people (either as anthropophobia or as erythrophobia) from the feeling that they may notice the blushing, we have also sketched in the cases of the singer and of the mechanic. We then mentioned also

Business fear. The anxiety experienced by some people on entering into business. Under cover of this anxiety are concealed criminal ideas such as burglary, robbery, murder, and similar phantasies. *Fear of thunder and lightning* (siderophobia) may likewise be traced to infantile experiences. During a thunderstorm the mother presses the terrified child to her heart, which engenders in it a mingled sensation of pleasure and trepidation. Some people become highly erotic in a thunderstorm. (*Casanova* in his Memoires describes how he overcame the resistance of a beautiful but bashful prude![1]) Combined with these erotic motives is the fear of God's retribution. Lightning is an ancient sex symbol and a mighty weapon in the hand of the Lord. The fear of thunderstorms more than any other phobia betrays the significant part played by religious influences in the mechanism of the neuroses. *The fear of falling down* (stasophobia) has the same motivation as the fear of height and may be figuratively interpreted as fear of falling into sin. *Fear of railway trains* is almost the commonest of all phobias and, in addition to its criminal root (inversion of criminal wish into anxiety!) it is closely related to sea-sickness, to *fear of water*, and *fear of boating*, etc. (rythmic shaking). It may be a disguised form of claustrophobia. It usually takes the form of fear of a railway accident, as punishment for a wicked desire directed against some relative. A person wishing for some accident to befall his rival, easily becomes a prey to railway anxiety.

Fear of animals (zoophobia) with fear of snakes, toads, mice, rats, cats, dogs, birds and horses is accounted for by the sexual animal symbolism, but also by sodomitic instinct, which is more wide-spread than is generally supposed. But my homosexual patient, who suffered from fear of horses, had been accustomed as a boy to ride daily upon his father's knee, which always afforded him intense pleasure. Repressed sodomitic tendencies may like-wise engender feelings of repulsion and anxiety, which Hirschfeld, mistaking repression, would call " Antifetishism." (Ueber Horror sexualis partialis. Neurol. Zentralbl., 1911, No. 10). Somewhat more obscure in its psycho-genesis is *Lyssaphobia*, of which, unfor-tunately I have only had the opportunity of observing one case, and that not thoroughly. It is probably of the same origin as

[1] *Virgil* in " Dido and Aneas " deals with the same motive.

Fear of dirt (mysophobia), *fear of germs* and *infection* (bacillophobia) and is associated with the self-reproach for having sullied oneself by masturbation and incestuous phantasy. Patients in this category often evince a pathologic washing-compulsion (see the case of the singer). The fear of dirt is the result of an inversion of the love of dirt (mysophilia !) Lyssaphobia proved, in my case, to be an inversion of an infantile phantasy of being a mad dog. This patient had the most pronounced cannibalistic instincts and in dreams used to represent a wer-wolf (Leukanthropophagia). The cannibalistic and necrophilian instincts play an enormous part in phobias, the significance of which we are only just beginning to realise. Syphilidophobia is a fear of moral dirt, mostly of incest. The incest-complex is substituted by the syphilis-complex. The instructive case of the young married woman, analysed in detail in Chapter XX., affords us an illustration of *topophobia. Hypochondria*, the fear of some definite disease, is revealed as a special form of anxiety-hysteria, compulsion-neurosis, or anxiety-neurosis. And to complete the list, we must mention *pantaphobia*, the fear of anything and everything. This consists in the transference of repressed sexual matter to all objects coming within the mental horizon.

Certain rare forms of phobia require individual analysis. For example, *Microphonophobia*, which was first described by Juhel-Renoy (Sur la peur des petits bruits. Bull. Soc. med. des Hop. 1892, *p.* 112). The *fear of deformity : Dysmorphophobia.* The fear of new formations : Carzinomaphobia. *The fear of glass splinters : Jalophobia.* The fear of pain : Algophobia (Odynephobia). The fear of a thought : *Phronimophobia.* The fear of depth. The fear of an empty room. The fear of the vertical position : *Atrimy*, or *Stasophobia.* The fear of insects. (Fear of fleas, bugs, lice, flies, bees, wasps). And the fear of some definite noises or persons.

(Germanicus could not bear the sound of cocks crowing. Tycho de Brahe fainted at the sight of a fox. Henry III. could not stand cats. Peter the Great could not cross a stream. Boyle fainted if water were sprinkled on him.)

The Great War is responsible for remarkable forms of anxiety. I allude to the *fear of poverty*, the *fear of starvation, the fear of hostile invasion, the fear of aeroplanes*, etc. The fear of poverty proved to be a transference of affect. It was fear of becoming destitute of love, and of dying a loveless death. Fear of starvation lead to all manner of food-neuroses, a morbid, insatiable hunger, which could generally be interpreted as love-hunger. Fear of hostile invasion, was, in many women a disguise for the wish to be violated.

The anxiety-hysteria of soldiers is worthy of special note. A witty scientist once called the Basedow a "petrified anxiety." This description is still more applicable to war-tremblers. Contrary to other analyses, I have scarcely ever found a sexual component of this class of hysteria. As already mentioned, it is always a matter of psychic conflict between self-preservation and military duty. In fact, my experience of War hysteria has convinced me that the monosexual ætiology of hysteria cannot be supported. Out of the vast material of a War-hospital I was continually finding evidence of the untenability of this one-sided standpoint. One thing is clear: the psychogenic root of all War-hysterias. All these maladies are parapathias.

We have seen, moreover, that occupation-neuroses are likewise parapathias, in which the repressed sexuality is carried into the profession. Yet it should be for the occupation to repress the sexuality. But the *repressed* matter becomes intermingled with the *repressing* forces. Innumerable are the phobias attached to occupation. The pianist who is afraid of breaking down, the violinist who is afraid of his hands perspiring, the speaker who dreads stopping, the doctor who is afraid of overstepping the maximum dose, the lawyer who is afraid of using a wrong paragraph of the law, the director who does not feel equal to his position and is afraid of the ridicule of his colleagues—these are only a few examples taken at random. Every age creates its own definite forms of neurosis. Before the advent of railways there was no railway-anxiety. But on careful analysis it is always found that, concealed behind the phobias are powerful repressions, that it is a question of anxiety-hysteria and compulsion-neuroses, which can only be cured when the deepest underlying psychic cause is discovered. Every phobia is a punishment exacted by the consciousness of guilt.

¹ Orthodox Freudians are of quite another opinion. " Zur Psychoanalyse der Kriegsneurosen." Contributions by Freud, Ferenczi, Simmel and Jones. (Internat. Psychoanalytische Bibliothek. Leipzig and Vienna, 1919.)

CHAPTER XXXI

HYPOCHONDRIA

THERE are many scientists, as is well known, who entirely deny the existence of "Hypochondria" as a separate disease and partly classify it under neurasthenia, partly under hysteria, and some even under paranoia. Wollenberg (Die Hypochondrie, Wien, 1904; Nothnagel, Spezielle Pathologie und Therapie) after an industrious investigation of the whole field of literature, has arrived at the conclusion that hypochondria cannot be considered as a disease in itself, that it represents a psychopathological condition, a psychic disposition of a specific nature.

The psychology of hypochondria is as yet an almost uncultivated territory, if superficial psychology is not taken as a standard. It was easily recognised that in the case of the hypochondriac his whole life had undergone a displacement by which it tended in the direction of displeasure feelings; but this conclusion after all is the essence of most definitions of disease. The best known definition is that of Jolly, supplemented by Hitzig : " Hypochondria is that form of melancholy condition (originating in a morbid change of self-feeling) in which the attention of the patient is concentrated permanently or temporarily upon the condition of his own body or mind."

Krafft-Ebing, on the other hand conceives hypochondria to be the hyperæsthesia and depression of the sense of general feeling, and lays stress on the fact that the hypochondriac experiences abnormal sensations as a result of a delusion, whereas the neurasthenic converts the primary sensation that he is conscious of into a nosophobia. The most valuable contribution towards the understanding of the nature of this malady has, in my opinion, been made by Schüle (Klinische Psychiatrie, Leipzig, 1886) who defines it as : " a psychic neurosis on the basis of hyperæsthesia of the sensory nerves of particular or of all the organic zones " with the " Effect of the ensuing *compulsion* on the whole psychic life."

This is the only author in whose works I have found the definition of the character of compulsion so clearly emphasized. Another noteworthy peculiarity described by many authors, is very aptly defined by Krafft-Ebing as : " The tendency towards the allegorical and often absurd elaboration of sensations." It is precisely the phantastic and bizarre element in the sensations of the hypochondriac which at once strikes the psychologist. These remarkable sensations have been very well summarized by Wollenberg in his monograph :

" The patients complain of general debility, tremulousness, weakness and stiffness. There is a burning, scorching, crawling sensation all over the body, or only in some particular part. The skin expands, contracts and seems to rise. Internally everything feels strained, too short, or too small. The body appears to shrink and become smaller and smaller until it is a ' mere skeleton.' The spine feels as thin as a bit of straw. There is a buzzing noise in the head, a twitching and burning. The skull expands and feels as if it were about to burst, hollows and channels seem to be forming within it. The brain tries to burst out at the top. The hair rises, becomes loose, threatens to fall out, and appears to be growing in unaccustomed places (imaginary growth of beard in women). The whole face is distorted, the mouth and left jaw crooked, the nose contracts, alters its form and size, and the ears deteriorate in like fashion. The eyes twitch, do not turn properly, become watery, are no longer firm in their sockets and rattle on movement. Hearing and sight become worse. There is a stabbing and hammering sensation in the ears, and an insufficiency of wax. The tongue becomes thick, withdraws far back into the throat ; everything in the throat is contracted, and it is impossible to swallow. In speaking unpleasant sensations manifest themselves. The lungs do not function properly, and an intense feeling of suffocation is experienced. There is a burning, oppressive feeling in the heart, it does not beat normally, and occasionally ceases to beat. The circulation of the blood is not satisfactory, it is either too hot or icily cold. It feels as if marbles were running in the veins in place of blood. The ' arteries ' stand out too prominently in one place, are too inconspicuous in others. The body is distended and swollen to such a size that the patient is scarcely able to sit down. Flatus is too weak, too strong or stops in the wrong place. There is a crawling, heaving, rolling, rumbling in the body which creates sometimes a feeling of mild disturbance, and at others a wild upheaval as if there were *an animal running about inside, or like the movement of a child.* The bowels are inflamed and strain in an upward direction, and the excreta and winds are similarly affected. The anus feels as if it were ' closed up.' There is a perpetual feeling of pressure in the stomach, the food sticks, is not digested, and, in that condition, is distinctly felt. The appetite is either too slight or too strong ; the stomach cannot assimilate anything. There is a burning, biting, twitching, drawing, tickling sensation in the penis, scrotum, vagina, womb, bowels, etc. The glans are quite cold, or inflamed, the præpuce sore, the whole organ is out of order, the member too flaccid, and altered in shape and size. The womb is displaced. The urine is described sometimes as too cold and sometimes as too hot. It is of a wrong colour and wrong substance. The excreta is too hard and too black, or too soft and too light. Perspiration is irregular, confined to the lower portion of the body, and attended by a feeling of intense cold. The tears are hot as fire. The flow of saliva is either excessive or insufficient. There is a continuous slight discharge of semen, etc. And lastly, as regard the psychic sphere, the head is empty, thought is impossible, the memory has suffered, etc."

I could supplement this list *ad infinitum*, but will confine myself, by way of illustration, to the account of a single hypochondriac of the feminine sex :—

" When I awoke to-day," the patient told me, " I felt as if my whole face were swollen to the size of a drum. My eyes had shrunk and were like two worms, and for a time they protruded from their sockets ; then there began a creeping, crawling, twitching and pinching sensation at the back of my head, and my whole head felt compressed as if a cord had been wound several times about it. This feeling then extended to the back, hands and feet (which became quite stiff until I couldn't move them)—and finally to the stomach which became *as hard as a board* and as heavy as if there were stones inside it. There was a rumbling, gnawing and pinching feeling inside me, as if a cat were running about there." (On closer analysis it transpired that repressed sexual phantasies were concealed behind these sensations.)

These bizarre sensations serve as the symbolic disguise for erotic phantasies, e.g., " I feel something moving about in my stomach like a hard stick." " My mouth feels full of phlegm, there is something sticky slipping up and down in my throat." Another example : " There is always something like a hard stout elastic substance in my anus." " In the flexura symoidea (in the case of a doctor) there is a hard cylindrical substance that will not go down."

Let us make a summary of the foregoing :

" The hypochondriac uses his psychic energy to observe his body, has a marked tendency to describe pathologic symptoms in phantastic allegories and feels predominantly unpleasant sensations."

If, however, we carefully sift the material, we shall find that the term " hypochondria " is only a collective term for the various very different diseases which are similar in their psychic structure but owing to their pathological grade represent different diseases.

We are obliged, therefore, to distinguish these varieties under four different forms of hypochondria :—

(1) The nosophobial form ;
(2) The hysterical form ;
(3) The compulsion-neurotic form ;
(4) The paranoidal form.

The various forms stand in the same relation to each other as anxiety neurosis, the phobias, compulsions neurosis and paranoia.

The first is the result of the ungratified demands of the sex-instinct. The second shows the psychic mechanism of repression ; and the formation of substitutes, and in the third the compulsion pheno- mena play the leading part ; and in the fourth a correction of the hypochondriacal ideas is impossible. The fear exhibits every symptom of hypochondriacal delusion.

Let us commence with the first form. It is probably the most frequent, and known to the practitioner under the eroneous title of " Neurasthenia." There are certain people to whom their health is a subject of abnormal anxiety. If they hear that a neigh- bour of theirs has died of pneumonia they become deeply depressed. Suddenly they feel a slight stabbing pain in their lungs ; their anxiety increases. The sinister foreboding has become a certainty. They immediately call in the doctor—he must come at once—it is a matter of life and death. They can hardly await his coming. When he arrives, can detect nothing amiss and reassures them accordingly, they draw a breath of relief as if they had escaped some great danger, and are immensely happy. But only for a short while. Some days later they are attacked by another com- plaint. They are the most profitable patients for the doctor, for they could not live without him. Neither could they live without some complaint or other. They project their anxiety on to any object. They actually go in search of a disease and are contented so long as it is not of a dangerous kind. They tremble at the idea of any serious new complaint (appendicitis) and welcome a harm- less fashionable one (uric acid diathesis). They populate the health resorts and hydros.

They all suffer from an anxiety neurosis consequent on a psychic conflict, generally between the moral ego and the sexual impulse. The " free floating quantity " of anxiety, the available affect charges any idea that happens to stand in the forefront of the mental horizon to which anxiety can attach itself. It may just as well be some business anxiety as fear of an illness. Freud says of it in his clinical work on anxiety neurosis : " Anxious expectation of course always has a trace of the normal, embracing everything that might be generally termed ' anxiety,' inclination to a pessi- mistic view of things, but as often as possible passes from this stage of plausible anxiety until it frequently becomes a form of compul- sion. For one of the forms of anxious expectation, i.e., that connected with the health of the individual in question—the old pathological term Hypochondria may be reserved."

Characteristic of the first form of Hypochondria, which, for want of a better term, we call " Nosophobia," is the fact that the hypo- chondriacal idea has not yet assumed the character of a compulsion and may be dispelled through the influence of the doctor, or by a reassuring explanation. The anxiety as such remains as a free floating element and again attaches itself to another idea. It does not disappear until the permanent sexual stimuli and desircs are assuaged by their gratification, or yield for some other reasons. The further we proceed with our analyses the rarer does this form become. It is, moreover, a form of *retributive* illness. We fall ill as a punishment for our evil wishes, and our illness takes the very form that we have desired for another, or for which we had not felt sufficient sympathy, but rather an inward malicious joy. This retributive hypochondria is very widespread. The reader will remember the case of the singer, Nastasia. She came to me with the fear that she was suffering from cancer of the throat. Her father had died of cancer in the rectum. These talion-illnesses are sometimes very easy to solve. A lady is suffering from heart neurosis. No doctor can convince her that her heart is sound. Her mother died of heart failure. A man suffers from frightful pains in the small of the back. His father had succumbed to a spinal disease. I could multiply these examples. They are, however, not all so simple. The death-thoughts are sometimes connected with some hated rival—a sister-in-law, a male friend—a female friend, etc.

No. 145.—Mrs. M. B. used to have a new disease every week. She was thirty years old, a healthy-looking, robust woman, who for the last four years had only allowed her husband coitus interruptus, from fear of children. She was very irritable, complained of headaches, giddiness, numbness in the arms and night sweats. She would appear suddenly in my consulting room and complain of violent pains in the appendicital region : then reassured, she was radiant. Or she would send urgently for the doctor while she lay in bed, suffering ostensibly from inflammation of the throat and high fever. If the doctor found her temperature normal and the tongue free from fur, she would jump out of bed and go to the theatre. When, despite the coitus interruptus, she happened to become pregnant, she was filled with anxiety during the first months :—she would never survive the confinement, she had certain premonitions, etc. When the anxiety-neurosis improved as a result of normal sexual intercourse, all her melancholy thoughts vanished and she faced the future with equanimity.

No. 146.—Mr. M. H., a merchant of forty-eight, had a sudden attack in November, 1910, as follows : He was seized with vertigo and had to sit down. Everything went dark before his eyes, and he broke into violent perspiration. He was overcome with nausea and vomited fifteen times in rapid succession.

Since that attack he felt very ill. He complained of lack of clarity and confusion in the head. Something seemed to be revolving in his brain. He was unreliable. He had a swimming feeling in his head, and a sudden stabbing sensation right down to the spermatic chord, like a shot. The right half of the body felt icily cold, the left, warm and glowing. He also complained of excessive heat on one side of the head which increased to a headache. The right side of the head was as if paralysed, there was an oppressive feeling as if his brain were being kneaded, or as if ants were crawling over it. He used to sigh day and night, and was subject to suicidal ideas. He was always in a lacrymose state and always thinking of death and dying. He slept very restlessly, and was awakened by diarrhœa. He had an aversion for meat, and had only taken a little poultry for months.

For twenty-one years, with the exception of four periods during which his wife was pregnant, he had practised coitus interruptus.

The condition had grown distinctly worse in the last weeks. He now suffered from a flight of ideas before going to sleep. He was haunted particularly by certain melodies. I questioned him about them, but he could not remember any special one. Eventually he remembered a melody, the words of which he did not know. I asked him to whistle it to me. The text was the same as the one that we met with in another case: "I am a widow, a little widow."

The psychogenic source of the trouble was then revealed. He had for years been in love with a neighbour, now a widow. Her husband died in November, 1910.

"On the day when you had the first serious attack?"

"A few hours previously. I was very much upset about it."

I will here give the result of my three hours' analysis. He thought at that time: If my wife were to die, I could marry my beloved. It occurred to him that a peasant had poisoned his wife with arsenic. Shortly afterwards he was seized with nausea, which gave symbolic expression to his poison idea.

His confused thoughts, the ants crawling about in his head, are the various criminal ideas. He lived in continual fear that he would commit some deed of violence on his wife. The coitus interruptus practised with an unloved woman thinking all the time of another was perhaps a contributing factor in the release of fresh anxiety.

The psychic mechanism of the second—the hysterical—form of hypochondria is of much more complicated character. This hypochondria is in effect a complicated phobia (parapathia).

It is recognisable from the behaviour of the patient in relation to her hypochondriacal idea, and in her attitude towards her health in general.

I have had various hypochondriacs under psychotherapeutic treatment. I was at first inclined to attribute the hypochondria, the nosophobia, to a pathological fear of illness. I was disposed to trace all hypochondrias to "anxiety neurosis," and my therapy consisted in enlightening the patients as to the groundlessness of their anxiety. This therapy proved to be without result in many cases. It was as if one were to assure a man suffering from agoraphobia that he had no cause to fear the open space, and that he should try calmly to cross over it. In such a case the patient would reply: "I know; but it is all the same impossible for me to cross over the space, there is some strange force holding me back." Schüle's pertinent observation that hypochondriacal ideas present the characteristics of compulsory ideas, indicates that these hypochondriacal ideas are "over-valued" and cannot be corrected without analysis.[1] *The hypochondriac is not of necessity always a nosophobic.* On the contrary he is in some cases of a positively light-hearted temperament, and I would emphasize, as a specially important point in the second and third forms of hypochondria the fact that *the anxiety of this hypochondriac only refers to a particular disease, and is of the nature of a phobia,* whereas its attitude towards other organic diseases is one of indifference or almost of heedlessness. *This indifference of the hysterical compulsive or paranoid hypochondriac towards an organic disease is never lacking in a genuine case, and is, in my opinion, the surest indication of the malady.* It

[1] Beard, who was an exceptionally keen observer, remarks very truly: "True hypochondria, i.e., pathophobia, cannot be cured any more than *morbid* fear of, any description by instruction and explanation of the symptoms." "Die Sexuelle Neurasthenie." Wien, 1885, Franz Deuticke.

is, of course, understood that the affected organ does not of necessity appertain to those zones with which a hypochondriacal delusion is associated.

An episode in my practice brought this remarkable fact under my notice, and once alive to it I was continually finding fresh evidence of this strange contrast between exaggerated anxiety and incredible indifference.

No. 147.—I had one of the most curious cases of hypochondria under treatment that I have ever come across. He used to lie in bed trembling with anxiety, and have the temperature of the atmosphere taken by his brother. If 15° were registered in the room he felt very well, and with 16 still better. But if the temperature had sunk to 14½°, a great change took place in him as soon as his brother had imparted to him the momentous tidings. He would become pale, begin to tremble, wrap himself in blankets and his teeth begin to chatter.

" I have caught cold," he would cry. " I have got cold shivers."

Doctors would be fetched, and antipyrin administered. He would spend the whole day in observing the temperature of the room ; this occupation was only varied by the close attention which he paid to his digestive organs, his stool, his food, and the effect of this or the other comestible.[1] Although, beyond a slight stomachic atonia there was nothing the matter with him, he grew as thin as a skeleton because he refused all solid nourishment ; he then underwent a fattening cure at a sanatorium and rapidly put on flesh ; but when left to himself, as rapidly lost weight again.

He would welcome every new doctor with enthusiasm, and complain about his last medical attendant who had " made a mess of him " ; but his enthusiasm would be quickly exhausted and the new doctor would be sent to join the rest and dealt with in a " collective abuse " of stupid doctors and their " ridiculous medicine," which could not even cure a catarrh of the stomach.

He was very indignant with me because a minced beefsteak that I had prescribed for him had done him out of the benefit of a strict dietetic cure.

One day—two years after my last treatment—I was called to his hotel. He was in bed with a fever and calmly showed me some blood in his urine— almost as if he were proud of being able to give a concrete proof of his illness. This time he was in reality very ill ; it was a case of acute nephritis. I gave him directions accordingly

" Can I not go to Meran to-morrow ? It is too cold for me in Vienna," said the patient.

" No," I replied, " You must remain quiet until there is no longer any trace of blood in the urine."

" Then I must not get up ? Would that be dangerous ? "

" Very dangerous ! You must stay in your warm bed and keep to the strict diet for the present." I then explained the gravity of nephritis : a chronic kidney complaint might develop, etc.

Judge of my astonishment then when on arriving at the hotel the next morning I was told the patient had departed. A letter informed me that he would never get well in " Vienna air." The warm air of Meran would cure his new disease much quicker. All my talk about the necessity for the strictest rest in bed, for constant warmth, and the prescribed diet, had been in vain, and my words had fallen on deaf ears. His hypochondriacal mania for air was stronger than any medical logic. His phobia, his fear of cold air and longing for warmer air had proved stronger than the doctor's art of persuasion, and the warnings of his brother, who had tried to frighten him

[1] Both of these bad habits were the result of the exaggerated tenderness and over-solicitous bringing-up of his mother. She used to take the temperature of the room and superintend his excretory functions.

by telling him that premature movement might cause hæmorrhage and he might die on the journey.

What strange tales could I tell of these anxiety hysterical hypochondriacs! Here is a man who alleges that he catches cold every other day. He wears two overcoats and woollen under-clothing, has his house heated on cool days in summer, and keeps it cool in winter for fear of getting over-heated, and goes to bed with a thermometer. Analysis of this case elicited the fact that he was a man afraid of love. He had once sustained a great disappointment and did not want to love again, although he needed a great deal of love. *He did not want to feel warm again for any woman* and this idea was converted into a dread of the illness that might result if he were to get *over-heated* and then suddenly *cool down*. He was perpetually reconstructing in his body the romance which had cost him his life's happiness.

Another hypochondriac, an officer, suffered in his fifties from a similar fear of catching cold. He was just going to his battalion when he was seized with the first anxiety attack in the street. He never went back to the battalion. He obtained a pension and lived like a prisoner in his house. The tendency of his hypochondria was to safeguard himself. He dreamed of a hypnotist who wanted to assert his will over his and force him to go out. He sought in hypnosis, of course unconsciously, homosexual violation. He was also in search of pleasure without guilt. He was, however, on his guard against all hypnotism. He went to a celebrated hypnotist in Sweden. He entered the consulting room, where he saw a woman asleep on a sofa. He at once detected the clumsy deception and " indignantly " left the astonished hypnotist, who did not guess that the man was fighting an heroic battle for his virtue. The second hypnotist was uncongenial to him, the third too weak, the fourth another charlatan, etc.

Self-reproach for masturbation and the injurious effects of youthful misbehaviour play an important part in the genesis of hypochondria. *Masturbation is a favourite dumping-ground for every sin. It is the store-house of the guilty conscience and is replenished from criminal, ethical and religious sources.* In these cases also there is evidence of a strange psychic mechanism in the development of the symptoms.

The anxiety of the hypochondriac is concentrated only on one or more definite " fixed " ideas. In organic diseases these compulsion-ideas induce him to behave light-heartedly. It is as if the fixed anxiety had left no room for other fears, as if the whole of the available anxiety were concentrated on one idea.

The hypochondriacal idea of this group is by no means identical with the nosophobia of timid, cowardly people and anxiety neurotics. How happy is the anxiety neurotic, who, on visiting the doctor after a sleepless night, is told that he is not suffering from " inflammation of the lungs " and that he is perfectly well. This feeling of exaltation, this relief at being freed from anxiety, is indescribable, says such a neurotic. He derives untold comfort out of the deliverance from the unpleasant feelings. The world seems a beautiful place to him now !

Very different is the attitude of the hysterical or paranoid hypochondriac ! He listens to the doctor's verdict with mistrust. He is never entirely reassured. He is the eternal doubter. Sometimes he is quite proud that the doctors know nothing about his illness. "It is a very rare complaint."

This is because his hypochondriacal delusion is based on repression, and the nosophobic idea is deeply rooted in the unconscious. But more of this later. Let us note as the first and most important symptom of this form of hypochondria, an anxiety towards certain illnesses, which is characteristic of a delusion and is in striking contrast with the indifference to other organic affections. This delusion may pass from the hysteric form to genuine psychosis or "paranoic hypochondria."

A second case of hysterical hypochondria : A nervous hypochondriac who imagined he was suffering from an incurable spinal disease came to consult me about pains in the small of the back. I examined him and found extensive bronchitis with fever.

"You have acute bronchial catarrh. You must go to bed at once."

All to no purpose. He could not be persuaded. He could not possibly go to bed ; he had important matters to attend to he only wanted something for the pains in his back. Then he would be quite satisfied. He would not listen to a word about his bronchitis.

I have observed many cases of a similar nature. Always this marked indifference to a real illness as long as it is not concerned with the hypochondriacal zone.

Now what is the origin of this hypochondriacal zone ? Is it mere coincidence that one is a stool-hypochondriac and anxiously inspects his evacuations, the other gazes daily at his tongue for fear that the anticipated cancer of that member should have already made its appearance, the third looks at his eyes and observes various alterations therein ?

From the remarkably compulsive character of the symptoms it is to be presumed that certain secret associations and powerful repressions are at work in the unconscious. Analysis confirms the assumption : that every hypochondriacal delusion has its logical foundation in the unconscious and can be resolved into its original psychic elements. The next example affords an illustration of these arguments :—

No. 148.—Mr. X. B. was seized with morbid anxiety that he would be afflicted with cancer of the tongue. But why specially cancer of the tongue ? The patient in question had an " evil tongue " and often used to think : " One of these days your evil tongue will be punished with cancer." As a critic he was notorious for his maliciousness. But this did not account for the hypochondriacal idea acting as a compulsion. Of far more importance is the fact that Mr. X. B. had before his illness made a declaration, had given a promise for which he could have bitten his tongue out. Had his tongue been silent on that occasion, he would have been spared much suffering. In a weak moment he had promised his mistress that he would marry her. He subsequently learned of her former life and could not withdraw his promise. A further detail : A man, standing in intimate relationship with himself and his mistress had died of cancer of the tongue. This patient was addicted to the perversity cunnilingus. His most intimate friend practised it. He himself often felt a great craving for it but had severely repressed it. But on one occasion he had yielded to temptation. His guilty conscience left him no peace. Would he not suffer the same consequences—cancer of the tongue ? As a child he had been very fond of sucking and was an extreme " gourmet."

We have then in this case three factors which are always to be met with in hypochondriacal delusions : (1) The transmutation of an erogenous zone into an object of hypochondriacal anxiety ; (2) The guilty conscience ; (3) The repression of ideas which are painful and unpleasant to consciousness.

No. 149 is a similar case to the last. Mr. D. Z., aged forty-five, suffered from a tormenting burning in the tongue. He used to visit a professor every week for fear of contracting cancer of the tongue. He had lost all pleasure in life and thought of nothing from morning till night but his tongue. This once jovial man likewise had promised his mistress, with whom he had had a liaison for fifteen years, that he would marry her. She kept him to his promise and was a strict, jealous wife. He, likewise, practised cunnilingus. In his dreams he revealed death-wishes against his wife, who had become a burden to him. She had a false tongue. After four weeks' analytic treatment all the abnormal sensations disappeared from the tongue. His joy in life returned.

Such are the " unconsciously " working hypochondriacal forces. The compulsory idea is due to the repression of perverse erotic impulses, in which important infantile roots can always be traced. The patients X. B. and D. Z. were suckers and gourmets, hence their tendency to cunnilingus. The tongue was here the erogenous zone, and, according to the talion principle, was destined to be the seat of the malady.

No. 150.—A hypochondriac, aged thirty-two, a robust looking, powerful man, came to consult me about violent pains in the back. The pains extended to the legs and testicles ; he felt jaded, tired, and incapable of any hard work. It must be cancer or spinal disease. He had tried every possible remedy without success. The objective examination produced a perfectly negative result.

I endeavoured through analysis to trace the origin of the hypochondria, and first questioned him as to his sexual life. Quite normal. At one period of his youth, it is true, he had masturbated for a short time, but there was no other irregularity. There was, however, one thing which he had almost forgotten. He suffered from frequent emissions which he found very weakening. After every emission he felt thoroughly worn out, and sought to " recover " his strength by much eating and drinking.

Frequent emissions are often only a sign of very active unsatisfied sexuality. Such was the case with him. He did not satisfy his wife, suffered from ejaculatio præcox, and in consequence rarely indulged in intercourse. He was positively convinced that coitus shortened his life, that it sapped his strength and made his " neurasthenia " worse. A celebrated psychiatrist had once told him that he must not have intercourse more than once a month (!) Since then he had feared the consequences of coitus.

This is an important factor in the psychology of the hypochondriac : the fear of the injurious results of the sexual act. (Sexual aversion). Yet there is a perpetual burning desire for sexual activity which manifests itself in endless phantasies. In fact many hypochondriacal affections are merely somatic translations of sexual phantasies.

Our hypochondriac was similarly troubled all day long by lustful thoughts. He undressed every woman he met, he pictured to himself the most daring erotic sensations, etc.

All this I, of course, only extracted from him by degrees. Then one day he remembered an incident which accounted to me for the pains in his back. While still a school-boy he once paid a visit to an aunt. A young student was living there, who led him into his room where they engaged in a variety of masturbatory manipulations. Finally the aforesaid student indulged in pæderastia with him (immissio penis in anum). He did not resist, for he experienced a pleasurable feeling thereby. This incident was several times repeated.

The fixation of this hypochondriacal zone was now explained. As a child he had suffered from constipation and always remained a long time in the closet. The evacuation of excreta always afforded him a pleasurable sensation. The anus and the lower dorsal region are erogenous zones. The remembrance of the unpleasant episode had been repressed. It lay in the unconscious like some foreign body. His sense of guilt in relation to his wife and his lost youth, his psyche oscillating between sexual desire and sexual anxiety all combined to form a typical picture of a hypochondriac.

I had occasion to see this man repeatedly. He is a latent homosexual and seeks to renew the indulgence which he enjoyed with the student. The memory of excessive lust has taken form as pain in the fork. To his wife he is impotent because coitus is to him no adequate form of sex-satisfaction.

Strange to say, his brother's case forms a pendant to this one. He is just such another hypochondriac with the same " anxiety-zone," hypochondriacally established, and the same symptoms. He has, indeed, had similar experiences with his aunt's lodger. This is again a typical example of predisposition caused by similar infantile experiences.

This case has brought us somewhat nearer to the psychology of the hypochondriac. We have seen that the dread means suppressed sexuality, that its origin and its control are psychic. With this is connected the remarkable attitude of the hypochondriac with regard to the sexual life. In the psyche of the hypochondriac two diametrically opposed forces are at work : sex-lust and sex-aversion. An overwhelming sex-lust that would embrace and enjoy everything, and an all-embracing sex-dread, which shrinks from every coitus as from a partial suicide. We see the same spiritual mechanisms at work as in the case of anxiety hysteria, only much more sharply defined.

With these patients the dread of sexuality does not mean dread of sexuality in general. This general dread serves only to conceal the dread of a *certain form* of amatory manifestation. Thus Patient No. 147 had no fear of loss of semen. No, he feared the homosexual act. Every human being who has made himself a system in which sex-activity is limited, is hiding a secret sex-goal, to him unattainable. A woman whose lusts tend to fellatio and who has victoriously combatted and repressed this practice will find that " intercourse " is injurious to her and after coitus she will feel faint and exhausted. And it will be just the same with a man who cannot satisfy his sadistic longings. *The dread of intercourse conceals their dread of a particular variation of sex-life.* With these hypochondriacs the anxiety is transferred to sexuality as such. They fear the injurious consequences of the sexual act. The dread is strengthened by the consciousness of having undermined the health through early indulgence in masturbation. All these patients that I have sketched were masturbators and full of remorse for the masturbation.

From this point of view the attitude of the hypochondriac towards the sex-act is explained in a quite remarkable way. The fact that it is almost exclusively men who are hypochondriacs is at once easily explained. The man is in the sex-act the one who expends life, who loses life ; the woman the one who receives, who gains. Only in the case of the man can an association of ideas between loss of life and sex-act arise, and only in cases where the woman is obsessed with the idea that she is expending part of her strength in the sex-act can a case of feminine hypochondria develop. As a matter of fact I have, in two cases of feminine hypochondria, succeeded in demonstrating this latent obsession.

No. 151.—Case of a forty-four year old woman, suffering for four years from all sorts of hypochondriac complaints. She believes herself to be constantly constipated. She has great pains in the bowel and in the fork. The stomach does not digest properly. She must have got some infectious disease. For three years there has been a discoloured discharge and this has been treated in hospital. The physicians ridicule her and say it is an innocent vaginal catarrh. But she knows better. She must have caught an infectious disease. She thinks it must be syphilis.

She has left off taking regular meals. She diets herself severely and is much reduced. In three months she has lost eight kilograms (17.6-lbs.). She knows that she has a cancer in the bowel. Nothing can help her. No doctor understands her disease. She has been twice to Carlsbad. There she was worse then ever. She has tried also a water-cure, Kissingen water, and oil cures, all without result. Her hands tremble for weakness. She will go the same way as her mother who has for years been suffering from paralysis agitans. The analysis of this case shows that as in all cases of hypochondria—it is only a peculiar form of a hysterical phobia. The tendency of those suffering from hysteria to manifold delusions is placed at the service of sensations of the various organs. The phantasies take on the character of a nosophobia. The delusions arise through the fixation of repressed sexual desires. Only that the dread is referred to the physical symptom which is placed in the foreground. Our patient states that four years ago she sat on a closet seat on which there was a piece of red paper. She must have got infected there. We find, however, that just at that time a married man made love to her. Dreading the consequences of coitus—her husband was away in the East—she refused to sleep with him. The man then made the cynical proposal—coitus in anum, which she indignantly refused as disgusting. The red paper came from a druggist's shop. The man had packed something in it. A medicine bottle ! She suspected at the time that she was infected. At once she was tormented with the thought : " Had he used you sexually, you would perhaps now be infected." Her imagination accepted this thought as true ; for the desire for sex-activity was excessive. She behaved as if she really had been infected at that time. The discharge and the pains in the fork and in the stomach appeared. She lost her appetite. Emissions weakened her to an extraordinary degree. " She lost so much of the body-juices in this way that her whole spinal marrow was empty."

She remembers that even as a child she liked to see other children at stool. Once she had even watched her father at stool. This had made a great impression on her at the time.

After the analysis she begins to eat again and regains weight in due course.

This was a case of short standing in which psycho-therapy has good prospect of success.

The central point of the illness was formed by the imagination, the coitus, sexual acts, masturbation and emissions carrying off the juices of the body.

No. 152.—A similar case with hypochondriacal dread is the following. It is specially interesting because it shows that behind the ordinary nosophobic conditions there may be concealed repressed erotic ideas. How widespread is the dread of appendicitis. I know a woman who after her twenty-two year old son had been operated on for this disease, suffered from such a violent dread of it that she ceased to take proper food. She began to select her foods with great care, and complained of violent stomach pains which occurred especially after taking foods difficult of digestion. She gave up eating bread, and consumed only finely chopped meat and very soft vegetables made into a purée. And among these foods she found some specially injurious. Potatoes were banished from the table. She would have liked best to give up eating altogether. She began to inflict the same diet on her children and lived in continual dread, which often rose to severe attacks of anxiety, and these caused her to call me in.

One day, after I had tried all the arts of persuasion, and after all the experts had in vain given the assurance that there was no danger of appendicitis, it occurred to me to investigate this phobia analytically.

And behold ! It was a remarkable surprise when I discovered a strange unconscious complex. The woman had lost her husband through pneumonia. The son took the father's place in the household. She loved him above every thing. As a child she had brought him up so susceptible to shame that when he stripped to the waist to wash himself she had to leave the room.

On the occasion of the operation, she had the opportunity as nurse to perform many services for her son. She handed him the bed-pan, helped him change his shirt, and so on. And it was a great pleasure to her to be able to help him in those anxious days, to wash him, comb his hair, rub in vaseline, and so on ; and she never had an unappropriate thought the while. After the operation there were of course no more of these little intimacies.

Then began the dread of the appendicitis. She wanted to be ill and to have her son nurse her. The thought of incest—a thought painful to her and which when it once occurred in a dream had made her quite ill—had never come into consciousness at all. Her thoughts were always of the appendix—a mere " transference " of course. For her thoughts were really concerned with the beautiful body of her son.

After the psychic solution had been attained the patient began to eat again and rapidly gained weight. The dread of appendicitus completely vanished.

In this case the hypochondria was just beginning. It manifested itself simply as a hypochondriacal delusion : the patient being in other respects cheerful and in general by no means anxious.

This case also exhibits all the criteria of a hysterical parapathia :—
The repressed erotic idea, thoughts of incest, conversion (stomach

pains) and the dread resulting from suppression of the erotic emotions; the consciousness of guilt and the psychic conflict were also not lacking.

This form of hypochondria is then only a special form of parapathia in which the dread is directed towards sexuality. It is a phobia; the object of the anxiety is the body of the patient and its functions.[1] All these hysterical hypochondriacs are very backward with regard to active sex intercourse. Mostly they reproach themselves for having in their youth dissipated their strength through ignorance. (The increased eroticism of youth corresponds to the acme of life which is a spendthrift of vital energy.) For the most part they experience after coitus all sorts of troubles. One feels exhausted and depressed, another complains of pains in the fork, a third of trembling in the legs, and so forth. To such a hypochondriac who suffered much from emissions I advised frequent coitus.[2] Every emission plunges him for a whole day into profound melancholy. The case was clear. In coitus he purchased an enjoyment with a proportion of his vital energy; by emission he paid this proportion without receiving a corresponding equivalent.[3] A very characteristic fact was that on the day of the emission he kept himself from suffering by a rich diet. He ate three meat meals, drank several glasses of milk or beer and took several eggs in addition. Naturally this over-rich feeding produced a proportionately higher sex-craving which expressed itself in fresh emissions. This increased nutrition corresponds to our popular view of the nature of the sex act. To this man, I recommended frequent coitus. He looked at me doubtfully and after a few days he came back to discuss the point further. " I cannot persuade myself that sexual intercourse does not injure me," he said : " I feel at once part of my energy passing out of me with every such intercourse."

One complains, however, only of a loss which has not been compensated by the gratification of desire. These men can easily renounce normal coitus. In fact they want something quite different.

Dread of the injurious consequences of coitus was stronger than his sexual need and my authority. All these people are inclined, from unconscious religious motives of guilt and penrance to ascetism and seek to find in hygienic considerations a rational ground for these ascetic tendencies.

There is also a striking tendency to use the hypochondriacal ideas symbolically. Dread of syphilis can take the place of dread of

---

[1] Freud now distinguishes between " Uebertragungsneurosen " and " Narzistische Neurosen." In the latter the lust has lost the capacity for possessing its object and is concentrated upon the body of the person experiencing the lust. Hypochondria is a narzistic neurosis.

[2] Really the only safeguard against emissions, which in many cases are only the *natural expression* of a very strong sex-instinct.

[3] The consciousness of guilt arose from the dreams accompanying emission, which were frequently dreams of incest.

incest, or, again, of dread of tuberculosis. I have a most interesting case of this sort.

The third form is the compulsion-neurotic. It is really a compulsion-neurosis and the hypochondriacal idea has been built up into a complete structure. Let us consider such a case.[1]

No. 153.—Not long ago there came to me in my consultation hour a simple, neatly dressed man, looking quite depressed. " Doctor, save me ! I am on the point of suicide ; I am in despair ; I cannot go on living if the pain does not get better."

" What is the matter then ? "

" I cannot urinate."

I suspect some organic disturbance, a stricture, a pain in the bladder, or a disease of the spinal column. On closer examination it appeared that the man was organically altogether sound. The urine was normal in quantity and in appearance ; and micturition caused no trouble. " Doctor," shrieked the patient in despair, " that is just what makes me so wretched. It is simply the *thought* that I cannot urinate which dominates me. It gives me no rest. I fall asleep with this idea, and I wake up with it. *I know well enough that it is nonsense* and that I really can urinate, but though I tell myself this a thousand times I cannot rid myself of the thought."

If one could for a time suppose that the patient was suffering from a lunatic idea, one was quite undeceived by the man's last statements. In this case there is a complete insight into the illness ; the patient knows that the idea is absurd. This distinguishes this idea from the delusions of madness, in which critical power and consciousness of disease are completely lacking. In this case we are dealing with a pure compulsion.

The man has already gone through several water-cures ; he has been treated with galvanic electricity at the Polyclinic ; has been dosed with opium and bromide at the clinic and is now, as he has just stated, at the point of suicide. He can think of nothing but " I cannot urinate."

He can no longer work, he cannot look after his family. " Yes," he cries, " even my little boys whom I so idolised, I can no longer bear to look at." (Let us accustom ourselves to pay attention to every word that the patient says to us. This sudden repugnance to his own child must certainly have a psychic basis.) We learn that the trouble began four months ago, was for a short time better, but has now become so much worse that the patient is tired of his life. In the first hour nothing more could be elicited from the distrustful patient.

Next day I questioned him in detail about his family life. He states that his is a most happy marriage, that he is highly satisfied with his wife, it is an *ideal* marriage ; his financial position is good, he has no cares and nothing special to excite him. I let him come daily for a week, and always tell me his trouble, maintaining that he has nothing more to say, that he has already told me everything. At the end of a week the ideal picture of a happy marriage begins to show itself in quite another light. He did not marry his wife for love at all. His brother came to him one day and said, " Look here, I know a beautiful girl for you, one who has money ; she's the one you ought to marry." He realises now that she is not the right wife for him. She is grasping, never satisfied, dirty and makes great demands on him. And so we have the true account of the happy marriage, about which he waxed so enthusiastic at the first interview. At the end of another week, after he had gained confidence in me, I learned for the first time the secret cause of his obsession. He was once sent by his firm to a lady to obtain payment of a small amount or to threaten her with legal proceedings. This lady, who evidently was somewhat free with testimonies of her favour, offered to grant him " everything " if he would wait another week. He succumbed to the

[1] From *Stekel* : " Zwangszustände, ihre psychischen Wurzeln und ihre Heilung." Medizinische Klinik, 1910, Nos. 5 to 7.

temptation. On the very next day the idea came to him : " *I cannot urinate.*" Originally only from fear that he had contracted disease. He went at once to several specialists who all assured him that there was no question of any infection. With regard to this his fears were set at rest, but the obsession, instead of yielding became stronger, so that in his despair the poor man confessed everything to his wife. He then became for a time somewhat better. He is a pious, faithful Catholic who looks on his adultery as a grave sin. Even the confessional did not alleviate his condition. Since his false step he has lost all love for his wife and *from that time has had no intercourse with her.*

We recognise now that the obsession " I cannot urinate " is a *substituted idea*. Really it should be " *I cannot have sexual intercourse.*" To a child micturition is a substitute for emission and is quite a sexual process and the neurotic man finds himself at the child's standpoint. His wife has no attraction for him and does not gratify his sexual desires. Since he possessed another woman his wife appears to him *revolting*. This thought which so tormented him, all this hatred of his wife which made him so miserable was repressed into the unconscious ; the strong affect was, however, split off from this idea and transferred to a *substituted idea*. When he said " I cannot urinate," this meant, according to the psychanalytic interpretation : " I cannot look at my wife ; she has no attraction for me ; she is revolting to me and even her child is repugnant to me. I can no longer live with her ; I would rather die."

From this example we gain an insight into the mechanism of hypochondriacal obsession. The affect of hatred against his wife was repressed ; the original idea, " I cannot have intercourse with my wife " was also repressed and in its place appeared the substituted idea : " I cannot urinate." Such substituted ideas are compromises drawn from the conscious and from the unconscious. They betray all that they seek to conceal. The repressed mental disturbance is then linked up with these substituted ideas. *In all neuroses there are disturbances of the affectivity.* Hereditary taint, inferiority feeling, degeneration, are only secondary considerations. As Otto Gross aptly observes they affect only the *activity* of consciousness not its *content*. ("Uber psychopathische Minderwertigkeiten." Vienna and Leipzig, 1909. *Wilh. Braumuller.*) We have seen that the *repressed* affect of hatred of the wife was the cause of an obsession. Further we can gather how false are the definitions of those German psychiatrists who maintain that it is just the *lack* of affect which is the very essence of obsessions. They suffered themselves to be deceived by the superficial picture presented by what appeared on the stage of consciousness and did not trouble to look behind the scenes.

In compulsion neurosis we have a very Triton among the minnows of compulsions. Among these the hypochondriacal compulsions play the greatest part. It is absolutely impossible to characterise this disease by an example. Here I will only try to indicate certain points of view. The patients show an exaggerated care for their own bodies and adopt strict regimes of all sorts. Many of these diet cures, air-cures, mountain-tours, etc., are disguised ascetic efforts. *Compulsion-neurosis is the disease of the criminal who denies his divinity in order to diminish his consciousness of guilt. Where there is no avenger there is no sin and no punishment. The compulsion neurotic is the pious man who is ashamed of his religion and is continually lying to himself.*

Thus I know a patient whose agitated care for his *body* revealed itself as a disguised care for the *salvation of his soul.* He underwent a severe fasting-cure. He became a vegetarian, and gave up smoking and drinking. All pennance and remorse! A good part of the modern abstinence movement depends on such obsession-neurotics who have transferred the conflict within them from the religious to the hygienic field. A patient who could eat no meat and nothing that was not bitten small, for fear he might get appendicitis, disclosed the following religious basis: He had received communion while harbouring sinful, impure thoughts. He had consumed the Body of Christ as a sinner. His whole neurosis was a series of punishments for this sin. But mark! The pennance was not recognised by him as a religious pennance. He trembled for his soul and was ashamed of trembling. He was indeed a free-thinker, an atheist. But he was not ashamed to tremble for his body and sought to strengthen it by deprivations.

Behind hypochondria also religion is often in the background as the power that determines the symptoms. More frequently than we imagine! The patients wish to live as long as possible so that the dreaded day of reckoning may be put off as long as possible. Their fear of death is fear of the Unknown, of what may come after death.

Let us hasten to conclude. We have succeeded in distinguishing among the confused features of the hypochondriac the following characteristic traits :—

(1) *The hypochondriacal idea has the character of an obsession. The hypochondriac is quite light-hearted with regard to any dangers except the one he fears.*

(2) *This idea is the substitute for a repressed sexual experience, or for a sexual phantasy.*

(3) *The hypochondriacal zone is always an erogenous zone.*

(4) *The hypochondriacal disease has arisen according to the principle of retribution (lex talionis) from a religious (or ethical) consciousness of guilt.*

(5) *The hypochondriac's dread of death transforms itself into dread of the sexual act. The hypochondriac avoids the normal sexual act because this does not afford him adequate satisfaction. His dread consists in fear of a perversion which his consciousness rejects ; and so he constantly oscillates like a pendulum between sex-longing and sex-aversion.*

The tendency to fanciful elaboration of the sensations has a psychic basis. For behind these fancies and allegories lurk sex-ideas, unrecognised, repressed sex-ideas. "A cat is running to and fro in my stomach." "A column is revolving in my stomach." "A pointed stake is sticking in my bowel." "Something is dragging at the nerve fibres," and so forth. All erotic fancies hidden in a symbolic form.

The hypochondriacal sensations are characterised by the fact that they are limited to erogenous zones.

While these forms can be attacked analytically and admit of psychic adjustment ("Redressement psychique") in the *fourth* form of hypochondria, "*hypochondria paranoides*" a cure is possible in the first stages only, perhaps quite impossible. Practical experience can alone determine this.

Here the hypochondriac idea, like the delusion of the paranoic, is incorrigible. The psychic mechanism of paranoia probably resembles that of hysteria. The analyses of Freud, Bleuler and Jung have proved this. But at present we do not know why in the one case hysteria, in the other case dementia præcox or paranoia results. Considerable light is thrown on the relations of homosexuality and the psychogenesis of paranoia by the notable treatise of Freud, "Psycho-analytical remarks on an Autobiographic Description of a case of Paranoia (dementia paranoides)" Jarhbuch für psychanalytische Forschung, Bd. III., I. Hälfte, 1911.

The *fourth* form of hypochondria is a grave psychosis and makes the subject completely unfit for life. For example, I knew a hypochondriac who through dread of the consequences of a non-existent infection with syphilis lost his post and spent all he had on consulting physicians. Finally he accused certain persons of having infected him and had to be interned.

Only fresh cases are fit for psychanalysis. When the hypochondriacal delusion is already old the analyst encounters great obstacles. The bridge which has been constructed between the unconscious erotic ideas and the conscious nosophobic ideas cannot be destroyed. So that, as I frankly admit, it is precisely all cases of hypochondria which oppose great obstacles to psychanalysis. The disease of hypochondriacs is their form of sex-activity without which they cannot and will not live.

Every hypochondriac and especially the paranoid hypochondriac throws discredit on every explanation, and his delusion is not to be destroyed. Hence old hypochondriacs are almost incurable and all the cures that can be effected are only apparent, i.e., the hypochondriacal delusion is temporarily dissimulating. And these hypochondriacs simulating healthy persons are met in countless numbers in life. For rudiments of every disease, of every neurosis can be detected in every normal human being.

The psychanalysis must therefore be made in the first stages in order to remove the secret consciousness of guilt that impels to pennance and asceticism. But in this stage it is the only method which offers any prospect of a lasting result.

CHAPTER XXXII

THE PSYCHIC TREATMENT OF EPILEPSY.[1]

THE relations of *epilepsy* to *hysteria* have long been clear, and the creation of an intermediate stage, the so-called " hysteroepilepsy " expressed this connection all the more plainly because it represented a sort of modest compromise, which without deciding between the one diagnosis or the other, attempted to do justice to both factors, the organic and the psychic. I am of opinion that a large percentage of the patients who are now diagnosed as " epileptics " are " neurotics " and, as I believe, a special variety of neurotics. *There is in them in the first place a great tendency to dissociation which manifests itself not only in attacks but also in other phenomena such as hallucinatory conditions, day dreams, temporary absent-mindedness, abstraction, abundant activity of phantasy, and secondly a most marked criminality which has been more or less completely forced out of consciousness by hyper-trophied moral inhibitory ideas.* In the epileptic attack the moral consciousness is overpowered by the unconscious criminality.[2]

Other observers have long been struck with the fact that epilepsy and criminality are intimately related, and the Lombroso school has greatly occupied itself with these relations as a phenomenon of degeneration.

In contrast to this school I can find no sign of degeneration or hereditary taint in three cases of epilepsy[3] each accurately analysed (and two of them healed) ; but I did find strong repression and *an amazingly complicated criminal complex.* Other observers had been struck with the connection of epilepsy with criminality especially in those twilight conditions known as pre- or post-epileptic madness. In pre-epileptic madness or in the aura of the attack epileptics may commit indecent assaults, or arson or even strike other persons down. (For example a peasant stabbed, in the pre-epileptic madness, his wife and three children). Kræpelin relates that an epileptic accused himself of manslaughter and indecent assaults, but the police were unable to confirm his statements. " I have occupied

---

[1] From the Zentralbl. f. Psychoanalyse, Bd. I., H. 5/6.

[2] I can find no better definition for epilepsy than the words of the young philosopher, Otto Weininger, who, shortly before his suicide, wrote : " Is not epilepsy the loneliness of the criminal ? Does he not fall because he no longer has anything to which he might hold on ? "

[3] Since first publishing this I have analysed sixteen cases, healed twelve seventy-five per cent.) and decidedly improved the rest.

myself with nothing else but murder and manslaughter " declared the patient. Then there is the remarkable aura, in which (it seems pretty well agreed) red veils, red cloths, and the like are seen, an indication of sanguinary phantasies. But blood and flames, too, are often seen by the epileptic in the aura. In post-epileptic delirium crime plays a great part and epileptics are known to be very dangerous. And according to Kræpelin the Malays when they run amok are suffering from a similar condition. According to the same author an epileptic accosted an unknown man with : " If you're a Jew you must die," and injured him severely.

Dr. S. Bruche described in the " Journal medicale de Bruxelles " (Les manifestations extérieures de l'epilepsie, 1908, No. 10) the aura of a patient whose attacks were introduced by a long series of painful hallucinations. " In the course of these hallucinations," says Bruche, " the poor wretch had a fight for life always with the same unknown man, a man of whom he could give no exact description. He lost consciousness and fell in convulsions just at the moment when after an obstinate combat he was about to plunge a knife into his opponent's breast.[1]

Such observations call for consideration and challenge investigation. I now submit the first three cases I have analysed to the consideration of my colleagues with a view to stimulating further energetic investigation in this direction. I would add a few words with regard to the differential diagnosis of epilepsy and hysteria. All cases of Jackson-epilepsy are of course left out of account because their origin is organic. Similarly tumours of the brain, lobular sclerosis, lues cerebri, encephalitic centres, abscess in the brain, in short, all forms of epilepsy of organic origin. Here and there one may come across a case whose ambiguous diagnosis encourages one to make a psychanalytic investigation. But I was cautious in the choice of my cases and observed some precautions presently to be mentioned.

How can one distinguish epilepsy of psychic origin (hysteria) from real epilsepy of organic origin ? All the details which have hitherto been made the basis of diagnostic differentiation are not absolutely trustworthy. Binswanger says : " The epileptic attack, especially the beginning of it, takes place with many patients for the most part in the night during sleep, the hysterical almost always in the daytime. If it takes place at night it is during periods of sleeplessness." Further, the series of hysterical attacks are said to lack the characteristic rise of temperature peculiar to the *status epilepticus*. The epileptic shows the initial pallor and utters the characteristic initial shriek, symptoms which in hysteria are only faintly indicated or are quite lacking. The epileptic falls down suddenly, the hysteric slips down slowly. With the latter the change of consciousness is gradual and incomplete. The epileptic exhibits

---

[1] The hero in Dostoievski's novel, " The Idiot " also falls in a fit when he is about to stab an adversary.

N

tongue-bite, *failure of the reaction of the pupils*, discharge of urine and fæces which are lacking in the hysteric. In the case of the epileptic a soporific state appears as after-stage, with periods of deep sleep of shorter or longer duration, and quite sudden awakening : the hysteric experiences rather exhaustion, headaches, nausea and so forth. The epileptic suffers from amnesia which in the hysteric is lacking.

None of these details of differential diagnosis will bear critical investigation. For tongue-bite, inhibition of the reaction of the pupils, foam, the initial shrieks, are observed also in the hysterical attack.[1] Karplus for instance, has shown that in the hysterical attack fixed pupils are found just as often as in the epileptic. Of the utmost importance is the sign of Babinsky.

L. W. Weber, in his short but closely-packed article, " Neuroses " (Diagnostische und therapeutische Irrtümer und deren Verhütung. Section III. Leipzig, Georg Thieme, 1917) states : " If the cramp attacks begin after the age of thirty this speaks against true epilepsy." He attaches great importance to tongue-biting and to scars caused by it, colour of the face (at first pale and then dark red and dark blue—almost cyanotic—during the tonic-clonic spasm period) involuntary discharge of urine (and fæces) on positive Babinsky (in coma or after the coma) on one-sided participation in the motor phenomena of the attack and scars on the skull. Petechia in the conjunctiva and in the retina and the cerebral character of the cramp in the muscles are mentioned by Jellinek.

Emil Redlich (Epilepsie und andere Anfallskrankheiten. Wience med. Wochenschrift, 1919, No. 13) follows Gaspero in noting the diagnostic importance of leucopenia before the attack, transformed after the attack into a leucocytosis (up to 10,000 and 12,000 with simultaneous increase of the eosinophiles) also the half side phenomena. Differences between the right and left sinew-reflexes, differences between the skin-stroke—and sinew reflexes, paresis of one side, left-handedness, family left-handedness, general signs of degeneration, asymmetric structure of the skull, micro-cephalis, hydrocephalis, and oxycephalis. All the authors mention the differential diagnostic importance of the psychic status.

What Binswanger says with regard to the psyche seems to me important. In epileptics we find a typical alteration of character and symptoms of spiritual degeneration which in hysteria do not occur in the same way. *In other words, the epileptic character is quite distinct from the hysterical and enables the psychanalyst to make a diagnosis without which the elucidation of the trouble would be full of difficulty.*[2]

[1] Compare Sadger " Ein Fall von Pseudœpilepsia hysterica psychoanalytisch erklart." (Wiener Klin. Rundschau, 14-17, 1909).

[2] An interesting hypothesis as to the psychogenesis of epileptic fits is due to Dr. L. Pierce Clark (Journal of Nervous and Mental Diseases, Vol. 42, No. 4, 1915). In a lecture delivered to the New York Neurological Society

According to my experience the hysteric actually suffers from hypermorality (which indeed must always be estimated relatively) whereas the epileptic has very pronounced impulses with a certain deficiency of inhibitory ideas.[1] Yet other factors seem to me much more important. Of true epilepsy we hear that the attacks have begun in the form of fits in the first years of life, and have recurred at certain periods throughout life. Or we know the preceding trauma. In the aura are seen the characteristic typical prodromi of Jackson-epilepsy. (Also in the case of fits following on a fall we have to look for a traumatic hysteria.) In the cases chosen by me for treatment the fits began in comparatively advanced age. Where the anamnesis was exact it transpired that certain prodromi had already appeared in childhood ; but these could be traced by analysis to psychogenic causes. I repeat then : *If in the absence of a fall or an injury to the skull fits begin in later life, and if it appears that the ethical condition of the individual is not disturbed, then we are justified in suspecting hysteria,* and in recommending the experiment of a psychanalytical treatment. On practical grounds the prognosis must be pronounced doubtful. The patient must be assured that it is only a question of an experiment ; an experiment which, seeing that our chemical and physical epilepsy-therapy holds out no hope, may certainly be ventured upon.

I would now record in the first place certain minor observations which plainly show the connection of the fit with the sexual and criminal complex.

No. 154.—A girl of fifteen comes home from school. The servant girl brings her a piece of bread and butter with the not very important statement : " Your mother cannot come in, she is busy in the kitchen." The sensitive girl, accustomed to a hearty welcome, answers : " Give mother my love ; if she cannot come to me, I will go to her." She takes the bread and butter and cuts off a piece with the knife. At this moment the " red " blood flushes her eyes ; she feels ill and that she is losing consciousness. She says to herself : " Now you must make haste to your mother in the kitchen." She falls to the ground with a fearful cry. People run to her and find her lying unconscious holding the knife convulsively in the right hand and waving it to and fro in the air at the risk of injuring herself. They try to take the knife away. Impossible. There is

he traces the fits to womb phantasies and this is confirmed by Dr. John T. MacCurdy. Indeed, MacCurdy who apparently is not acquainted with my work, considers Clark's views the most important advance in our knowledge of epilepsy. Clark sketches the epileptic character as egoistic, badly adapted to its environment, with which however, it is much pre-occupied, a bad workman, no spiritual refinement, free from scruples and from doubts with but little restraint of the animal instincts, often in conflict with the outside world, in lust self-centred, stiff, crude, no true friendship, no reasonable conception of the universe. These are the traits of the true epileptic while affect epilepsy presents a very varied, much more pleasant picture.

[1] Compare Maeder, " Sexualität und Epilepsie " (Jahrbuch für psychoanalytische Forschungen, 1909, Bd. I.).

nothing else to do but to make her hand fast until, at the end of half an hour the attack has passed, without its psychogenesis having been made plain. She simply repeats that she wanted to go to her mother to ask for help.

Up to the nineteenth year no second fit occurs. Then one day she is left alone with her pianoforte teacher. He begins to caress her, a tempestuous scene of mutual kissing follows, then—there was no one in the house—he lays her on the sofa. After a quarter of an hour she wakes up and does not know what has happened.

The further course of the trouble was that gradually a grave compulsion neurosis (combined with epileptic fits) developed in the centre of which stood—doubt. For example: whether she had shut the door; whether she had said good-bye; whether she had sent the letter open or closed; a doubt which extended to all the incidents of daily life. In the analysis there appeared as the most obvious source of this doubt, the fact that she did not know what had happened to her in that quarter of an hour, when she had lost consciousness. She doubted whether she had remained untouched, and this had grave practical importance for her, as she rejected several good matches for superficial rationalised motives and persistently chose objects for her affection which were unattainable for her (an archduke, married men, Court actors). In this choice of lovers appeared a repetition of a typical infantile constellation. She saw in her mother the rival who had interposed between her and her ideal. In addition to the typical constellation, father, mother, child, the analysis showed also that later in life a similar constellation had appeared, which confirms the law, discovered by Nietzsche, of recurrence of the same thing, as an important principle in the origination of neurotic conflicts (psychic parallelism). When she was fifteen years old (a month before the scene with the bread and butter took place) she was with her mother at a watering place, where they made the acquaintance of a gentleman who found favour with both of them to an extraordinary degree. The girl noticed that the gentleman courted her mother, thought, indeed, that she noticed something more than this, felt herself put in the background, fell violently in love with the handsome " uncle," and looked on her mother as the spoil-sport who stood between her and the loved one.

The further analysis showed that there were thoughts of murdering the mother, which during the bread and butter scene had developed to a direct impulse. Cutting the bread with the knife called forth the association of stabbing. The girl felt impelled to go into the kitchen with the knife and to stab her mother. This painful thought was rationalised even before it could rise into consciousness. She wanted to go into the kitchen to tell the mother that she felt bad. But even in this rationalisation the original thought breaks through; she wanted to tell her mother that she, the mother, was bad, that through her she had been robbed of her beloved. What more she wanted to do is shown by the convulsive grip of the knife, by the way she moved it, and by a series of dream-analyses which need not detain us here. I would only add that in accord with the principle of lex talionis she has long reproached herself with thoughts of suicide. As a sequel to the scene with the pianoforte teacher an obsession arose that she had left an account unpaid. That means in reality : she has a debt.[1] [2] The analysis showed that very strong criminal thoughts of poisoning the wife of the pianoforte teacher had established themselves. A friend also, a lady who was happily married, was doomed to the same fate. Finally, criminal plans could be traced back to early infancy. Poisoning, stabbing, setting things on fire, leaving the gas turned on were her pet phantasies. She had a hypertrophied consciousness of guilt. She constantly believed herself " guilty " of something. She had an incredible tendency to day-dreams, and could sit for hours half-conscious.

Here the fits served for doing of the unbearable, and for the execution of the murder plans rejected by the consciousness.

No. 155.—The second case is also a transition case. It was a matter of temporary loss of consciousness which befel a gentleman of thirty-two during dinner when he was cutting up meat. The attack did not always take place, but periodically, and then often several days in succession. According to the accounts of eye-witnesses it developed as follows :—Mr. N. cut into the meat with the knife. Suddenly his right hand began to tremble and was shaken as by convulsions ; he became deathly pale, his heart beat violently and for two or three seconds he lost consciousness. He remained seated at the table and was able to continue his meal. The last fit had taken place when he had had the evening before a violent quarrel with his wife. He wanted to attend a choir-practice, and this provoked his wife, who feared being left alone, to violent reproaches. Some weeks later he read in the newspaper that a young man had stabbed his mother, and he became anxious lest he might do his wife a mischief. He came under my treatment, but gave it up at the end of a week. The short analysis showed plainly thoughts of murdering his wife, the chief motive being a strong partiality for his niece. She was sent away from the house in the first days of the analysis. I had the opportunity of seeing him again a year later. The short elucidation seemed already to have done its work, for Mr. N. states from that time he never had another attack. This good result he ascribes to staying four weeks at Lahmann's institute.

[1] She followed a very common compulsory action with children : she would remain for hours watching the clock. The analysis showed a connection with the " account," namely, the words of Tell, " Make thy account with heaven, Governor, thy watch has run down." Looking at the clock usually signifies " How long will he or she live ? "

[2] Schuld = debt—guilt.

No. 156.—The third case I will give somewhat more in detail. Although the therapeutic result is not specially brilliant, yet this particular case affords a deep insight into the psychogenesis of the pseudo-epileptic fit. Mr. Lamda came under my treatment four years ago, not on account of his epileptic fits, but on account of a paraphilia which had already several times involved him in awkward situations. He was an urolagnist, and the impulse was expressed in the following manner. He tried to sneak into a woman's water closet, or from the men's closet to watch the micturition of women. This sight alone aroused a strong lust in him, which forced masturbation, or showed itself in an emission. Also he would manage to get into the women's closet, and then if any urine was left in the vessel he would get it out with his hand and drink it up with the most pleasurable feelings. Another way of satisfying his paraphilia was to wait behind bushes until some passing woman eased herself there. He rushed then to the place, licked up the excreta with his tongue, and felt most pleasure when any earth remained sticking between his teeth so that it crunched. (Be it noted, by the way, Mr. Lamda stated that he had noticed with regret that he had several like-minded competitors who all knew each other well!) With women he was before the treatment impotent, from prostitutes he demanded micturition, but only very rarely tasted their urine. Bloody urine disgusted him. This patient suffered from severe fits, which mostly occurred at night. According to his father's account, they ran their course as follows:—He uttered a piercing shriek and began to strike out frightfully with hands and feet. The attack was often followed by a "twilight," half-conscious, apathetic condition lasting several days, which I had repeatedly observed in this case. He then appeared like one slightly intoxicated, and always behaved as if he was in a certain year of his youth. It was not always the same, but the time between eleven and fourteen years of age was always reproduced in the half-conscious state. This patient had been diagnosed as epileptic by various experienced psychiatrists. He was so reduced by large doses of bromide when he came under my treatment that he was incapable of work of almost every kind.

The analysis acted at first like a charm. This brilliant action I attributed not only to the unburdening of the mind, but to the cessation of the bromide doses. His acne vanished, his appetite improved, he began to look flourishing, and everyone was struck by his calm composed manner. It is not possible for me to give here the whole analysis. One thing manifested itself as certain, that he was probably the strongest sadist that I had found in my analytical practice. He revelled in blood curdling ideas of sadistic content, which, as always happens in such cases, were varied with masochistic ideas of being fettered, beaten, martyred, burnt.

Before the treatment my opinion was : Since the paraphilia is so strongly established, then in the fit, if it is a case of repressed impulses, there must develop a much graver crime, a much stronger paraphilia. In other words, the paraphilia of urolagnia had established itself as an offshoot of a much stronger pathogenic complex ; the eruption of the whole complex produces a fit, since the complex is rejected by the consciousness.

The dream-analyses brought to light a vast number of sadistic impulses, among which for a long time there was nothing definite until finally, as the result of a dream, a long repressed memory of childhood was resurrected. He was five years old and had at home in the garden a little deer to which he was greatly attached. One day there came a man who also played with the deer ; suddenly he drew a knife (he was a butcher) and plunged it into the animal's breast, then disembowelled it and threw the genitals to the boy with a foul remark.

His favourite food was at that time a cake made from baked goose blood. In his memory this incident was fused with the favourite food to one picture, as if he had eaten the bloody genitals of the deer. The attacks had first occurred in the year when the story of Jack the Ripper was in all the papers and attained a great popularity. The further analysis showed that one had to do with a typical woman-murderer, who in the fit killed his mother or some other woman in order to devour her genitals. The urine had taken the place of the blood, the urolagnia took the place of the thirst for blood. The crunching earth was the substitute for the crunching flesh (Mother Earth). Long before he knew of these explanations he had become potent through the analysis. I hoped by leading the sex impulse into the normal path to put an end to the thirst for urine. This did in fact constantly become weaker, but in the presence of prostitutes he always had the feeling that he must run away before something frightful should happen. Once he had a clear vision of a lust-murder. Thus was gained a deeper insight into the psychogenesis of his disease. The attacks became more and more rare, intervals of up to three and four months occurred, but to further analysis the patient opposed immense resistance. Weeks went by without this breaking down. For weeks together he heard tones, voices, sentences without being able to lay hold of anything definite in them. His mental capacity rose so considerably, that he was able to take up a difficult and highly responsible post and to do it full justice. Urine drinking impulses became much rarer, and he could more easily master them if instead of running to the park he went to a prostitute. The fits too occurred at ever greater intervals.

There is not the least doubt that the fits occurred in the service of his criminal sadistic nature. I had occasion to analyse him immediately after an attack, and to prove the presence of his criminal phantasies. The time recalled in the post-epileptic delirium was analytically difficult of access. Finally we came upon two definite traumas : a murder, in which he was indirectly a witness, and the reading of a tale of horror, which occupied him for years, and isolated scenes from which returned to him in dreams. Some dream-analyses of this case are given in my book : " The Language of the Dream." '

The last case I shall report here is remarkable because it concluded with complete success. I give here the history of the illness of a patient who for years was treated as an epileptic, a history composed by himself. I will not give the wearisome methods and dream analyses which elucidated the case for me, but only the results.

No. 157.—The patient, who was born in 1879, is a simple, very intelligent man of strongly pious disposition. This piety was encouraged by his surroundings. It was his mother who urged him to pray. A strong impression was made on him by the teacher of religion at the elementary school, who threatened the little children with all the terrors of hell if they were not pious and had sinful thoughts. The analysis showed that the patient had a fit when only a boy. He was then twelve years old, and made confession at five o'clock in the afternoon. The catechist then addressed the children and admonished them to take care that until the morning when they were to receive the Communion, they should have no sinful thoughts ; otherwise God would punish them, they would suddenly die, or some severe illness would befall them. He remembers that he was terribly excited, and finally, when he received Communion the next morning he fell down senseless and was taken home.[1] From that time, i.e., from 1886 to 1904, he had had no more fits. The analysis shows further the presence of strong incest thoughts directed towards his sister. In spite of strong resistance, a scene was brought to light which developed as follows : One evening, when he was eighteen years old, he was alone with his sister. She was leaning out of the window ; he approached from behind and attempted an assault, which she fiercely repelled with the words : " Have you gone mad ? " He is sure that he can remember how at sixteen years of age he was afraid he might render his sister pregnant because she bathed in the same water in which he had masturbated. Later appeared obsessions that his sister might become pregnant through washing his linen. He exhibited several compulsory actions. He had to brush his coat for hours together. If he saw a particle of dust he brushed round it the whole day, washed his hands innumerable times, in short, he wanted to be " clean." Then these phenomena ceased, and he remained in fairly good health, until in 1904, four years after his sister's marriage, the fits began. Through several dream-analyses it was brought to light *that he nursed thoughts of murdering his brother-in-law.* (Compare in my book, " The Language of the Dream," the chapter, " Crime in the Dream," Dream

[1] In all my cases of pseudoepilepsy I was able to demonstrate a strong religious complex marked by much feeling.

No. 447). And now the psychogenesis of the fits and the different symptoms at once became clear. I will mention here only what is most essential for the comprehension of the origin of the attack.

The following anamnesis has been placed at my disposal by the patient :

The Record of my Illness.—" I was born in 1879[1] of healthy parents, and before the fits I was always free from all complaints. Up to the year 1904 I was an essentially healthy human being. At that time I lived in X, near a stone-mason's yard. Our kitchen opened on a courtyard, and the above mentioned stone-mason's yard adjoined this courtyard. At that time we had our meals in the kitehen to save the dining room, as we kept no maid and my mother did all the housework alone. Now, when I came from my work in the afternoon and sat at table in the kitchen *I often noticed that the knocking of the stone-masons irritated me immensely, so that I had to shut the window, which in summer was open.* I did not attach much importance to this at first, and was of opinion that this sensitiveness was caused by the worries of my work, for at this time I had had for some years a very difficult, strenuous and irritating job. and both my predecessors in this post had urgently and energetically begged to be transferred, saying that they could not perform the duties any more, as they were in constant excitement, could not sleep, nor eat, etc. I was in the habit of resting for some time after a meal, and then the nervous feeling caused by the knocking of the stone-masons again passed off.

" But soon the sensitiveness to noises increased and the noise of the street was terrible for me. My office was only a short distance from home, about four minutes. In order to avoid the noise to some extent I always chose my route through other streets, and so reached my house by a great détour. In the morning when I went to the office I noticed the worry less, but most when I came out of the office. This lasted a considerable time. Now one day I went in the afternoon after my meal from my house to my barber, who lived in the same street. During the shaving, as I sat with my head bent back I felt rather queer, and was glad when the shave was finished. From the barber I wanted to return to the office to work. *Then as I stepped from the barber's into the street I suddenly noticed the noise as never before.* The different traffic noises let loose all sorts of thoughts in my head, wherein arose a fearful hammering and heaving. I could no longer think of anything, and finally I felt as if my head was absolutely empty (this condition can hardly be described) and I only tried now to get to the office ; it would have been only two hundred paces, but I could not manage it ; in the open space before the office I collapsed. (This was the first attack.)

" I was much depressed about this, but I laid the blame partly on stomach trouble, as we had had at dinner a dish which I did not much like the taste of.

N*

" Soon after this we went with mother, who was very poorly, to N., to stay for the summer.

" *Now it was the travelling on the railway which on many a day reduced me to despair.* Apart from this I was quite all right, but the journey was for the most part terrible. I now lived in constant dread of again collapsing. Some days I was better, some again worse. *During a journey, and also walking along, I would read, as I had observed that this distracted my attention from the street noises.* So passed the summer, and we moved back to Vienna. To my worry about my condition, was now added a much stronger anxiety concerning my sister, who had undergone an operation in the spring and now began again to complain. Before the operation she had been sickly for some years, and as we at that time lived in the same passage and met each other daily, I was compelled to notice this all the time, *and this cost me sleepless nights.* To this constant feeling of anxiety, which made it impossible for a happy mood ever to visit me, I must in great part attribute the cause of my condition.

" The fits did not recur often, every two or three months, with sometimes a yet longer interval. So I thought, surely it will leave off again. After every attack I hoped it would be the last. For each one I found a special cause—one time great excitement, then a physical strain, or again stomach trouble, so that after all I always managed to console myself.

" So one and a half years went by. Then a fit seized me as I was riding home from the office in a tram. At this I was really upset, and I consulted Dr. B. After I had described my condition to him, he found that my kidneys were inflamed, and also that there was albumen in the urine. I was now four weeks sick at home, took medicine, for several weeks ate no meat, and for a much longer time white meat only, and for quite a year avoided alcohol in every form. The hoped for result was however lacking. After some months there was, indeed, another fit. In the summer I obtained six months' leave, which I spent in W. On the whole I kept well while in the country, but when I returned to Vienna the effect of the street noises was as before. The attacks began again, and I was more discouraged than ever before, because the belief established itself that I was suffering from epilepsy. This disease had always seemed to me the most dreadful because it is incurable. I now began to quarrel with my fate, said that I had committed no such serious crime in my life as to justify such a punishment, doubted the justice of the Almighty, and was filled with thoughts of suicide. In the evening I would lie for hours on my bed before I fell asleep, and prayed fervently to be freed from my sufferings. But nothing availed. Then I went to Professor X, who diagnosed ' Epilepsy.' He prescribed for me a mixture of the bromides of sodium, potassium and ammonium dissolved in water to be taken three times a day. But every few months the attacks recurred.

I now imagined *that some substance was always collecting within my body*, until after some weeks or months it exploded. The spectre of epilepsy I could not banish.

" Next summer I obtained four weeks' leave. In his certificate the physician wrote : ' Attacks of dizziness with epileptiform fits.' I had now altogether lost heart. It seemed to me, or I imagined, that the cause of the fits lay with the heart. I now consulted Dr. N., who found neurosis of the heart, and prescribed drops with a penetrating smell ; he said, ' When you have taken one phial you will be cured.' In course of time, however, I took not only one phial, but about six without result. The physician ordered also the upper part of the body to be washed in cold water of an evening.

" So time went on ; once, after a long interval, hope returned, but vanished again and gave place to complete discouragement. When a fit occurred again, I took sanatogen for a long time, and I ordered stuff called ' anti-neurasthin,' but all with no result. I carried for a long time three chestnuts in my pocket, as I had heard this praised as an infallible cure. Very often when I went to the office in the morning I suffered from fearful urgency to relieve the bowels, no doubt the result of anxiety. For a long time (and to some extent even to-day) I was of the opinion that smoking, especially a cigarette, would cause me to go off. In short, I worried myself with the most incredible ideas.

" In the spring of the present year I went, in consequence of the advice of a comrade, to Dr. W. He also spoke of epileptiform fits, and treated electrically my spine, heart and head ; also he talked of a heart neurosis. In the summer he sent me to a sanatorium. There, too, I receive electric treatment, and had cold baths ; this physician also spoke of epileptiform fits ; he said : ' There are more people who have epilepsy than you think, even in the highest circles.' This was, however, not much comfort for me. When I returned from the sanatorium to Vienna to the street noises, it was the same thing over again. I had a fit almost every week."

The patient gives us also a description of a fit : " I come out of a closed space (dwelling-house, office or the like) feeling quite well, and think, ' To-day it will be all right.' Then when I have walked along for a while, after a distance sometimes longer, sometimes shorter, the thought suddenly shoots up within me, ' I may have a fit.' This happens especially when I have to walk a good distance where there is no house door, and also when I have imagined that I was getting on especially well. Then suddenly comes the thought that it is really presumption to suppose that I am now proof against fits, in short, I can, so to say, not believe it ; I fear *that heaven will soon show me that in reality I am a poor worm*, and so forth.

" Now when these thoughts come, there is no more peace. The traffic noises fill my head with every possible nonsense. *Words*

*come into my head whose sound seems to harmonise with the noise of
a carriage, the clip-clap of the horses' hoofs, the whistling of the trams.*
When I have got hold of such a word I have to keep repeating it,
then comes a second, a third and more still ; a confusion arises in
my head and I cannot grasp any reasonable thought, a feeling of
immense dread arises, a heaving in the head, and I have only one
longing : ' If all was over.' Then I run to reach the entrance to
a house, a closet, or any closed space. Now suddenly my head
becomes as if quite empty ; I feel as if I can no longer stand. In
the *left* leg in the region of the calf I feel cramp and I sit down.
Then I notice too that the sight on the *left* side is contracted, and
I feel as if my mouth is quite out of shape and that my breath
begins to come heavily. I draw my tongue back as I have
already nipped myself several times ; and then I lose my
senses."

Analysis.—The beginning of the trouble was the irritation which
he experienced at the stonemasons' knocking. The explanation is
simple enough. Simplex sigillum veri. (Simplicity is the seal of
truth.) He thought, " When will they be hewing the grave-stone
for my brother-in-law ? "

The scene at the barber's has also a criminal basis. He wanted
to cut his brother-in-law's throat. From similar motives he
always felt ill when he put on a necktie. Unconsciously he thought
then of strangling the hated rival. The railway was especially
unpleasant for him ; he wanted it to take over the hangman's
job ; the same with the street traffic (motors, electric cars, omni-
buses, cycles, etc.). In the street it was especially the closed
vehicles, e.g., the ambulance van, a coach, a dust-cart that
troubled him. All these vehicles (besides having other meanings)
represented the *hearse* and the coffin. The street noises were for
him the symbols of the voices of his inner self which cried out
for the death of his brother-in-law, and of the voice of conscience.
The anxiety for the health of his sister was the rationalisation of
his incestuous cravings, as was also the fear which constantly beset
him that his sister might have another child.

*The fit represents the assault on his brother-in-law which he wants
to commit.* " Words come into his head, whose sound harmonises
with the noise of carriages, the clip-clap of the horses' hoofs, the
whistling of the electric railway." Let us analyse some of these
words. First, a sentence which has no sort of similarity to the
noises of the street : " *It is possible !* " The solution is, " It is
possible that the brother-in-law may be run over." Another word :
" *Crefeld.*" This stands for *Krähenfeld* (crowsfield). Ravens and
crows are the true death-birds. And this reminds him of the
cranes of Ibykus, which just represent his bad conscience. A
third word, *Piasavabesen*, has apparently no meaning. The analysis
shows that it is connected with the religious complex (Pia) and
with the brother-in-law, who was born on the river Save. Finally,

a fourth word that reminded him of the trampling of hoofs, " *Massapust.*" This word contains two desires directed towards the death of the arch-enemy with whom in actual life he was on very friendly terms. " *Massa* " in the Slav language, means " flesh." Let the brother-in-law be trampled into a formless mass of flesh under the horses feet ! The syllable " *pust* " expresses another kindly wish : Let the brother-in-law catch small-pox or syphilis and die of it ! Criminal ideas, active and passive, are his incessant pre-occupation. In the street the impulses to commit the crime grow ever stronger and stronger. It is as if the voices of the street cried out to him : " Do it ! Do it ! " Finally he escapes by means of the fit, in which he commits the crime.

Especially in his dreams the criminal motive is clearly expressed. Note the following dream : " *I was walking through a park (probably the Kaipark) with my brother. Suddenly behind us I saw a suspicious-looking individual ; my two companions also saw him and fled, leaving me alone. I turned round, the tramp then came up to me and, saying that it was unjust that we should live so well while he had nothing, he drew a knife and scratched my* left[1] *hand. I fell into his arms and he became quieter. I looked him sternly in the eyes, and that seemed to cow him. I pulled out my purse and gave him a shilling, whereupon he made off ; the knife I did not return to him. Meanwhile my companions returned, and my brother also gave him a shilling.*"

This dream—apart from its homosexual meaning—becomes comprehensible only when one substitutes for the brother the brother-in-law, with whom in fact he had " drunk brotherhood." The tramp with the knife is himself. The crown symbolises the sister. For him she is the crown of creation and the queen of his heart. She is his chief treasure ! (his purse).

If, however, anyone should be doubtful as to the incest-phantasies of this patient, the next dream would teach him better.

" *I was in a little cottage (like the houses of the market gardeners in Simmering). At my right hand stood my sister. Soon a strange man appeared, who related several doubles entendre in a way that caused me sexual excitement. My member became stiff, and I could help myself only by pressing against my sister, the upper part of whose body was now bare, so that an erection followed. Thereupon I awoke.*"

The strange man is the brother-in-law. Evidently the fulfilment of a wish !

This dream refers to the above mentioned traumatic scene with his sister, the only one which he can clearly remember.

The next dream betrays necrophilic tendencies. At the same time it shows an identification of the mother and sister which renders comprehensible many of his criminal fantasies.

" *It appeared to me that my mother had died ; I saw the coffin*

[1] Notice the prominence of the *left* side as an expression of criminality, .e., of what is not right also in the aura of the fit.

with the body in it. And yet I knew that my mother had died long ago ; next, I think it is my sister who is lying in the coffin ; and yet on the other hand it seemed to me that the corpse in the coffin did not at all resemble my sister. I did not know what to make of it."

Within these narrow limits it is impossible for me to give any idea of the hell which raged within this man's breast. He was eaten up with sombre thoughts of vengeance against the man who had " robbed " him of his sister. His brother-in-law was temperate. This he interpreted as avarice. The frugality of the petty official he called being sordid. All this, however, only in thought, for in fact he lived with his brother-in-law to all appearance on the best of terms.

I had the opportunity once to observe a fit. (Cf. " The Language of the Dream," *p.* 506.) In this fit, which occurred during my treatment, he kept on repeating one word " Kasten " (chest). Often he uttered it also with the Viennese pronounciation, " Kosten" (cost). Also several times, one after the other, " Kasten—Kosten." I knew his dread of the closed carriage, and referred these words to his desire for the death of his brother-in-law—for having taken him away in a coffin (Kasten). A month later a dream showed me the overdetermination of these words. He dreamed that he wanted to hire his sister a new house, in which was a large chest. The house was, however, already let, so that he was inconsolable, and woke up in a flood of tears. The affect continued long after waking, and for a long time he could not regain his tranquility.

The analysis gave the explanation of this strong emotion. The brother-in-law is, as I have mentioned, a very worthy, but frugal and economical man. His sister has two strong desires, which, in spite of her begging and praying, the brother-in-law has not yet fulfilled. She feels cramped in the little dwelling, and has no room for her clothes. She has urgent need of a *chest*, for which, however, she can find no room. Also she would like her daughter to be taught the pianoforte, and has no room at disposal for the " *tinkle-chest*," as the brother-in-law called the piano. The couple had many quarrels, until finally the husband promised to get a piano, which could be accommodated in the old dwelling. In spite of the promise, months went by, and the piano did not appear. He was afraid of the cost (Kosten) of the two chests (Kasten). This experience gave him an apparent justification for his hatred of the brother-in-law. What ! His beloved sister is not even to possess a chest. In the murder scene he hurls at his rival the vengeful word " Kasten." " That for your meanness for not buying my sister the clothes' chest and the " tinkle-chest." Also the " *Kosten* " are concerned. The brother-in-law was always talking of the high *costs* of moving.

Thus the words " Kasten " and " Kosten " betrayed the rationalising of the motives for his criminal phantasies. He was a very pious man. Therefore, these criminal ideas had to be entirely repressed, by forcing them into the unconscious. Before the analysis he had no idea that he hated the brother-in-law so savagely. The whole conflict proceeded in the conscious. The fit was a compromise between two emotions. It served as the punishment of God and also for the execution of the crime. The fits came for the most part when he was on the way to the brother-in-law. We are far from having exhausted his criminal impulses. We are able to give only a few indications of them. The result of the analytical elucidation was absolutely startling. The fits came more and more seldom, and finally ceased altogether. His deep piety played a great part in bringing about the neurosis. The remorseful thoughts had occupied other positions, but in the end they made his life unbearable.

In almost all my cases I have found a close connection between *masturbation* and *epilepsy*. In most cases of " affect epilepsy " we have to do with a sex crime. (Rape, lust murder, child rape, necrophilism, cannibalism, vampirism, incest and so forth.) It could constantly be demonstrated that in the masturbatory acts parts of this phantasy (sometimes the whole phantasy) could become conscious. In coitus also fits occur, if during the coitus the phantasy of a crime creeps in.

Féré says : Coitus can bring about epilepsy. Sauvages instances a man with whom a fit resulted every time ; Zimmermann knew a young man who had a fit every time after masturbation.[1] Krafft-Ebing tells of a fetish-worshipper who had epileptic fits on onanising, and also on touching the shoes of the women in whose service he was. Hammond mentions a pederast who had a fit during the act. Maurice[2] (sic) mentions a dog which showed epileptic symptoms every time he copulated. Guersant mentions an infant who had an attack of convulsions every time when his mother, who was of an excitable disposition, gave him the breast *after she had indulged in connubial joys.* Moreover there are persons in whom both in the sex act and in the epileptic fit certain phenomena of the sensorium, erythropsis, coloured visions and subjective sensations of the olfactory organ are developed ; and certain impulses manifesting themselves in phenomena are common to both conditions of excitement. Often the epileptic symptoms and the venereal excesses develop simultaneously ; the former begin and cease together with the latter. [3]

The following observation by Féré on the connection between masturbation and epilepsy is specially noteworthy :

No. 158.—The patient, like his brothers and sisters, began to walk and to speak at the normal age, and was also clean at an early age. He had scarlet fever and measles without any nervous symptoms. At nine and a half years he had in the course of six weeks four convulsive fits with swooning and micturition, tongue-biting and subsequent numbness. He has no recollection whatever of these fits, and it is not known whether they made themselves noticeable beforehand by any subjective phenomena.

[1] Esquirol Mentale Krankheiten. Vol. 1, *p.* 301. L'Instinct Sexuel, Evolution et Dissolution, by Ch. Féré. (Médecin de Bicetre) Paris, 1899, Ancienne Librairie, Germer, Bailliere et Cie., Felix Alcan. Editeur.

[2] Ch. Maurice. (sic. Trans.) Onanie und sexuelle Excesse (Dict. de med. et de chir. pratiques, 1877. Vol. XXIV. *p.* 528.)

[3] Morel, Lehrbuch der mentalen Krankheiten, 1860, *p.* 176. Ch. Féré, Sexual Excesses and Epilepsy. (C. R. Soc. de Biologie, 1897, *p.* 331.)

When he was freed from worms the convulsive fits ceased, but were succeeded by fits of dizziness, which the child described, and still describes very precisely. Suddenly, usually in the small hours, *every object about him appeared red*, in a moment the intensity of the colour rapidly increased and he saw nothing but red ; all forms vanished. He had a sensation of nausea and threw up with hiccoughs two or three mouthfuls of a clear liquid. The whole lasted about a minute ; he did not lose consciousness, heard what went on about him, but was very pale and looked much terrified.

These crises of erythropsis developed two or three times a day during two months, and suddenly ceased without any reciprocal effect, or the application of any remedial measures. In the interval he had several times been given vermifuges, but no worms were passed. For two years the child enjoyed perfect health. He had no nervous disturbance of any kind ; his sleep was peaceful. One night, about two o'clock, his father was awakened by a fearful cry ; he rushed to his son's bed and found him uncovered, holding the penis with both hands and writhing with pain. A very strong erection was noticeable, the glans was quite distended and tinged with violet. Almost instantaneously a complete relaxation set in. It was light in the room ; the father had sprung up immediately he heard the cry ; he was much surprised at this sudden attack, the more so as the child did not seem to notice his entrance. In spite of the child's crying, he was in doubt as to the cause of the phenomenon or rather he was convinced that there was some external stimulus and then a phantasy with pains. The child was carefully watched, without any trace of bad habits being discovered. A month later the same scene took place, at about the same hour ; fourteen days later the same about two hours after going to bed. Two hours later the child gave a remarkable cry and was found in convulsions and foaming at the mouth. After two or three minutes he fell into a deep sleep from which he awoke next morning stupid and quite worn out. He had wetted the bed and bitten his tongue. Six weeks later he seemed to have completely recovered, when, at breakfast, his face suddenly became distorted, he turned pale and he seized his genitals with both hands and shrieked ; the same violent erection was seen, which after not more than two minutes suddenly ceased. The child had not lost consciousness.

He has on several occasions described the phenomenon as an abrupt and terrible shock, extending rather suddenly and very soon becoming painful.

Some days later the child began a bromide cure : during the following six months he had no more attacks of cramp or priapism, but often fits of dizziness with fainting, which cause one to estimate the result of the cure only with reserve, yet help to confirm the diagnosis.

There was no local irritation of any kind : neither constipation, nor intestinal worms ; nor any injury to the penis or the urethra. Urination is easy and normal ; the foreskin is not narrow and its mucous membrane as well as that of the passage and of the glans show no signs of any irritating lesion, the testicles have their normal weight and position and cannot be pushed back into the groin passages. Every sign of puberty is lacking whether in the genitals or the larynx ; nothing abnormal in the region of the breast.

These facts show us the infantile origin of the trouble and the connection between masturbation and epilepsy.

I intend to deal with this highly important subject in a special volume of this work. I cannot but wonder that medical literature has taken no notice of my first publication (1911). I have been able to observe a considerable increase of this epilepsy during the War, because the War has of course mobilised all the wild instincts in man. I succeeded in curing several cases, among them a man forty years old who had two severe fits a week, and wanted to take his life.

The splendid success in a case so grave and so near to suicide bids us investigate in every case of epilepsy whether we have not to do with pseudo-epilepsy. In all these cases, which are really parapathia we shall be able to confirm the views here set forth. I will state them once more :

(1) *Epilepsy is more frequently than we had hitherto supposed a psychogenic disease.*

(2) *In all cases it shows a strong criminality which the consciousness rejects as unbearable.*

(3) *The fit is a substitute for the crime, or, it may be, for a sexual act which is a crime (Self-protection).*

(4) *The fit often results from dread of the punishment of God and symbolises guilt, punishment and dying.*

(5) *Pseudo-epilepsy is curable by analytic psycho-therapy. It requires long periods of treatment, as the condition of divided personality has advanced to an extraordinary degree.*

[1] Dostojewsky suffered from so-called epileptic fits. How aptly he recognises the nature of his epilepsy when he states : " The depression which in my case succeeded the epileptic fits had this characteristic : *I feel like a great criminal ; it seemed as if some unknown guilt, a criminal deed oppressed my conscience !* " (Quoted from Otto Hinricksen, " Zur Psychologie und Psychopathologie des Dichters." J. F. Bergmann, Wiesbaden, 1911.)

This crime of the mighty poet seems to me to have been child-rape. Evidences of this are to be found not only in " Raskolnickow " but also in the fact that among his literary remains the detailed description of such a crime was found. This description is said to have been so realistic and horrible that his literary executor has not yet had the courage to publish the work.

It is interesting that the Romans caused epileptics to drink as a medicine the warm reeking blood of the slaughtered gladiators. Probably the motive of this remarkable therapy was a dim recognition of the thirst for blood of these patients. (Stemplinger, Sympathieglauben und Sympathiekuren im Altertum und Neuzeit. Munich, 1919.)

CHAPTER XXXIII

ON THE BORDER-LINE OF PSYCHOSIS
(BETWEEN PARAPATHIA AND PARALOGIA)

MELANCHOLIA is the psychosis best known to the practitioner. In spite of this, slight cases are often overlooked and set down as " nervousness " or " nervous depression." (Cf. Ziehen, " Die Erkennung u. Behandlung d. melancholie in der praxis." *Carl Marhold*, 1907.) A sudden, unexpected attempt at suicide then all too late makes the diagnosis plain.

However, we do not wish to speak to-day of the clinical aspect of melancholia. For us this disease is of interest because like other grave psychoses, e.g., "epileptic insanity," it often begins with serious conditions of anxiety (raptus melancholicus) often in the midst of apparently undisturbed health so that one might be tempted to think it a simple neurosis.

Little is known at present of the psychic bases of melancholia. *The ideas of having sinned*, the perpetual reproaches of the patients that "they have committed grave faults " were looked on as the *consequence*, not as the cause, of the disease.[1]

[1] For example, while Kræpelin originally classed melancholia under the psychoses of the advanced age he now sees it only as a stage of insanity with depression mania. (Cf. his preface to Dr. Georg L. Dreyfuss' " Die Melancholic ein zustandsbild des mannisch depressiven Irresein."

To be sure in the case of melancholia in particular, the majority of psychratists find it impossible to exclude the view that for the occurrence of this disease psychic causes are the first to be considered. Obersteiner estimates the proportion of psychogenic cases at forty per cent. (Das psychische Moment in der Ætiologie und Therapie der Seelenstörungen. Vierteljahrsschrift für Psychiatry, 1897.)

The importance of psychic causes is maintained with special warmth by Gaupp (Die seelischen Ursachen d. Melancholie, Münchener med. Wochenschrift, 1905, No. 2) and Albrecht (Die seelischen Ursachen d. Melancholie, Monatschrift für Psychiatry and Neuralgic, 1906). The latter shows that the hereditary causes are less important than the psychic. He estimates the psychogenic cases at seventy per cent. To be sure the psychic disturbances act according to him by physical processes, namely by irritation of the vasoconstrictors. In his little work, " Melancholie und Schuld " (Stuttgart F. Enke, 1884), published more than thirty years ago, Dr. Carl Krausold opens up important points of view which in some respects very much resemble my own. The case of the middle-class woman of C. (*p.* 36) shows great similarity with the first observations here published. Reimann (" Die hysterischer Geistesstörungen," Fr. Deuticke, 1904) analyses a number of varieties of hysterical melancholia and bases his diagnosis of hysteria on the " hysterical character " and the " Suggestibility." At the height of the disease any one " would have been obliged to diagnose melancholia without the least doubt without knowing the genesis of the trouble and without personal acquaintance with the patient."

Up to the last ten years our knowledge of the psychogenesis of the psychoses was slight to the point of absurdity. The somatic facts were in all cases conscientiously noted, the *endogenic* and *exogenic* causes, hereditary influences, toxins, derangements of circulation and assimilation were all sought out, but the most important thing, the mind of the patient, was forgotten. I will publish here a modest contribution to the solution of this question. I have not the slightest doubt that with the aid of Freud's procedure we shall succeed in penetrating the riddle of certain psychoses, e.g., of paranoia, and dementia præcox ; perhaps also of "maniacal depressive insanity." A beginning has already been made ; we possess two paranoia analyses[1] by Freud, and a considerable work by Dr. Jung, "The psychology of dementia præcox."[2] In this latter, proof is given that in dementia præcox also we have to do with repressed complexes. Then, too, we have contributions by Bleuler,[3] Abraham,[4] Gross,[5] Maeder.[6] It is true that there is still an immense amount of work to be done, and Jung is quite right when he says that it is far beyond the powers of a single person to perform in a few years all the preliminary experimental work. The call to this great work goes forth above all to the practical physicians who have the opportunity to observe how the psychoses arise from their first beginnings and to get an insight into the psychic genesis of the disease.[7]

For most psychoses come before the nerve specialist only when the symptoms make the patient a nuisance to his surroundings ; when the repression has gone so far, the psychosis has so far obscured the clear consciousness that an exact analysis of the case is quite out of the question. Such cases usually enter the clinics and hospitals when the disease is at its height and one has to content oneself with helping the patient over these bad times by means of tranquillising procedures and of watching.

I am in a position to give the psychogenesis of three psychoses, three cases of melancholia, which are connected with our subject

[1] Analysis of a case of chronic paranoia (Collection of short essays on the doctrine of neuroses). In the course of these discussions I shall have occasion to return to Freud's second paranoia contribution.

[2] Carl Marhold, 1907.

[3] Bleuler, Freudsche Mechanismen in der Symptomatologie von Psychosen. Psychiatr-neurolog. Wochenschr., 1906, and his celebrated work, " Schizophrenia," also the " Allgemeine Psychiatrie."

[4] Abraham, Ueber die Bederetung sexueller Jugendtraumen für die Symptomatologie der Dementia præcox, Centralblatt für Nervenheilkunde, 1907, No. 238.

[5] Das Freudsche Ideogenitätsmoment in manisch-depressiven Irresein,

[6] Maeder, Psychologische Untersuchung von Dementia præcox-Krunken. (Jahrbuch, Vol. II., first half).

[7] Since the second edition the literature has grown so enormously that I cannot record it here. I can only refer to the wonderful work of Bleuler on Schizophrenia and to the contributions of the Vienna school (Pötzl, Schilder and others).

in this respect that they developed on the basis of an anxiety neurosis and that in both cases the anxiety occupied a central position in the illness. Conditions of anxiety among those mentally diseased are in fact something uncommonly frequent and attain degrees of intensity which far surpass those of ordinary neurotics. Very frequently the psychosis begins with an attack of anxiety which may be so violent that it drives the patient to suicide. (Cf. Dr. Stelzner, "Analyse von 200 Selbstmordfällen." S. Karger, 1906.) Cleptomania, too, and arson begin with a fit of anxiety. The poor patients evidently stand in dread of themselves. Suicide then signifies a punishment. " Better kill myself than become a murderer ! " So runs the secret reasoning of the unconscious. Every anxiety is the endopsychic recognition of one's own criminality. But in the case of psychoses this anxiety is distinguished from neurotic anxiety because clearly-marked uncorrected hallucinations are mixed with it. Transitory delusions may also develop. But they are very soon corrected. It seems to me to be established beyond doubt that the anxiety of the mentally diseased springs from a secret consciousness of guilt. It is always the " guilty conscience " that expresses itself in violent attacks of dread. Let us then begin with a description of our first case, one which has been several years under observation.

No. 159.—About eight years ago, Mrs. J. L., forty-five years old, consults me about palpitation of the heart and sleeplessness. I deduce an anxiety-neurosis and recommend her husband to substitute for the coitus interruptus which he had hitherto practised the coitus condomatus. Thereupon the condition of this lady is greatly improved, but the complaints do not altogether disappear. In fact she is not always satisfied by her husband with the coitus condomatus. Moreover, he is a rather frivolous person who all too frequently seeks his pleasure outside the house, so that he is good for very little with his wife. The anxiety-neurosis improves when the lady occupies their summer residence and remains for some months separated from her husband. Some years later, however, occurs a violent exacerbation of the disease. The patient becomes very much excited and irritable, sleeps badly and suffers frequently from palpitation so that I recommend her a water-cure in an institution. After a four weeks' stay in a sanatorium she comes back considerably improved. After two more weeks the lady is hardly recognisable. She looks blooming, almost youthful, increases in weight and experiences in some degree a second youth. I see her from time to time because I am treating her husband. Each time I am glad to see that the wife, now cheerful and full of life, no longer needs my help. One day, however, she again calls on me unexpectedly with the request that I will examine her heart very " thoroughly." She says she must certainly have something wrong with her heart ; she cannot sleep again ; the least noise frightens her so that she collapses, also she has no proper appetite, no more any real joy in life. I examine her carefully, find that her organs are perfectly sound, and recommend her the same sanatorium in which she had such excellent results on the last occasion. It was a great surprise for me when with great emotion she raised a violent opposition to this. She says she will not enter that place, the physician is quite unsympathetic to her and does not take any real pains. Can I recommend her any other institution ? I do this. She travels a good way from Vienna to the Salzkammergut. The further the better, she thinks. However, in a week she is back again. Meanwhile her health has become much worse. The neurosis is gradually transformed into psychosis. She is seized with a continual unrest. She can hardly remain seated on a chair for a few minutes. If she is at home she wants to be driven to the house of a friend. At this friend's she remains only a very short time, a few moments, gives a distracted look round the room and rushes away as quickly as she came to seek another friend. They try to influence her by distraction. In vain. She remains in no café more than a few minutes. She leaves the theatre in the midst of the first act ; she can hear no music because everything excites her and she wants to cry more than anything. She complains frightfully of feelings of anxiety. She knows that she is lost, that she has an incurable disease, not only is her heart affected, but also something will go wrong in the head, and she will be obliged to be sent to a lunatic asylum. She does not sleep a single night ; she torments those about her in the most frightful fashion. Her husband or her daughter must always sit by her bed and hold her fast by the hands. As soon as they go away such a terrible anxiety overwhelms her that she begins to shriek. In spite of the presence of her dear ones she suddenly cries out loudly and unexpectedly. Then she drives everyone away from her, husband and daughter too. She begins to strike the people about her. She hurls herself unexpectedly on her husband and gives him a blow. She can only be restrained by force from beating the servant girl especially. At the same time she develops a pathological avarice. No medicines must be bought because she is convinced that they are now quite impoverished and will soon have to go begging. She tells me a long story : her husband had had a partner who had made away with their whole property. This rogue had reduced them to beggary. They had not even enough to live on for half a year. The narrative was only partly true. As the husband explained to me the truth was that he had indeed suffered great losses through the partner. He had, however, enough money left to live on without anxiety and even without work. But still every day she bemoans her poverty. The psychosis increases from day to day. She never has her hair done and cannot be induced to buy a new hat or a new dress. The lady whose dress and hair were formerly so well cared for now makes a perfectly miserable, neglected impression. In a few weeks she has become an old woman. She wears her oldest clothes when she goes out, and instead of a hat an old black cloth round her head. She refuses all food because she has no appetite and because everything sticks in her throat. One evening she implores me with uplifted hands to give her poison so that she may die at once. She is a wicked sinner. God has punished her for her grave sins. She has only one wish—to die ! While I am making a friendly effort to talk her out of all this, she rushes at me and gives me a blow on the breast. The next day she attempts to commit suicide. She attempts to jump through the window, but is held back in time. We have her watched by an attendant. The patient, however, is cunning enough to succeed, in spite of this, in inflicting a considerable injury on herself with a fork. She has to be taken to an institution where she is fed with a tube because she refuses all food. There for the most part she speaks not a word, lies in a corner as if bereft of her senses, and in spite of chloral, veronal and trional she spends sleepless nights. In the intervals hallucinations, pracordial anxiety, ideas of her sinfulness. When she visits her husband she comes to life again, falls on her knees before him and implores him to take her home, she is getting worse in the sanatorium, she will quiet down at home ; so that the man quite upset takes her back home the next day. There I treat her with great doses of opium, packs, and general massage of the body, and succeed in attaining some degree of tranquillity. The fits of anxiety become less frequent. The patient begins to sleep a few hours at night and is also induced to take small doses of milk and food preparation. At the same time I try to get light on the psychogenesis of this disease and behold ! my efforts are crowned with success. From scattered indications given by the patient I infer that the partner had something to do with it. Thus she once said : " This fellow has eaten and drunk every day at our house and then he shamefully deceives my husband." The story of the partner as given by the husband was as follows :—A young man was recommended to him as an extremely capable merchant. He thought he could get a son-in-law for his daughter, then seventeen years old, and they opened a factory together. At first this went pretty well. He took to the young man so much that he invited him to take his meals at his house so that they never went out without him. He was always with them. Gradually, however, the business began to get worse, and the partner announced to him that they were, so to speak, on the point of bankruptcy. Frightened at this he withdrew from the business as he did not want to appear before the Court. The partner promised to return the capital he had invested in small instalments. He would do his utmost to save the business from bankruptcy. If, however, they should go bankrupt he would bear the responsibility alone. This procedure turned out to be a skilful swindle which quite deceived the honest man. A short time after the dissolution of partnership the partner married quite privately a very rich widow, with whom it seems he had had relations for a long time and the factory began to flourish in such fashion that it was plain the manufacturer would soon become a millionaire. The man had borne this shocking behaviour fairly well because he possessed besides the factory a small business from which he could live decently. Also he had at his disposal a little capital which he had not touched. Moreover, the money he had put into the business was repaid by the partner after his marriage. But the wife behaved as if raving mad. Hence it occurred to me that there must have been something between the wife and the partner and I tried at several meetings to induce her to speak. She said, however, that she had nothing to say and mostly refused any answer. But in the course of the treatment when by a rather large dose of opium a considerable temporary tranquillisation had been achieved she put more confidence in me and I simply risked it, *and asked her direct what had taken place between her and the partner.* At this she became much excited, burst into tears and confessed to me as follows :— She made the man's acquaintance at the sanatorium to which I had sent her the first time. She was interned in the institution while he lived close by. The unsatisfied woman at once succumbed to his seductive arts and formed with him a firm liaison. It was terribly painful for her when her husband spoke of having chosen this man, whom in the meantime he had got to know, as partner and as son-in-law. She had always pointed out that her daughter was too young, that there was plenty of time to think of marrying her and so forth. The arrangement as partner was very welcome. She hoped by this means to attach the young man permanently to herself. The partner was her daily guest and came very often when he knew that her husband was not at home and that his daughter was engaged outside. Not only did the liaison continue but she supplied him with considerable sums of money which she had saved in the course of years. All her savings and a part of her weekly allowance went into the pockets of the lover. She loved him more than her husband, than her daughter, than her own life. She loved him with that fanaticism, with that blind infatuation of which only women who are getting old are capable. And this man to whom she had sacrificed everything one day cast her off brutally and then cheated her husband in such shameful fashion out of the fruits of his honest work.

Her despair, her disillusionment, were beyond description. Besides, the emotion was to some extent repressed. She could not give rein to her rage. She would have liked best to hurl herself upon the faithless man and to strike him down. That is why she struck her husband, her daughter and the servant girl. These were acts of compulsion arising from repression of the tormenting thought. At times she hated her daughter because she had been her rival. Her avarice, too, was easy to explain.[1] She reproached herself because she had given him so much of her savings.. But what caused her the greatest suffering was that she could not speak of all this to any human being. It is true she scolded and stormed about this "rascal." But to no one could she tell the real truth and declare what a criminal this man had been. Hence she ran from friend to friend, from physician to physician, because she always intended to confide the secret to *one* person in the world.

After this revelation her health improved in the most striking way ; she became more and more tranquil, increased in weight and with very small doses of opium slept five or six hours. In the course of some months the psychosis gradually disappeared. To-day, after two years, the unextinguishable traces can still be observed. All the distrust has been transferred to the servants. At every opportunity she accuses them of theft. No one stays with her more than a few weeks. She is filled with a morbid distrust and her frugality, if no longer pathological, yet appears in striking contrast to her former careless way of living. Her excessive tenderness to her husband is also very striking. He is tended like an infant, and if anything can change her meanness into extravagance it is her concern for her husband. For him she finds nothing too dear. Moreover, the woman who was formerly enlightened and quite free from prejudice has become very pious and goes to church daily. As I learned later she has also done pennance for her sin and received absolution.

I do not venture to conclude that the open confession hastened the good result. Perhaps time completed the cure. At any rate the improvement after the confession was remarkably quick.[2]

The second patient's history is very similar to the above case. No. 160.—One evening I was called to Mrs. K. B., whom I found sitting in bed and suffering from a violent fit of anxiety. When I entered she cried out : " There, they're coming already, the men, the black men, who want to fetch me. Go away, go away, go away ; you shall not catch me ! " She sprang from the bed and made for the door. I took her by the arm and said to her kindly : " Do you not know me ? I am your friend, the doctor." " You, too, are my enemy," she cried again. " I don't want anyone near me, I will have quiet. Get out, away with you ! You are come to put me into a lunatic asylum, I know." With a great deal of trouble we succeeded in quieting the patient, and getting her back to bed, where after a cold pack and a good dose of brom-chloral-hydrate she very soon seemed quite calm. She slept fairly well in

[1] It had also a symbolic significance and served retrospective " tendencies to annul." She grudged her gifts and kept her purse tightly closed. Avarice as symbol of hoarded love. . . .

[2] Supplementary, after two years : I saw the ex-patient some weeks ago. She is perfectly healthy only rather depressed and subdued.

Ten years later : Completely cured. After the death of her husband a second marriage of the rich woman with a younger man.

the night and had only twice violent but transitory fits of anxiety. The next day I found her somewhat quieter and more composed. She wished to speak with me alone and begged me to give her some poison, she could no longer live with such agonising attacks. She was continually in dread that men were coming who wished to attack her. Every time during our talk when the door creaked she collapsed and almost lost her senses with terror. Interspersed with the sensibly conducted conversation she uttered many confused disconnected things. She felt herself persecuted by enemies. That was the punishment for the errors of which she had been guilty.

I knew the previous history of this case and knew exactly how this psychosis had arisen. As long as six years before she had sought my medical advice. She then suffered from palpitation of the heart, dyspnœa, sleeplessness, feelings of terror, dizziness, irritability and worry about the future. That is to say, from a typical anxiety neurosis. The cause was also known to me. Her husband had become completely impotent after an apopletic fit. The woman, still quite strong and passionate, and moreover ten years younger than her husband—at the time of this treatment she was forty-one years old—had a great sexual need. As to the objective evidence there were even at that time slight signs of a Basedow—marked goggle-eyes a slight struma and trembling of the hands. (Early photographs show, however, that this bulging of the eyes already existed when she was a girl.) To be sure she was nervous even as a girl, so that one might assume a certain *forme fruste* of the Basedow as basis of her neurosis and psychosis. At that time her health improved very quickly upon her forming a liaison with her music-teacher. This man—let us call him Adolf —was later to play a great part in her hallucinations. I knew further that in nursing her husband when he was very ill she had somewhat overstrained herself. The man had died about two months before, after she had nursed and watched him for two years, far from Vienna, it is true, and under circumstances very unfavourable and exciting for her. She lived in Gmunden with a step-daughter who shared with her the nursing of her husband, and who was attached to the father with a great and enthusiastic love. It was known that her husband had been able to save a great deal and had left her very well off. He had in his life-time repeatedly told his friends that he would leave his property in equal shares to his wife and to his yet unmarried daughter by his first wife. All the more remarkable appeared the almost boundless despair of this woman after the death of her husband which at first related solely to one point : she was afraid she would not be able to live on the remaining capital. She continually cried, " Oh, poor woman that I am, he has left me a beggar ! There is nothing left for me to live on." When it was explained to her that after all for the last eight years of his life her husband had earned nothing and had lived on his investments and that the property was certainly so large that she and her daughter could live comfortably on it, she shook her head, burst into tears and repeated her stereotyped cry, " Oh, poor woman that I am, what shall I live on ? " An absolutely pathological avarice took possession of her, so that e.g., she would not suffer anyone to call the doctor or fetch medicine from the druggist. I had to assure her that I charged " not a kreuzer " for the treatment, and made her believe that on my recommendation the medicines also were given her free from the chemists. Only in this way could she be induced to let me observe her and treat her.

In view of this remarkable motiveless excitement, it was at once clear to me that this was simply a case of the consequences of a guilty conscience. Evidently she reproached herself bitterly for having deceived her husband with Adolf, for, in one of the next fits of terror in which she ran madly about the room and then wanted to run into the street in her shirt (raptus) she suddenly cried, " Adolf, beloved Adolf, come and help me ! " So that the long guarded secret of her love was betrayed to everyone about her. Now Adolf had just before the death of her husband married one of her well-to-do nieces. That she had played with the thought of marrying Adolf after the death of her husband she disclosed in a second hallucination, when she cried out, " There he stands, the good-for-nothing, the wretch ! He is come to fetch me ! " Asked who the good-for-nothing was, she cried, " Adolf, the rascal." Then she looked distractedly about her and said : " What have I said ? I must have been talking great nonsense."

A few days later I found her senseless on the ground. In order to end her torture she had drunk Lysol. Although I had instructed her family to watch her most closely and had recommended immediate internment in an asylum, they still believed it was only a case of excessive grief for the loss of her husband. And so in an unguarded minute, while her nurse had gone to the water-closet, she was able to drink a considerable dose of Lysol. I observe that I did not get the diagnosis, lysol-poisoning, from those about her, who thought it was a " nervous " attack, but that I was convinced it was a case of suicide by the profound unconsciousness, the stertorous breathing, the weak pulse and some little blisters on the lips and face. The people about her refused to admit the diagnosis of poisoning.

In the evening the patient felt somewhat better, complained only of great pain in swallowing and groaned : " *Now I am disgraced for life.*" She denied emphatically having attempted to take her life. After a week during which her behaviour was completely negative, the consequences of the lysol-poisoning disappeared. She could hardly be got to move in order to take a little milk, gave no answer to any one but only stared indifferently, almost apathetically into a corner. After a few more days she got up and wished to take advantage of a free moment to leave the house.

She ran into the street in her shirt to throw herself under the electric car. But the attendant followed her in time and brought her back. At length the family (an old father and the step-daughter) yielded and she was taken to an asylum. There she wept for weeks together or sat sadly in a corner and when she was asked why she was so sad, she said : "*Because I am disgraced for all time.*" She meant the scars on her face which, however, had begun to heal and were of a quite superficial nature. In the asylum they diagnosed "maniacal-depressive insanity." After some weeks there followed on a melancholy stage a period of great excitement. She called herself a bitter sinner. Her sins could never be expiated. She began to have hallucinations again, talked a great deal, told the attendants she had received a visit from "the Empress Maria Theresa " and so forth. These phenomena too, passed away and she made a violent demand for the step-daughter. When the latter appeared the patient wept and wanted to kiss her feet. This was all the more striking because during the whole time she had got on very badly with the step-daughter. At this visit also I was present. and she implored us to take her home, she would be quite quiet. I was able also to make her a communication which exerted a great and evident beneficial effect upon her. I told her the will was already published ; she was to receive a small sum with which with a little good will she could live in a modest way.

Here I must add something. It had struck me that her husband, who was known to be well-to-do should have left her a compara-tively small amount. As appeared later, and as I already knew at that time, the wife had already in the life-time of her husband had part of the property written down to her name, another part deposited with relations. What she had feared the whole time was this : on the one hand the official would come down on her for this fraud and impose on her a heavy penalty for evading taxation. On the other hand the step-daughter might take legal proceedings to claim a judicial division of the property according to her father's intentions. For by this procedure the step-daughter had been deprived of three-fourths of the considerable fortune which was rightfully due to her. From this consciousness of guilt arose the patient's dread that "men " would come ; she was afraid of the law. The motive which influenced her may have been in the first place the love of Adolf, whom she wished to buy for herself with this money. When I informed her that the business of the inheritance had been settled in a satisfactory way (the step-daughter behaved with remarkable generosity about it) it made a visibly tranquillising impression on the patient. In a few days she was able to be moved into a quieter division, and in the course of some weeks she came home much improved.

Meanwhile a new drama developed. After some quiet weeks the condition grew worse and the patient presented at home the picture of a heavy psychic depression. She took no interest in anything, would not go out, could not be induced to change her clothes, she was completely apathetic. In one point certainly she was still constantly interested : this was the expenditure again. She was always checking the accounts, and all household expenses had to be reduced in the most absurd way to suit her. She wanted to reduce her establishment, to send away the servant girl, to give notice to leave her home and so forth. In the meantime I gained her confidence, and one day I directly tackled the ticklish subject. I gave her to understand that I had seen through the psychic conflict. She broke into tears and confessed to me her great mental sufferings and her fears. Also she expressed remorse for not having fulfilled the last will of her departed husband and for having defrauded his daughter out of the inheritance. What should she do now to attain peace of mind ? I comfort her and recommended her to consult a barrister who was a relation of hers. He advised her to come to a private understanding with her daughter which should completely pacify her conscience. After completely regaining her health she might make her step-daughter heiress of the whole property ; i.e., after her death everything would come to the daughter, so that she would only have deprived her of the interest, which after all did not so much matter as the daughter was about to marry and was in any case well provided for. This suited her very well, she joyfully agreed to the proposal and the grave psychic condition improved in such striking fashion that she went out again, visited friends and made a few purchases. She increased in weight, and began to take an interest in things. Six weeks later, however, she again fell ill with nightly anxiety attacks and an internal unrest which tormented her to an extraordinary degree. She constantly accused herself of having committed grave sins. She was again incapable of making a decision, e.g., she had given notice to give up her home and was quite wretched about it. She ran to the landlord and besought him to cancel the notice[1]. When he promised this she regretted this in turn and informed the landlord that he might let the notice hold good. And this was repeated twenty times a day. She took apartments elsewhere and while she was moving in she gave notice to leave them. In short, she had to fight all day against her lack of will-power. Each time it was a mistake which she had made. Her condition again deteriorated. One day she threatened her old father, who had hastened to tend his child, with a great kitchen-knife. Occasionally, too, she would strike him violently so that she had again to be put into an observation room. Neighbours who were sorry for the old man had informed the police. But she dissimulated there so skilfully that no one would have suspected that she was suffering from a serious mental disturbance. At the entrance examination by the hospital physicians her father himself denied that she had threatened him

[1] She wished to cancel a sin. Evidently the wish for the death of her crippled husband.

with the knife, denied the blows, and declared that it had all been done as a joke so that she got out of the asylum again. Then I witnessed a tragic scene which at once made plain to me, the reason of the new attack. The daughter had married in the meantime and the son-in-law defrauded of part of her dowry, demanded of the mother-in-law that she should recognise in legal fashion the claims of his wife to her father's property. If anything should happen to her to-day, "and after all she was only mortal," the property would go to the State and the daughter would get nothing. At any rate she might consent to make a will. Of a will that should be valid in law there could be no question. But the patient had herself the day before expressed the wish to make a will—that would restore her peace of mind. I thought she should wait a bit till she was quite well. She insisted, however, on fulfilling her desire. Now I believe that it had all been arranged among the relatives and that it was only by chance that I was a witness of this scene. To my astonishment the patient now refused on account of her excited state to make a will and I was not a little surprised when the patient's grey-haired father jumped up and cried, "Who is my daughter's heir? The heir can only be the father and no other. I will suffer no new will. Here is a will; it makes me the sole heir." It was now clear why she had kept on striking him and why she had attacked him with the knife. She had purchased her peace of mind by resolving to bequeath to her daughter the illegally acquired property. But the father had induced her on the evening before to make a will in his favour or rather in favour of his three other daughters. This new psychic conflict was too much for her. The daughter at once broke off all relations with her, without going to law about the matter. The poor woman's condition became daily more and more grave. The anxiety attacks grew more frequent and one day it was found she had hanged herself from the cross-bars of the window.

Here we see how an anxiety neurosis and a melancholia develop on the basis of a Basedow.[1] It was an atypical melancholia. In fact, when the psychic conflict was first settled, this brought about a rapid cure. In the final conflict between her and her father I was powerless to intervene, all the more because the father looked askance on my visits and regarded me as an adherent of her stepdaughter. I should have exceeded my rights as physician if I had made the slightest attempt to influence her in favour of the daughter. Moreover her mental condition forbade her to execute a legally valid deed. The so-called will—a scrap of paper—she had torn

[1] Giran ("Zur Frage des myseödematösen Irresein") Communications from the Hamburg public hospitals, Vol. 7, Part 1) points out that in the case of adults, thyroid gland diseases are often hidden under the appearance of a psychosis accompanied by what looks like dementia (which is rather inhibition), hallucinations and imaginary persecutions, and that these yield to specific treatment with thryoidine tablets. Levi and Rotschild (Archiv de neurologie, 1907, No. 8, p. 141).

to pieces before her death. I believe that it was not only a bad conscience, and dread of the law and of legal proceedings which drove her to her death. In the first place it was the loss of her beloved for whose sake she had done everything. Later all that lost its value for her and she took refuge with her first love—the father. She dreaded the punishment of God and executed on herself the death sentence.

To those ignorant of the psychic roots of this disease this psychosis would be just as much a riddle as the delusion of paranoia or the stereotyped words of one sick of dementia præcox. As, however, Jung and Bleuler prove, here too the psychic roots of the disease can be demonstrated. I will not deny the constitutional components. In one case it was the slight Basedow. But only the exact knowledge of the psychogenesis secures us the complete understanding of the symptoms. The fear of not having enough money to live on corresponds in fact to that fear which drove her before the death of her husband to set aside part of the money so that it should escape the sharing. It was the inner motive of her crime, which, however, was only committed to capture Adolf. Further, the understanding of the money neurosis is facilitated for us by the circumstance *that money always symbolises guilt.*[1] *The patients fear guilt and express that through their dread of debts.*

The great suffering caused by the death of her husband was the reaction against her sinful wish when she was nursing him. " Oh, if he would die so that I alone might secure the money and marry Adolf." She threatened her father with the knife because he had incited her to the new conflict by persuading her to deprive the step-daughter of the money thus to make good or expiate a part of the sin. He compelled her to keep for her family the ill-gotten Rheingold to which clung a curse. Her incapacity to come to a decision arose simply from the doubt : " To whom shall I give the money, to the step-daughter or to the father ? " On this point she was undecided.

But she projected her indicision into all the other questions of life. She accused herself to all her friends and to her physician of having committed grave errors. That was the truth. Only the errors had been committed many years before. And through everything the erotic complex had permeated. It was her greatest dread that she would never be able to make any more conquests, and this showed itself repeatedly in the wish that she might marry if anyone would have a woman who had so disgraced herself.

Since the first edition of this book I have repeatedly had occasion to analyse in detail various cases of melancholia. Always, with more or less trouble, I was successful.in laying bare the psychogenic basis. To be sure, I constantly found also a deep religious tinge which caused the feelings of sin and guilt. The suicide which is so frequent in cases of melancholia is the punishment which the

[1] In German Schuld = guilt and also debt.

neurotic inflicts on himself. For this reason I find unjustified Freud's reproach which he makes in the discussion on suicide. According to my analyses the motive for suicide in melancholia is no longer a mystery. Here, too, holds good the secret principle of the talion. Freud considers that the emotional processes in melancholia, the fate of the libido in this connection, are completely unknown to us and that the permanent emotion of grief has not yet been made comprehensible psych-analytically (" Ueber den Selbstmord, insbesondere über den Schülerselbstmord." Discussions of the Vienna psycho-analytical Union, J. F. Bergmann, 1910). We have been able to see from the first records of patients that my utterances in this discussion (*no one kills himself who did not wish to kill another*) have solved the deep problem of suicide in melancholia. *What drives the patients to their death is guilt.*

In a very interesting article, "Trauer und Melancholie" (Int. Z. f. P.-A., Vol. IV., 1916-1918) Freud compares the two conditions, and says : " Grief is the loss of a beloved being, while melancholia represents *the loss of the capacity for love.*" The melancholic loses his capacity for love. That is correct. But we have seen that also melancholia is for the most part the reaction that follows on the loss of a beloved being. Of a being, it is true, that has been lost in life and through life not through the inexorable fate of death. Freud says that to the melancholic the object is " unconscious." For some cases that is true, but not for all. Just as little is Freud's contention generally valid, that the complaints of the melancholic are really accusations and are directed against some person in the entourage. All reproaches which they make against themselves should really go to another address. The essence of melancholia Freud sees in a regression of the libido to the ego. Hence would ensue an extraordinary impoverishment of the ego. " In grief the world has become poor, in melancholia the ego itself."

I must confess that I conceive melancholia only as hate-neurosis and guilt-neurosis. The anxiety of the melancholic is dread of himself, dread of killing another, dread of committing a crime. The avarice is the symbolic expression of avarice with love. The melancholic sees himself prejudiced in his love. The hatred enlisted by defiance dominates his ego. At the same time the unconscious has already in mad fashion done away with all pleasure in life.

The important researches of Herschmann and Schilder ("Träume der Melancholiker, nebst Bemerkungen zur Psychopathologie der Melancholie," Z. f. d.g. N. u P., Vol. III., 1920) which show that melancholics have remarkably many pleasurable and cheerful dreams give as result : " Our own material gives no decisive proofs for the hypothesis of Freud that the contradiction, the denial is directed against another person."

I should like to refer very briefly to some more cases.

No. 161.—A lady, forty-six years of age, falls ill of melancholia and has to be interned for a year in an institution on account of several attempts at suicide. The case was typical : ideas of sins committed, self-reproach, fits of anxiety, refusal of nourishment, sleeplessness, and the like. In the analysis, which proceeded smoothly enough, it came to light that the patient had fallen in love with the brother-in-law and had desired the death of her husband. The outbreak of melancholia was preceded by a severe inflammation of the lungs of the husband. His cure apparently did not correspond to her (unconscious) wishes. For in the prayer which she offered in thanks for the marvellous recovery of her husband, there happened to her a misfortune which she only confessed to me after a six weeks' analysis and then only with great resistance. At the end of the prayer she had the misfortune to let a flatus. Involuntarily there slipped from her the blasphemous words : " Tady mas " (Czech for " There Thou hast it "). This crime had oppressed her the whole time and she had not had the courage to make confession of it. On the contrary ! Although she is very pious, she had after this incident not trusted herself to go into the confessional chair for fear the priest might say to her that she had once for all wrecked her chances of salvation. In this case I played the part of analytical diplomatist. I applied to a priest of my acquaintance, Father Sch., a very humane, amiable gentleman, and told him the peculiar story. He caused the lady to come to confession and absolved her from the sin. After some months I received from her husband a letter which informed me that the improvement which had set in slowly had advanced rapidly and that the patient was again finding joy in life and in her household.

No. 162 shows us melancholia as preventive of the marriage of a passionately loved daughter. (Refuge in illness.) A woman well over sixty years, falls ill of melancholia in the midst of the preparations for the wedding of her remarkably beautiful daughter. The preparations are interrupted. No one may mention the wedding to the old lady. She always objects : " So long as I am so very ill, I have no head for the wedding and cannot bother myself about the preparations. The wedding must be put off till I am quite well." At night she can only lie quiet when the beloved child lies by her. She holds her like a vice and never lets her go for a moment. Describing the night the intelligent lady says : " I tell it you without any extenuation. I seize her wherever I can catch hold of her, behind or before. What I should like most of all would be to creep right into her." Here the unconscious strong homosexual love is felt as heavy guilt. She knows that she has selfishly ruined the life-happiness of her child. The engagement was broken off because the impatient bridegroom would not wait so long. Naturally the lady reproached herself that she had ruined the happiness of her daughter. The suicide of the bride-groom aggravated the illness to such an extent that attempt after attempt at suicide followed and the dear little old mother had to be interned. Some months later a stroke put an end to her life. Of course the question arises whether in this case the melancholia was not to be interpreted as a retrogressive phenomenon in consequence of arterio-sclerosis. But even admitting the participation of these organic factors, the psychogenic basis was so clear that it could not be left out of the reckoning.

This case shows us the importance of *homosexuality* in bringing about psychosis. The emotion of grief must also have a component in the circumstance that these impulses carry in themselves the stigma of hopelessness.[1]

It is Freud's great merit to have discovered this point of view for the psychology of the psychoses. His second paranoia publication, " Psychoanalytische Bemerkungen über einen autobiographisch beschriebenen Fall von Paranoia (Dementia paranoides) " in Vol. III. of the year book, is a landmark in the history of psychiatry.[2] For psycho-analytical investigation a new shaft has been sunk which promises the richest yield. The new researches will make plain to us the great importance of homosexuality for the life of the human soul.

A grateful task for psycho-therapists is presented by the cyclic depressions which for the most part start from the basis of fear-hysterio. Here occur forms representing the transition stages to typical cyclothvmio. After periods of more cheerful mood come severe depressions in which the patient withdraws from all the world and struggles against suicidal impulses. This trouble is much more frequent with women than with men and is amenable to psycho-therapy. Generally at the beginning of the treatment a severe depression breaks out. The results are various. A few cases prove to be incurable in spite of the treatment. This is connected with the nature of the disease. Every depression represents mourning for one's own chastity and the answer to a sexual renunciation. We have mostly to do with highly erotic people to whom their passionate desires are not known. Psychoanalyses can here, according to Freud's apt expression, only convert hysterical misery into ordinary misery. My greatest success was with an author who after having had brought into consciousness

[1] I have brought together my latest experiences in the article " Depressionen : ihr Wesen und ihre Behandlung " (Therapy of the present day, 1920). This article was included in the second edition of Vol. II. (Appendix). I mention there the importance of homosexuality in the psychogenesis of the depressions. Also in cases 150 and 151 I see retrospectively that I quite overlooked the homosexual components (in the first case love of the daughter ; in the second, of the step-daughter).

[2] Already there are confirmations of this, all of which have been published in the *Centralblatt für Psychoanalyse*. This the work of Ferenczi, " Pathogenesis of paranoia " (I. Vol.) and the work of Morechan-Beauchant (Poitiers) " Homosexuality and paranoia " (Vol. II., Section IV.).

his sexual and criminal phantasies and after the bringing to light of infantile dreams has been for three years in almost perfect health " But for little inconsiderable morbid moods," he writes, " moods such as a normal person might have, I feel perfectly well."

On the other hand, with women I have already had some ill-success which, however, may be due in part to the defective technique. The transference manifests in these patients an incredible strength and almost degenerates to passion if not at once and energetically counteracted. With these women any advance of a friendly nature is dangerous because they mistake it for love ; and therefore the greatest strictness seems to me to be called for.

That various other forms of the psychoses may be affected psychanalytically is becoming more and more certain in the light of numerous researches. Dipsomania is only a special form of cyclothymia. The criminal impulses are reduced to silence by drinking, whereby in certain cases that happens which was to have been avoided : the crime.

For this psychosis also the beautiful words of Jung hold good : " To the feeble and sensitive soul of the patient the problem seems insoluble,[1] hence the emotion waxes insuperable ; thus from the psychological side the mental illness appears to us. The series of apparently senseless incidents, of so-called lunatic tricks has suddenly acquired a meaning ; *we understand the sense in the senselessness* and thus the mental patient seems nearer and more human to us. He is a human being who suffers as we do from the human problems common to all and he is not a brain machine that has fallen into disorder. Formerly we believed that the mentally afflicted showed us in his symptoms nothing more than the senseless abortions of his sick brain-cells. That was pedantry, reeking of the midnight oil. But when we feel our way into the human secrets of the sick man then even his lunacy reveals its system and we recognise in the mental disease simply an unusual reaction to emotional problems in which there is nothing strange to us."

All the observations which I have mentioned show on analysis the logical psychic motive. One may perhaps doubt the diagnosis " melancholia," and think rather of a hysterical mental disease. Names are noise and smoke (Goethe Faust). And who knows whether the future may not astonish us by showing that melancholy is only a variety of a parapathia.[2]

[1] " Der Inhalt der Psychosen." (Schriften zur angewandten Seelenkunde. Deuticke, 1908).

[2] Further publications on this subject are : Jones, " Psychoanalytic Notes on a case of hypomania." Americ, Journal of Insanity, October, 1909, *p.* 203 ; Maeder, " Psychoanalyse bei einer melancholischen Depression," Centralblatt für Nervenheilkunde and Psychiatrie, No. 302, Part 2, 1910. Brill, " Ein Fall periodischer Depression psychogenen Ursprungs," Centralblatt für Psychoanalyse, Vol. I., part 4, *p.* 158, 1911. Stockmayer, " Zur psychol. Analyse der Dementia præcox," Centralblatt für Nervenkrankheiten, 1909, October. Schwarzwald, " Ueber hysterische Dämmerzustände," Journal für Psychologie and Psychiatrie, 1910 (Brodmann). Nelken, " Analytische Beobach-

Is it not strange ? The crimes of the patients who suffered from anxiety hysteria were not committed. The bad thoughts remained fettered monsters of the underworld. The two melancholic women, whose fate occupied us at first, burdened their conscience with heavy guilt. Does the leap from the repressed thought to the sinful deed open for us the chasm which divides the neurotic from psychosis ? Or does the neurotic take refuge in psychosis to escape the deed and insure through insanity the impunity of his forbidden wishes ?[1]

The path of the psychiatry of the future must travel is clearly indicated : it leads into the wonderland of the human soul. The key that opens this wonderland is psychology.

tungen über Phantasien eines Schizophrenen " (Jahrbuch, IV. Vol., 1912). Grebelskaja, " Psychologische Analyse eines Paranoiden " (*ibid.*). Landaner, " Spontanheilung eines Katatomie " (Int. z. f. P.A., 1914). K. Tausk, " Ueber die Entstehung des Beeinflussungs-apparates in der Schizophrenie " (Int. z. f., P.A., 1919). Pötzl, " Ueber einige Wechselwirkungen hysterie-former und organisch-zerebrall Hörungsmechanismen " (Jahrbuch f. Psych. u. Neur., 1917). Schilder, " Wahn und Erkenntnis " (Berlin, 1918). Nunberg, ' Ueber den Ratatonischen Anfall " (Int. z. f., P.A., 1920).

[1] To the somatic prevention consisting in a disproportion between the skull contents and the skull which has been rendered incapable of expanding by the complete growing together of the sagittal suture, I have referred in my pamphlet, " Poetry and neurosis," *p.* 11 " Dichtung und Neurose (Grenzfragen des Nerven und Seelenslebens,",J. F. Bergmann, 1909.) In this paper I proposed for the first time to name nervous disturbances " parapathia " in contrast to the psychoses which should be called " paralogia." At the same time I am aware that in the case of the psychoses also the disturbances of the emotional life are the primary thing. But in addition to the disturbance of the emotionalism there is the disturbance of the intellect, the " paralogia."

THIRD PART

GENERAL

CHAPTER XXXIV

GENERAL PSYCHOLOGY OF FEAR

FEAR is the will to immortality. Cowardice perhaps only the striving for immortality. The immortal is the infinite. The infinite, however, is for us the inconceivable. And every thing that is inconceivable is a source of fear. *Fear[1] is the expectation of a displeasure.* In the widest sense! In the narrowest sense, fear is aversion to death. Every fear is fear of death. It is true there are persons who do not fear death and who even long for it and seek it. Either these persons have the hope for an eternal life, that is for immortality or they defy the higher powers and throw away a life whose limit seems to them frightfully short in contrast with the infinity of creation. They are the " proud sons of the Gods " (Vischer) who will not accept anything as a gift.

Fear is the expectation of the unknown. We fear only what is new. What has become familiar to us loses the capacity to produce fear. *Death, too, is to us the absolutely new and unknown.* For one should be able to die but once. To be sure there are neurotics who die every day or at least play at dying.

Man endures everything, but not the unknown whose characteristic symbol is the dark. Faith fulfils a great mission by setting up a positive affirmation in place of the great question mark. *Religion is the symbolised mastery of the unknown.* God descending to the children of men becomes human. " Mekadö, the Lord of the earth, descends for the sixth time, that he may become like unto us, and feel with us pleasure and pain." The thundering God of the Greeks, Jupiter, also became a man and showed human weakness. In this way the Greek religion lost a great part of the feelings of fear.

The God of the Jews was the abstract unknown. It was forbidden to make oneself an image of this God. He was the God of

---

[1] In the first chapter I have already set forth the psychologic differences between fear and anxiety.

wrath and of punishment, and was feared. In the Book of Job there is a significant passage which lays bare the root of this fear : " Because I saw faces in the night, when sleep falls upon the people, there came fear and trembling upon me and all my bones were afraid. And as the spirit passed before me the hairs stood on end on my body ; there stood an image before my eyes and *I knew not his form ;* it was still and I heard a voice : How may a man be more just than God ? or a man purer than He Who made him ? " (Job iv, 13 to 17.)

Here the relation is clearly expressed. Job does not know the form and he trembles. The God who is known is already a human being, who only after his death, that is to a generation to which he is unknown, can become a God. Only the unknown are pronounced holy.

It was a wonderful thought to give men a religion of love. Only a God could do that who was known to men and mingled with them. A man who became god ; a martyr whose image spoke of human sufferings. But this new religion also could not dispense with fear. It compelled love *through fear of hell*, which again is only an " unknown."

Lombroso maintained that all men suffer from fear of the new, that is, the unknown. He called this phenomenon " *neophobia.*" This discovery collapses if fear is already fear of the unknown. Then one may say more simply : *All men suffer from fear.*

This is an insurmountable fact. Fear accompanies us all through life and lies hidden within us. The brave man hides it more cleverly and often from himself also, which is the most difficult, the fearful man lets it be openly seen. " Fear is the prolongation of life," says Leonardo da Vinci. Fear is really only the longing for its prolongation.

Fear can never exist by itself alone. Indeed all phenomena of the soul appear *bipolar.* What is the counterpart of fear ? Möbuis calls fear the most important manifestation of the self-preservation instinct. The opposite is, however, the desire for annihilation, the death impulse or the longing for death. The more important is the sex instinct, perhaps the power which will exert itself to insure the immortality of the species if one wishes to think teleologically.[1] *Fear, dread of destruction, and the sex instinct, the longing for creation cannot be separated. Both appear in company with the death impulse. Dying and living are equivalent factors in the great symbolic equation of the infinite.*

There can be, then, no anxiety which does not tell of life, and no expression of life which is not accompanied by anxiety. Pleasure can become anxiety and anxiety pleasure. Fear of pleasure resembles the wish for pleasure. And the death-impulses may culminate in an act which is called suicide and really represents the last sexual act, the last expression of an instinct which embraces equally death and life.

[1] Schopenhauer.

Having thus discussed the question of the fundamental conceptions of fear we will consider the different stages and varieties of fear. *Distrust* and *care* represent the first stage of these displeasure feelings. Both are displeasure feelings related to something unknown. I worry about a future whose consequences are unknown to me. Whether it is a question of blame, shame or poverty, in the background lurks fear for existence.[1] *Distrust* has to do with phenomena which are unknown to us. A boy of my acquaintance said to a gentleman who spoke to him in the street : " How do I know that you are no robber ? " The same is true of shyness. One loses shyness when one becomes acquainted. Uneasiness and anxiety express half conscious " objectless " feelings of fear and also occur when we are confronted with unknown incidents and results. The uncanny is the rendering objective of the strange and unknown. As a child with its mother we feel at home. A new person is always sinister to the child.

E. Jentsch, to whom we are indebted for the first study of the uncanny, emphasises two points : The uncanny regresses to the well-known, the long trusted and it is always something with which one is not familiar so that it seems to arise from an intellectual uncertainty. With his accustomed ingenuity Freud[2] investigates these opposites (the old and the new) and attempts by means of psychanalysis a deeper explanation. The investigation of language shows at once the double sense of the word " heimlich " (homely) in almost all languages. Now Freud shows in connection with a tale by E. T. A. Hoffmann, " The sand man " that esentially it is a question of the " castration-complex." The uncanny person is the father who seeks to take vengeance, or threatens with castration. More generally : The uncanny is experienced when repressed infantile complexes are revived through an impression or when primitive beliefs which we have outgrown again appear to be confirmed.

I must confess that Freud's ingenious arguments, convincing as they appear for the example chosen, have not convinced me of their general validity. The uncanny is a preliminary stage to a feeling of anxiety. The uncanny arouses in us a timid feeling as if there existed a danger for our life and our ego. Our ego can maintain itself only in a world which it understands and finds natural. To the simple person a bright form at night will seem uncanny because it reminds him of a ghost and the ghost seems to be beyond the bounds of his existence. Let me now illustrate the feeling of the uncanny by two examples. In the cool of a summer night we are walking home by moonlight. Suddenly everyone halts. Near the churchyard wall stands a long pale form like a shadow. The women feel it " run cold down the back," they shriek and refuse to go on. Some of the men, too, lose courage. I go up to the spectre and find that the shadow of a figure has been so projected on the wall as to give rise to the impression described. General laughter changed the uncanny and incomprehensible into the natural and matter of course. In vain may we seek for a castration-complex. It is true we encounter the infantile belief in the marvellous, supernatural and magical. (Are there then ghosts ?

[1] Hoche (" Pathologie und Therapie der Nervosen Angstzustände." Verhandlungen der Gesellschaft deutscher Nervenärzte. Leipzig, C. W. Vogel, 1911), who otherwise stands utterly without any solution in face of the whole problem of fear (like all investigators who do not wish to know and to recognise Freud) states : " To my taste in language, worry would have to stand in some degree as a lasting form of fear, having to do on the whole with the further future, quantitatively perhaps weaker, often with specific allied sensations, such as are denoted, e.g., by the expression " gnawing worry."

[2] Imago, 1919.

Is there a world beyond this visible world ?) The spectre is always an ambassador from the kingdom of death, and causes the shudder of the fear of death. The women all felt only fear. I, the sceptical and enlightened one, had a feeling of the uncanny. But I must mention that as a child I would go home alone from my friends' house although the way led past a churchyard, because I never had any dread of ghosts.

Yet more remarkable was another experience. We were sailing on a beautiful August day into a Norwegian fiord. The scene was framed by high steep rocks whence clear waterfalls plunged into the deep. The little vessel ploughed its way through the green water. Then happened the marvel. Did I dream or was I awake ? A little boat, like a toy, so insignificant, steered towards us. In the boat rowed a being that seemed as big as a Hop-o'-my-thumb. This lasted some minutes. The toy skiff came nearer and only quite close to the ship could I realise that it was a normal boat and a quite ordinary human being. It was an optical delusion brought about by the disproportion between the gigantic rocks which being so near to them I had under-estimated and the little man. I confess that I felt something uncanny. Why ? Because during some seconds the world of wonder and legend had opened to me. In this sense Freud may be right. But here, too, the inexplicable and marvellous were the uncanny. Therefore I should rather agree with Jentsch's explanation. Analysis will perhaps discover new bases of the uncanny. They will be in essence the bases of every anxiety.

I had a dog which for the first few days was in great fear of me. I was strange to him. He never came up to me except crawling. Soon he learned to like me, had thrown off all fear and was very trustful. One day he was lying on the ground when I went to the piano and for the first time began to play before the dog. I have never seen such another remarkable sight. First he put his head very much on one side, opened his eyes wide and suddenly ran from the room with a mournful howl. The noise was " uncanny " to him. Later he preferred to lie under the piano when I played and accompanied all passages in E-major with a remarkable singing.

Here we have yet to mention *respect*, which besides fear expresses social differentiation and recognition of superiority. Persons who are inclined to blasphemous behaviour (hatred of the authorities, libelling royalty, slandering God) suffer from overwhelming feelings of reverence. The blasphemous behaviour represents a reaction and an attempt to free oneself from the tyranny of respect. That *disgust represents fear of a contact* I have shown in detail in Chapter IX. *Shame*, according to Havelock Ellis ("Die biologische Bedeutung des Schamgefühls." Stuber, Würzburg) is made up of two components of which one represents an inherited repellent attitude of the female except in periods of heat, the other fear, disgust and repugnance to excitement. I consider this view as artificial and *see in shame fear of sexual excitement and its consequences.*

Shame is often sexual excitement itself expressed in a negative form and as inhibitory feeling against sexuality is highly valued. The more shame and disgust the man has to overcome the greater is his triumph and his libido. By the magnitude of the shame she has overcome and the disgust she has conquered the woman measures the magnitude of her love. (How I love thee if I do all this for thee!) I will not dispute that fear of seeming contemptible to the man is one of the weightiest of the woman's inhibitions. But this phenomenon occurs with girls and women who are free from shame itself. Shame is the confession of sexual excitement and fear of unknown sex processes. That is, again, fear of the unknown. When women know a man well they lose shame in intimate intercourse and maintain only so much of it as they require to satisfy their internal and external need for respect.

Awe is fear of unknown higher powers, of unknown phenomena exceeding the limits of the finite. Shuddering is the foreboding of the infinite ; horror a heightening of the shudder through the threatened annihilation of life. While *fear* is the chronic state, terror, fright, horror, abhorrence, dread, represent acute fear of annihilation, remembering that abhorrence is not fear but is to be classed with the disgust feelings and betrays the strongest negative erotic mood.

Cowardice and *lack of courage* are results of an over-estimate of life and its finite phenomena. They may also betray the tendency to prolong the finite in order to escape the problematic infinite and a possible testing.

The normal readiness to fear of every human being may rise to "anxious expectation." This "anxious expectation" is really only the increase of the self-preservation instinct in presence of the threatened danger. The soldier, e.g., finds himself when in the field of battle in a state of anxious expectation. The latent readiness to fear becomes manifest and expresses itself in heightened excitability and irritability.

Seif ("Zur Psychopathologie der Angst." Int. Z. f. ärztl. P. A., Vol. I., 1913) describes anxiety expectation as follows : "What strikes one at first among the psychic phenomena is the enormous prominence of the emotional factor ; a mixture of discomfort, displeasure, unrest, embarrassment, tension uneasiness and uncertainty, an increasing and ever more dominating feeling as if something fearful and terrible, horrible must happen, as though a dark unearthly danger threatened, as though one were losing one's reason, one's consciousness, one's self-control, as though one were falling a prey to madness or to sudden death. The characteristic is the feeling of expectation of an unknown something, dark, vague, threatening. The process of thought is either accelerated or slowed down ; we have all stages from the most frantic rush of thoughts to perplexity and incapacity to think at all. The faculty of observation is more or less strongly lowered."

This perplexity results from the affect. I call it "affective imbecility."

There is no human being who may not be entirely filled with fear. In cases of sudden fright one sees what great fear can be set in motion with incredible power. The affect of fear is infectious. But it can only be so because we all *live prepared to fear*. Panic, panic fright, is the sudden letting loose of these fear-feelings. It is self-evident that such immense emotional masses must destroy the equilibrium of the soul and rob the individual of his reason. This every affect does: anger as well as envy; jealousy as well as love. But fear awakens all the instinct of self-preservation. Fear is indeed the most important expression of the instinct of self-preservation.

In contrast to the other fear-phenomena the psychology of panic is fairly evident. We have to do with a mass reaction based on the rapid transference of a latent affect. This affect is the readiness of people to fear expressing itself in shrinking together and in the flight-reflex. Anyone may experience this readiness to fear himself when the pneumatic tyre of a motor car bursts in the street with a loud explosion. The crowd is ever ready to yield to the atavistic instincts. In the crowd the individual soul-life succumbs uniting itself with the mass-soul. The mass easily falls to the level of the lowest; it exalts itself with great difficulty to the highest. The reactions of the mass are infantile, it behaves like a child, it lets itself go, overcomes all inhibitions; it follows the primitive instincts and primitive reactions of mankind. In panic the self-preservation instinct of men expresses itself, and fear must be regarded as its most primitive expression. The reactions mostly lack all meaning. That condition sets in which I have called "affective imbecility." Panic is a mass parapathia. The reactions are mostly senseless (running away, throwing oneself on the ground, shrieking, crushing together, running over each other, rough treatment of one's fellows who may be in the way, and so forth). All ethical, moral, religious and social inhibitions vanish.

There is then no state in which man is free from fear. Freud says that phobia with its limitations and precautions makes the patient at last free from fear. I will give his views in the words of Hitschmann, whose little book, " Freud's Neurosenlehre " (Leipzig and Vienna. Franz Deuticke, 1911) gives the real views of Freud better than this work which in many respects deviates from the great master: " In anxiety-hysteria there is from the beginning onwards a continuous psychic effort to put in psychic bonds the anxiety that has been set free, but this effort can neither effect the reconversion of the anxiety into libido nor link up with the same complexes from which the libido arises. There is then nothing left for this effort to do but to block each of the possible occasions for anxiety by ' a psychic screen ' in the nature of a precaution, an inhibition, a veto; and it is these protective structures which appear to us as phobias, and so far as we can see make up the essence of the disease. The nature of this inhibition whether it is a derangement of the gait or of the oral zone (impediment in eating or speaking) etc., will depend upon the constitutionally emphasised and erogenously aggravated organic function wherein the anxiety may concentrate.

The anxiety becomes a phobia when it, so to speak, crystallises in a definite complex."
But has the patient really become free from anxiety through the phobia (in the sense of Freud and Hitschmann)? *No! he has only converted the manifest anxiety into a hidden anxiety. He stands in constant readiness for anxiety.* The anxiety starts at the least occasion. In fact he thinks of his anxiety all day and constantly produces it in small quantities. *A phobic never becomes anxiety-free.* His dreams betray how grievously he is continually suffering from the development of his anxiety.

To be sure, he avoids all possible causes for fear. He becomes a reactionary and dreads all change. He abandons all aggression —which really means the conquest of the new—and falls back on the old and trusted, on his youth.

I have already shown that all of us fear only the new. Lombroso calls this " misoneismus," and thinks that only geniuses, fools and criminals love the new, are " neophils." *Misoneismus* shows itself, according to Lombroso, in customs, laws, institutions and languages. Now this is certainly a very one-sided point of view. For customs alter, laws are repealed, and language undergoes constant change. Lombroso has disregarded the bipolarity of all phenomena. All mental phenomena have a two-fold aspect. Corresponding to the *" dread of the new "* which certainly plays an important part in human life, there is a " passion for the new " which everyone has, and which we may also call hunger for sensation and need of change. In reality this passion for the new is the greatest power in human life. We crave variety. Joy makes us long for pain. " A god may enjoy himself thus, but I am subject to change," sings Tannhäuser. We are all subject to change, and we should always strive only for change if fear of the unknown *new* did not restrain us.

From this standpoint fear is seen to be an essential part of our mental equilibrium. It is true that genius seeks and finds the new. But the average man would also gladly find and seek it and many a genius suffers from dread of the new and achieves his great conquests only because this fear is more than counter-balanced by an almost morbid joy in creating the new. And so the geniuses love to shut themselves off from the world and to pass their days in the midst of old familiar sensations. Shall I here call to mind Grillparzer, who distinguished himself by strong conservatism. Even Gœthe knew these moods when he was disinclined for anything new. Mörike says in a letter : " In my present state it is a really painful feature that everything new, even the smallest, most trivial thing that comes to me from without, even a person not well known to me, if he only approaches me for a moment, throws me into the most frightful, the most anxious state of uneasiness and worries me."

Stanley Hall, an American psychologist, has attempted to solve the problem of fear by a great mass-investigation. His " Study of fears " (1896), has been made accessible to the German public in the "Ausgewählte Beiträge zur Kinderpsychologie und Pädagogik " (published by Oskar Bonde, Altenburg, 1902) in the translation of Josef Stimpfl. The questionnaire was answered by 1,701 persons who described 6,456 objects of fear. Of these people the majority feared "heavenly phenomena " ; thus 603 thunder and lightning ; 143 storm, etc. ; 532 darkness ; only 203 ghosts ; 483 reptiles (i.e., snakes !) ; 365 fire. Further : 436 feared strangers ; 153 robbers, and only 299 death and 241 diseases. Besides these there was a number of special objects of fear which we cannot discuss, because they are accessible only to a psycho-analytical interpretation. From our investigations we know, of course, that in most people fear is symbolically expressed. We have investigated in detail all that may be hidden behind the symbols. But Stanley Hall's questionnaire has been answered by normal persons also. It can therefore give us correct information.

Stanley Hall sees in all these phenomena inherited instincts of self-preservation.[1] Fear of the water, of violent winds, of heights and of falling, are based on the instructive vestiges of the mind which are derived from the time when our forefathers lived on the sea and were exposed to its storms. The fear of hairy animals goes back to the time (he says) when we had daily to fight such animals. As proof that the fear would otherwise be motiveless, Stanley Hall says : " Night is now the safest time, snakes have long ceased to be among our worst enemies ; strangers are not dangerous ; the fear of heavenly phenomena befits the heaven of ancient superstition, but not the heaven of modern science." Here Stanley Hall appears to be unaware that many objects of fear are only symbols. And these symbols are known to us : the snake is the symbol of sin, the wild animal of a passion. And yet in a certain sense Stanley Hall is right. *The kernel of truth in his doctrine is the fact that fear is in part inherited.* It is, of course, unthinkable that fear should not be inherited through the flight of ages. Millions of years of fear certainly do not remain without influence on the brain. And I believe, indeed, that one kind of fear alone is propagated

[1] Hatschek ("Zur vergleichenden Psychologie des Angstaffektes." Verhandlungen der Gesellschaft deutscher Nervenärzte. F. C. W. Vogel, Leipzig, 1911) is of the same opinion : "We must then adhere to the view that the fear-emotion is based on the primitive instincts of flight and defence inherited through countless ages. The vaso-motor, visceral and muscular reactions, originally very purposeful and useful are caused by external stimuli and it is simply the perception of these reflex manifestations which constitutes the anxiety affect." This is supposed to lend new support to the familiar theory of James and Lange which was thought to have been refuted. The somatic phenomena of the affect called forth the anxiety. Anyone who has read this book carefully can see in numerous examples how an "amoral" idea, a sexual emotion rejected by the consciousness has caused an anxiety anxiety. The *first thing* is always an idea, the affect of anxiety is a reaction caused by this idea.

and this is the fear of God and His punishment. Thousands of years of faith cannot be overcome by intellectual force alone. *We cannot break the threads that bind us to the past.* Though invisible they endure and their hold on us is stronger than we think. Stanley Hall's questionnaire seems to me so valuable because it really confirms the fact that people fear the punishment of God.[1] There is, perhaps, no other psychic fear whatever. To prove this will indeed be my task.

From numerous analyses I have found that every one who suffers from fear of thunderstorms, fears the punishment of God. The 996 objects of fear which Hall describes as " heavenly phenomena " betray even by their names fear of the divine power. Let us not forget (besides the vast prehistoric past which manifests itself as instinct, i.e., an unconscious memory) the historic past of the man, his childhood. Then we heard wonderful stories, how God blasted the wicked with His lightning, how a rain of sulphur destroyed a sinful town and a flood annihilated every one but Noah. The 203 persons who feared ghosts feared supernatural phenomena. *Superstition is only a degenerate faith.* Often only a disguised faith. To fear ghosts means to fear God and to believe in the supernatural. Darkness, too, is the domain of the supernatural. In the night appear the messengers of good and evil. In the night awake the evil thoughts that one fears. Why do ordinary persons fear sin and crime ? Only on account of the punishment of God. Morality for its own sake, the ethos of noble minds exists only in rare exceptions. If we consider the details given by those who answered the questions, we are certainly struck by the religious symbolism, as well as by the more or less plainly erotic. No. 32 fears falling through the cracks in the earth left by the drying up of puddles.[2] In another form this fear is not at all rare. It is based on the

[1] It may seem to be contradictory that in this book I have always described anxiety as the fear of oneself. A closer examination will show that this contradiction is only apparent. An official e.g., is afraid of fire-arms and will not buy himself a sabre or revolver for fear he might " accidentally " shoot his wife or child. The analysis shows that the man is full of unconscious notions of shooting his wife and the children in order to marry his parlour-maid. This patient feared himself. He will have no weapon in order that he may not fall into temptation. He has an obscure intuition that accidental deeds execute the commands of the unconscious. He fears with justice that he might suddenly execute such a command. But why does he fear himself ? Why does he not shoot his wife ? The answer is simple : his moral ego opposes it. But if we analyse further we find that the Simplizissimus is justified when it declares : " Morality is the fear of what may happen to us." He fears the earthly judge, he fears the Heavenly Judge. He must be an uncommonly exalted mortal if he fears only " the God within his own breast." Noble human beings are the few who do good for the sake of good. These negligible exceptions apart, one may safely admit that all fear of oneself really conceals fear of the punishment of God.

[2] The sexual significance is too clear. But it seems very probable that all sexual symbols have religious meanings and vice versa. Cf. Jung's paper : " Conversions and symbols of the libido " (Jahrbuch, Vol. III., 1911 and 1912).

[3] Simplizissimus is a German comic paper. Tr.

unconscious idea that the earth may open and swallow the wicked sinner. So Korah and his troop were swallowed by the open mouth of the earth because they did not believe in Moses. The fear of falling symbolises—as we already know—the fall into sin, which plays so great a part in the Bible. Representations of the fall of the evil spirits into a horrible abyss contribute to fix the picture in the child's mind. Similarly the fear of snakes receives a religious colouring from the Bible. The snake is a symbol of sin. The fear of losing oneself, again, is derived from the fear of departing from the right way and wandering in the path of sin. The fear of being shut in always betrays (besides a womb-fancy which is also present) the criminal basis and the fear of judgment which hides the ideas of the heavenly judgment and the last judgment when the good shall be divided from the wicked. Fear of the water is derived, apart from its enuretic basis from the Flood. Only the neurotic who has desired the death of another by drowning falls ill with this fear. One of my patients fell ill of water-fear after his hated father had made a long sea voyage. Suddenly he who had always been a splendid swimmer, could not trust himself in the water. Of course, behind the retribution, the Talion, there was a retributive power (" With what measure thou measurest, it shall be measured unto thee again. An eye for an eye, a tooth for a tooth). Some examples from Stanley Hall show plainly the religious motivation. No. 28 imagines that she must drown when there is heavy rain, and often when there is thick fog (the Flood). No. 19, five girls fear violent downpours of rain which lead to a general flood. The fear of storms, too, shows the same basis. One fears that the wind will blow an acquaintance away ; another thinks of storms at sea. A third believes and fears at times that the wind will sweep the earth flat, so that the inmost forces of nature will break forth and everything will be thrown into chaos.[1] The fourth thinks the wind is the wrath of God ; the stronger blows the wind, the greater is the wrath of God.

In the fear of heavenly objects the questionnaire shows an abundance of religious pictures. The clouds form themselves into frightful pictures of savage men, beasts of prey and mythological monsters. Thus in the heavens themselves is waged the war between religion and eroticism. There is also an eruption of religion unadulterated : So. No. 11.—Since she heard of the flood, she cried at every violent rainfall, because she believed the world would come to an end. No. 12 sees the crucifixion in the clouds. No. 15, heavenly triumphal cars. No. 17 takes the most beautiful cloud to be the garment of God. No. 23 is overwhelmed by the feeling of his own nothingness and the omnipotence of God. He does not pray because he thinks himself too insignificant to be noticed by God. Two children think the rain is tears of heavenly

[1] I would again remark that all these phenomena are determined in several ways. She fears the breaking forth of her inner nature.

spirits who have been naughty, and fear punishment, another fears horrible signs of the zodiac.

Fear of fire is also permeated with religious motives (Sodom and Gomorrah). One lady believes that every fire-alarm means the beginning of the end of the world. No. 13, when she was alone, was afraid even by day of the flaming sword of the angel who was represented in the Bible as guardian of paradise. (Very fine fusion of an erotic and a religious symbol.) No. 15 was always thinking how frightful the tortures of hell-fire would be.

The realm of the supernatural begins in the dark. Hands appear which symbolise the hand of God ; awful dream-faces affright the poor patients, fear of ghosts infects even the enlightened. Fear of ghosts is stronger than ever at the present time and expresses itself as spiritualism in which reasonable people can only believe because they must believe something. And a storm by night lets loose every fear to which the soul is subject. God the Father thunders and demands the reckoning for all sins.

The " devil," too, still plays a great part. We must have the courage to look the truth in the face and admit that men are more pious than they themselves know.[1] They are ashamed of their piety because they feel it to be something foreign to them and something the intellect cannot grasp. But the power of the inherited fear-instincts overcomes the intellectual. Then comes the fact that we train our children to be fearful. We do not train them with love but with fear, which is certainly more convenient. Fear is, of course, the foundation of the social system. Training to and through fear begins in the earliest years of childhood.[2]

[1] Fear of the devil is fear of sin. Since this anxiety, as I have shown, corresponds to an inward craving and really expresses the wish for the devil, we can understand that the devil plays the chief rôle in the erotic fancies of the Middle Ages. He it was who at midnight sought out the terrified nuns and raped them. In Boccacio's novels the phallus is expressly called the devil, and a priest who wishes to seduce a young girl sends the devil to hell as a punishment. He calls the vagina hell. What wonder that the girl wanted to punish the devil every day ! We shall understand, however, that the pleasure which is linked with the pain, only corresponds to the repressed wish. There is no somatic conversion of anxiety into pleasures. Anxiety is the longing for pleasure and as representative of this longing may become pleasure.

[2] Hattingberg (" Analerotik, Angstlust und Eigensinn," Z. f. ärztl. psychoanalyse, Vol. II., *p.* 145, 1914) proposes to distinguish sharply between pleasurable-anxiety and masochism and gives a number of examples of anxiety heightening libido and bringing about an orgasm. In many cases of pleasurable-anxiety he was able to demonstrate a pronounced anal and urethral eroticism in Sadger's sense, so that he thought there must be a co-operation of constitutional and psycho forces. Pleasurable-anxiety he holds to be a mixed emotion. In children inclined to pleasurable-anxiety there was an over-excitability of the sympathetic, increased mechanical excitability without simultaneous spasmophilism. According to my experience this co-operation only holds for certain cases and perhaps represents that often mis-used constitutional predisposition which Freud is so fond of emphasising when he reaches the borderland of the psychic. The experiences of the world war have shown us how enormously widespread is this constitutional pre-disposition to neurosis and in fact that it may be left out of account.

Leo Hirschlaff remarks in his paper, " Ueber die Furcht der Kinder " (Zeitschrift für pädagogische Psychologie, 1901 and 1902) :— " Experiences and horrors communicated in stories and readings contribute far more to the creation of fear than those actually encountered." Mosso says truly :—" He who trains a child is responsible for its brain. Everything ugly that he says to him, the bitter words, the pictures of horror, are so many splinters which he leaves in the child's flesh and which cause it life-long injuries. Mother, nurse, maid-servant and man-servant should no longer try which of them can most terrify the growing children with the beloved bogies, were-wolves, scare-crows, magicians, black men, with legends of witches and evil spirits and countless other things. That this fetishism of fear, that is the custom of filling children's fancy with fear-images by means of nursery tales, horrible stories (e.g., of hell and the devil) and preposterous reading (back-stairs romances and penny dreadfuls) is one of the most important causes of fear, is shown by a table of Scott's on the origin of the fear of death in which are mentioned, as the first rubric, the tales one has heard, newspapers, the Bible, etc."

Freud says that every child would hear of such stories and yet they have a lasting effect only on neurotics and make no impression on the healthy child. That is certainly a weighty objection. But precisely because the neurotic child is very sensitive to these tales it must be protected from them and given courage and enlightenment. As a little boy I went home alone in the black night ; and I liked playing in the churchyard. But then my mother always told me : " There are no spirits ; there is no devil. Bad men are devils. See that you become a good man ! "

How greatly are children sinned against in this respect ! If the child falls and bruises itself that is " God's punishment," because it has romped about too wildly. If it has done anything mischievous, it is told that God sees and notes everything. The devil is also utilised for educational purposes. The grampus with a huge birch appears to the naughty child. I would instance also the patient's history on page 232 which shows us how the ineptitude of a minister throws a child into the gravest conflicts. How helpful it would be for ministers of religion if they would avail themselves of the lessons of psychanalysis.[1]

It is important to know whence comes the exaggerated devoutness of the neurotic. I have my own views as to this.

To me it is clear that the neurotic, like the artist and the criminal,

[1] I would refer here to the excellent writings of Rev. Dr. Pfister, of Zürich, one of the foremost advocates of psychanalysis. Especially worthy of mention are " Psychoanalytische Unterschungen über die Psychologie des Hasses " (Jahrbuch f. ps. F. Vol. II.) and " Die Frommigkeit des Grafen von Zinzendorf " and " Wahrheit und Schönheit in der Psychanalyse " (1919, Rascher & Cie, Zürich). Further, the great work " Psychoanalytical method " (Leipzig, 1913). A collection of his scattered works is given in the latest book, " Zum Kampfe um die Psychanalyse " (Vienna, Leipzig, Zürich, 1920).

is a "retrogression phenomenon." But I do not conceive this to be "degeneration." With more justification we may speak of "regeneration." If humanity wishes to create something great, it must ever plunge deep into the reservoir of the past. There result then persons with strong impulses, and if they must and can live according to these impulses they become asocial criminals. Lombroso has pointed out that the criminal shows striking recklessness and equanimity in face of death. He simply does not know fear. The neurotic is the bipolar opposite. With similar impulses he is always full of care and trembles before death. The poet has artistically sublimated the destructive impulse of the criminal. He tears down the old. But he has more than compensated the destructive impulse by an immense urge to creation. He creates new values. The neurotic with his atavistic instincts is not adapted to our culture. He must hold the instincts in check with fear. He fears himself and falling into sin. But behind this fear there is as I have shown, the fear of the punishment of God. For the religious instincts, too, are more strongly marked in these retrogressive-phenomena. This explains the fact that so many geniuses cannot get away from the religious problem. They attack God (Nietzsche) or submit to Him (Strindberg) or they take their place among the prophets (Tolstoy) and found new sects. The special need of our time is a religious faith. The vast consciousness of guilt comes from religious sources. Even the various modern hygienic movements are nothing but disguised asceticism. The whole abstinence movement, the various vegetarian reforms and hunger cures are pennances for secret sins. The modern abstinence apostles are the successors of the fanatical Savonarola.

How many of the neurotic symptoms are only a punishment of God anticipated by the unconscious? The arm of the rabbi (No. 97) loses all feeling because he gave his hand to a strange woman whereupon a stream of burning lust rushed through him. That is of course clear and comprehensible. The priest (No. 98) cannot read mass because he has sinful thoughts the while. But many cases of paralysis and most phobias are also only the punishment of God. A self-dictated punishment, it is true, and all the more cruel for that, but executed in the name of God.

In a most ingenious parallel Janet has compared the hysterical paralyses and contractions with the phobias. The similarity is in fact striking. I have shown elsewhere that neurotics have the peculiarity of thinking and acting in symbolic equations. Thus they suffer under the imperative "I cannot." This inability will show itself in various forms from fear of an act up to complete paralysis. The kind of paralysis or of contraction will always betray the nature of the act which the neurotic cannot perform. The arm which would murder remains paralysed, or the fist which would strike some one down remains clenched, so that the patient cannot open it. Janet says: "The contractions are systematised like the paralyses. This is often overlooked because the contractions are not noticed at the outset and with time they spread and lose the systematic form which they had in the moment of origin. Such contractions permanently preserve a definite attitude reminiscent of an act or an emotion. After a transport of anger the arm remains raised, the fist clenched and menacing ; a woman gives her child a box on the ears and—her arm and hand remain fixed, as by the punishment of Heaven, in the position they were in at that moment."

A young girl who was learning the violin has the left arm paralysed in the position of violin playing ; a woman walks for years on the tips of her toes, unable to bend her feet. They are drawn up as by cramp in the position of the crucifixion. This was a patient who suffers from ecstatic crises and who imagines herself crucified like the Saviour.

In these cases it is pretty clear that we are dealing with self-punishment from fear of the punishment of God. The paralysis expresses the same thing as the contraction, " I cannot."[1]

The various phobias, like the fear of crossing an open space, express the incapacity to perform an act which is always a sinful one and one rejected by consciousness (the *moral* consciousness). For example, the open space fear may express the incapacity of absconding to America after a fraud. (Case No. 1). The patient remains standing before an open space begins to tremble and cannot cross over. " To all appearances," says Janet, " the function of motion is not suppressed. The patient believes that he can use his limbs perfectly well, and even begins to execute the motion quite correctly. But at this moment he feels all sorts of perplexities and derangements ; he feels himself filled with the strangest fancies, and shaken with the most incredible thoughts. He tries all possible movements ; his heart begins to palpitate, he loses breath and is seized by anxiety. These derangements paralyse his courage, and he stops, disheartened. Every time before an open space this fear returns so that finally he gives up the job, just like a lame man who absolutely cannot move his legs."

We see the effect is the same as with paralysis or contraction. Fear paralyses physically or mentally. The most important point is that the sinful act remains undone.

There are in fact anxiety conditions in which there can be no movement whatever (akinesia algera of Möbius). But the analysis will always show that that is a case of a forbidden act. It is true that the patient expresses this in remarkable fashion. He remains in the room, e.g., for fear of getting a chill or for some other " rationalised "[2] motives. If we investigate further we find that the patient is not sure of himself. He has therefore voluntarily condemned himself to prison.[3]

---

[1] Really ; I will ; but I cannot because I ought not.

[2] The apt expression originates with Jones.

[3] Baron v. Berger in his wonderful novel, " Hofrat Eysenhardt "

I will close this discussion with a practical example which will show the importance of this new point of view.

No. 154.—A thirty year old highly educated and enlightened philosopher suffers from a remarkable fear. He has the fear of losing. If he has to open a purse he does it in fear and trembling. He might lose a few coins. If he takes his handkerchief from his pocket he must carry out laborious investigations to make sure that he has not lost anything. He always counts the things that he carries about in his pocket. He repeats to himself : Knife, key, handkerchief, purse, pocket-book, note-book, etc. So you have everything. You have lost nothing. This fear tortures him on all possible occasions. He cannot read a book, or attend a concert but he must constantly assure himself that he has lost nothing. —A dream enables me to explain this strange phenomenon, for which all previous solutions had been worthless. This dream runs thus :—

A great number of people, men and women, are going up a mountain. I try to get ahead of everyone else, and I succeed. I come to the bank of a stream. A dark ferry man stands beside a small boat, a cutter. The boat is divided in the middle. There was much water in the boat. The ferryman and I bale it out. I think that in the meantime the others will certainly overtake us. Then it seems to me that I have already made the crossing. I stand on the bank, look into the boat and see the articles that belong to me. A letter from my mother strikes me. All saturated with water. I wonder that I have not the least fear of losing anything. Also when I took out my purse to pay the ferryman I had no fear of losing anything.

Let us leave on one side the details of the dream, whose solution would take us too long, and confine ourselves to the main points. Why had the dreamer no fear of losing in the dream ? One might say this was just the fulfilment of a wish, which the dream brings. But the dream brings the fulfilment of the wish in a certain situation. What is the meaning of the situation ?

We can understand this dream only if we know the death symbolism which plays a prominent part in all dreams. What lies

(Deutschösterreichischer Verlag., 1911) relates the fortunes of a judge who is really a criminal by nature. His sentences are known for their draconic severity. His sadism betrays itself in the artful way in which he convicts the accused and makes them confess. Finally he himself commits a crime and shoots himself. On his writing-table is found a document :

"IN THE NAME OF HIS MAJESTY THE KAISER !

" I have committed a grave crime and feel myself unworthy to continue to " discharge the duties of my office, or even to live. I have condemned myself " to the severest punishment, and I shall execute it next minute with my " own hand."

This novel deals with an incident which actually happened as the poet has described it. It shows its truth in every line. The neurotics, too, condemn themselves to the most severe punishments. But in the name of the highest justice.

on the other side of a stream is the kingdom of death.[1] The ferry-man in this dream is Charon, to whom the dreamer must give an obolus. Years ago he had a tormenting obsession after crossing a ferry. He thought he had not paid the ferryman. The neurotic always confuses symbol and reality. So the real ferryman became Charon (to whom he had not paid the obolus). Now we understand the baling out of the water. His life-ship is laden with guilt. It is the tears of his mother. She had written him a letter on which the traces of tears were to be seen. The boat contains also his father's tears. Indeed, it is divided into two parts. The recognition of what his fear of losing means comes to me in a flash. He fears losing eternal salvation. Since in the dream he is a Greek and drinks Lethe he need not fear any more. The serene religion of the Greeks knows nothing of the guilt which attaches to sinful erotic thoughts.[2] The patient remembers presently that his illness dates from a confession in which he did not confess having masturbated.[3] He intentionally suppressed the most important thing. Thus according to his religion he heaped sin upon sin and was justified in his fear of losing eternal salvation. Of what avail now any earthly success? He ceased to study. He wished to make his way upward as in the dream where every one was struggling towards heaven. He wishes to get ahead of all the others. He wants to be first and to sit by the throne of God. With this solution the obsession of losing collapsed. Enough of this example! It shows the decisive import of religion in bringing about the neuroses. We see that the conflict between impulse and inhibition is waged mostly on the religious field.

But how do these observations bear on Freud's hypothesis on the fact constantly re-confirmed by me that repressed libido becomes fear? Are then all anxiety neuroses only faith neuroses?[4]

I believe that besides the dubious physical results of frustrated excitations which I have detailed in earlier chapters the psychic components come into consideration. The man who is hungry will have criminal thoughts. The person who is sexually unsatis-fied seeks in fancy for ways of achieving libido. These ways enter the realm of the forbidden. For it always stimulates people to overcome difficulties and to set their powers to work. A pleasure that is permitted loses the character of pleasure on account of the lack of resistance. Therefore even when there is normal satisfaction,

---

[1] Cf. "The Language of the dream," p. 373.

[2] Since neurosis also contains his secret religiosity, the "fear of losing" means also the fear of losing the neurosis. Cf. in my book, "Disguises of Love" (Kegan Paul, London) the chapter, "The Will to Disease."

[3] The consciousness of guilt which attaches to masturbation is of very complex nature. The masturbation covers a number of "forbidden" fancies and lustful ideas among which the criminal (amoral) ones play a great part.

[4] Heinroth (Lehrbuch der Störungen des Seelenlebens, Leipzig, 1818. Fr. Chr. Vogel) traces all mental disturbances to the "conscience."

anxiety neuroses arise if the sexual object has lost its stimulating power. The cravings creep into the domain of sin and then begins the religious or ethical conflict.

In this discussion I have tried to give only some small contributions to the psychology of fear, and to call the attention of psychotherapeutists to the great importance of the religious problem.

CHAPTER XXXV

GENERAL DIAGNOSTICS OF ANXIETY CONDITIONS

THE diagnosis of a violent anxiety affect (anxiety attack) is mostly gained from the lips of the patients and betrays itself in the patients' characteristic expression of face. They receive the physician with the words : " Help me. I am so terribly afraid," or " I am in such a state of anxiety." The eyes starting from the head proclaim their fear of death. But the fear is not always so easily recognised as fear. Indeed, we have seen in our discussion of the anxiety-equivalents of anxiety-neurosis that the subjective sensation of anxiety may be thrown quite into the back-ground, and that particular symptoms of anxiety may be repressed. Something similar happens also in other attacks of anxiety. The patients moan about cramp in the neighbourhood of the heart, lack of breath, palpitation of the heart, etc., without directly complaining of anxiety. Often nothing remains of the anxiety but the frightful excitement and the torturing unrest.

We will try to recognise an attack of anxiety by certain objective signs. The symptoms are, of course, known ; the patients complain of pressure in the region of the heart or of palpitation. One finds a small and very rapid pulse. The face becomes pale and the eyes start out because the lids are opened to the utmost. The legs totter. The hands tremble. The hair stands on end. The pupils dilate. A cold sweat stands on the forehead (anxiety-sweat). The patients report dryness in the mouth and throat, and great thirst. Further, in extreme cases, we notice diarrhœa and even involuntary stools, urine urgency, violent screaming or speechlessness.

Sigmund Kornfeld has drawn attention to certain objective symptoms of attacks of anxiety. He found in all his cases a marked rise in the blood pressure and an alteration of the pulse curve. " This consists in a diminution of the rising limb of the pulse-wave that synchronises with the systole of the left ventricle." I have already mentioned the acute dilatation of the heart in acute anxiety conditions. Max Kaufmann[1] was able to demonstrate small quantities of grape sugar in anxiety conditions of paralytics as also of women at the climacteric. (Also in anxiety neuroses.) Since anxiety neurotics also usually complain of dryness in the mouth and throat, great thirst, ravenous hunger, and pruritus, a confusion with diabetes is very easily possible.

[1] Münchener med. Wochenschr., 1908, No. 12.

But for quick diagnosis by the practising physician these objective signs are of little importance. They have considerable theoretic interest. More important is the dilation of the pupils which Kornfeld[1] always noticed. I too can confirm this observation but could not always find a difference in the pupils in Fliess's sense (only in certain cases). Fliess found (as stated) the left pupil dilated to the utmost *before* the attack. In any case this statement should be kept in view as, if confirmed, it indicates a premonitory symptom of much diagnostic value. Sommer draws attention to a characteristic curve of fearfulness.[2]

The symptoms of anxiety attack which have been sketched may be taken as typical but they have not the constancy of a law. Thus Kornfeld observed a child who in an anxiety attack became as red as a lobster. (Apparently a combination of anxiety and anger.) I know anxiety attacks with a great flow of saliva ; and so on.

There are also innumerable variations and transitions.

The diagnosis of " anxiety " as such is easier than the recognition of the trouble caused by the anxiety.

One must always ask oneself the question : Is this a symptom of a parapathia or is there an organic illness behind the anxiety ?

In discussing anxiety neurosis I have always had regard to the differential diagnosis and therefore refer to those particular chapters.

Especially must it be borne in mind that certain acute intoxications (atropine, hyoscine, cocaine, pyramidone, trional, etc.) are accompanied by violent anxiety. Also in chronic poisoning (nicotine, alcohol, morphine, cocaine) feelings of anxiety frequently occur. More frequently as abstinence phenomena, probably caused by the anti-bodies. Feelings of anxiety also accompany the phenomena of " Maphylaxy."

The similarity of anxiety neurosis with certain chronic alkaloid poisonings has already been mentioned. So that all organic causes must be excluded before one pronounces the diagnosis "neurotic anxiety."

The fact that acute infectious diseases very often begin with sensations of anxiety is also important. Kornfeld mentions a case of lyssa in which most acute anxiety was the first symptom. " A psychic reflex," says Kornfeld, " was excluded, as the patient did not know the nature and the danger of his condition."

I have very often found anxiety dreams as the first symptom of an infectious disease. It is high time to take into account the dream

---

[1] Dr. Sigm. Kornfeld. Jahrbücher für Psychiatrie and Neurologie, 1902.

[2] Sommer (Lehrbuch der psychopathologischen Untersuchungsmethoden. Urban and Schwarzenberg, 1899, Vienna and Berlin) took phonographic records of the various forms of expression in speech, and found in great anxiety monotones, repetition of certain tone series and of certain rhythms together with long-drawn moanings. The pulse curve of fear sensitiveness taken by this author (reaction to sudden noises) is also interesting. The psycho-galvanic reflex (veragouth) also comes within the scope of these investigations.

life in diagnosis. Näcke[1] has pointed out the diagnostic importance of sexual dreams, though without regard to the interpretation of dreams. Much work will still be needed to distinguish the various specific forms of anxiety dreams and to make use of them for diagnosis.   Typhus is indicated with special frequency by an anxiety dream. Also accumulated fear dreams are observed long before the outbreak of the fever (i.e., in the incubation stage).

No. 134.—Some days before the outbreak of spotted fever a lady dreamed the following dream—a mixture of sexual desires and fear of death :—
" I dreamed that I was on a visit to my parents in the town of my birth. The day was just dawning and I was sitting in my parents' bedroom as they lay in bed. Suddenly in the courtyard of the house a trumpet sounded. Everyone hurried to the windows and we saw a black horseman in helmet and armour with his sword drawn. He dismounted and to the astonishment of all came straight into the house where he looked round as if seeking someone. Suddenly he pointed at me, and said : ' Since there is no one else here who can go to the war, she there must go.' My parents began to wail, I clasped my hands, fell at his feet and begged him with tears to let me live as I was so young. However, he consoled us : ' Weep not, I will bring her back to you.' "

Of diagnostic interest is the following case from my own experience :

No. 135.—A twenty-three year old youth cries out in his sleep for several nights. Suddenly his parents are informed that their son is mentally deranged ; that he has made an uproar at the Town Hall and demanded to be taken to the Burgomaster. At the end of a week the diagnosis of hebephrenia is altered to typhus ambulatorius. In six weeks complete cure. From this we see the importance of taking the temperature in an attack of anxiety, or immediately after it.

But for the sake of completeness we must mention that the anxiety conditions in melancholia and the anxiety deliria of epileptics are often accompanied by considerable increase of temperature. There is also the important fact that derangements of the hypophysis and of the thyroidea (Basedow !) and for the rest all disturbances of internal secretion may be accompanied by sensations of anxiety. These indications of organic causes of anxiety conditions may suffice.   Only investigation can decide between anxiety of organic and anxiety of neurotic origin. In both conditions the symptoms are the same.

In the judgment of nervous anxiety conditions we shall try to distinguish sharply between general nervousness and attacks of anxiety. This distinction is, however, not always practicable and in many cases the general nervousness increases to attacks of anxiety. *General nervousness of indefinite character combined with irritability is found especially in the pure uncomplicated forms of anxiety neurosis.* It may refer to personal health and then we call it hypochondria ; it appears almost justified in the case of exaggerated carefulness in business and finally as the expression of a refined conscience in the fear of breaking religious or ethical laws.

[1] " Der Traum als feinstes Reagens für die Art des sexuellen Empfindens." Monatschrift für Kriminal psychologie, 1905.

I need not here repeat the symptoms of anxiety neurosis. Very characteristic are the anxiety dreams in which there is much dreaming of the dead. Relatives appear, who are already long dead ; one sees living persons in coffins, or one attends a funeral procession. Next to death dreams, dreams of rape predominate as anxiety dreams. Robbers and thieves appear and throttle the victim. Knife, revolver, sabre, cross-bow, fire, water, narrow ravines, sudden falls, play a great rôle. Also wild animals, bulls, stallions, raging biting dogs. Criminal thoughts of poisoning, arson, etc., express themselves in characteristic anxiety dreams which I have discussed in detail in my book, "The Language of the Dream."

In these cases we shall often be able to detect some injurious form of sex life ; it may be coitus interruptus, abstinence, vain excitements during betrothal, etc., a loveless marriage, disgust and repugnance to the consort, a suppressed perversion. The diagnosis is then confirmed by the rapid success of the therapy, so far as the conditions admit of a therapy. For differential diagnosis, Basedow's disease has also to be considered, for its attendant symptoms, dizziness, headache, increased sensitiveness, restlessness, sleeplessness, palpitation, sweats, occur also in anxiety neurosis. Also I have already pointed out that in anxiety neurosis and anxiety hysteria one very often finds a greater or lesser struma. Many "formes frustes" of the Basedow are nothing but anxiety neuroses. The struma is in fact the expression of the somatic predisposition for the neurosis. For genuine Basedow the familiar symptoms are : the constant, strengthened, and accelerated heart action, the acute struma, the exophthalmus, the incomplete and infrequent winking (Stellwag), the insufficient convergence capacity (Möbius), the absence of movement of the upper lid on lowering the glance (Graefe), and finally, the characteristic trembling motions. If the anxiety symptoms vanish after putting the sexual life on a hygienic basis, then the success of the therapy gives the diagnosis—anxiety neurosis. That infantile nervousness is always connected with a sexual excitement I have shown in detail in discussing the anxiety neurosis of children.

However, there is a certain nervousness which is not conditioned by any neurosis. It is the consequence of an abnormally developed instinct of self-preservation or the product of a deficient education. Yet this "fearfulness" as it might be called has always a corresponding psychic motive. Pathological nervousness is a painful affect of expectation which attaches itself to a definite object, the most interesting at the moment. There is a certain disharmony between the affect and the cause of it which calls for the diagnosis—neurosis.

I will discuss this with the help of a few examples. A lady is constantly afraid that she has forgotten to turn off the gas-meter. This fear is readily comprehensible, for an open gas-meter involves a certain degree of danger to the house. Gas may escape, an explosion may result, the children may be suffocated, etc. Now we must never rest satisfied with the obvious motive for " fear." We must always ask further whether there is a neurotic anxiety, a hidden psychic conflict, i.e., a derangement of the affective life (parapathia). investigate further. We learn that there are peculiar habits attached to this gas-meter notion. The lady goes out every evening before retiring and turns off the meter. After that the servants have to work with a paraffin lamp. Still comprehensible enough. The husband gives us further details. They are lying in bed. Suddenly the lady declares that she cannot go to sleep, she keeps thinking the gas-meter is open, the husband must, for God's sake, go out and turn it off. Till then she would get no rest. The husband has to give way and go out, whereupon the wife becomes more tranquil. But she may yet wake up and ask, " Did you turn off the gas-meter ? "

This demands a closer analysis. We learn that in Vienna the word *gas-meter*[1] has a second meaning. As a girl this lady once heard her parents speaking of her brother. The father had just heard from a colleague " that Emil had a new gas-meter, and that often instead of going to school he was going about with the gas-meter." We learn further that this lady is much dissatisfied with her husband's performances. It is true he practices the *coitus reservatus* in such a way that she is satisfied. But he maintains that this mode of love is very injurious to him. For weeks at a time he does not cohabit with her. She is very irritable, and suffers from nightly sweats, diarrhœa, anxiety dreams. Her fear that the gas-meter is open indicates a repressed wish for sexual activity. It is as if she would exclaim to her husband : " Take care ! My gas-meter is open. Make haste and close it or I shall get some one else to do it ! "[2]

Thus a fear with inadequate motive may on closer analysis betray neurotic anxiety. Just in the same way we must estimate the fear of burglars, robbers, thieves. It corresponds to a repressed wish " to be suddenly fallen upon."

The little every-day phobias of which we take no notice often render possible the diagnosis of an anxiety neurosis, phobia or compulsion neurosis. A woman cannot go to sleep before all the doors are shut. Certainly a very usual act of fear. Several times, or in slight cases only once, she jumps out of her warm bed, tries the door and tests the lock. (Doubt is a characteristic symptom of compulsion neurosis). This fear, too, has a symbolic significance. He who wishes to possess her would be forcing " an open door." It is, of course, the hyper-moral, the so-called "virtuous" women whose unsatisfied craving thus expresses itself. One of my patients reported to me that at the time of a liaison with a friend of her

---

[1] = Girl.

[2] With the experience I now possess I should in this case have sought also for criminal factors. Had the woman played with the thought of killing herself or her husband by turning on the gas ?

husband's she never had any sexual enjoyment, although he was a very potent man. She was constantly dominated by the idea : " The doors are not locked. My husband will surprise me." Even when she had several times tested the lock she could not rid herself of this fear. So she gave up the liaison, and then, in contrast to the experience she had been through, she slept with—open doors.

In men also an anxiety neurosis with a small admixture of compulsion neurosis and hysteria, which seems hardly ever absent, may show itself in slight every-day derangements of function. I give only a few examples : the fear and doubt whether one has properly locked the door, the anxious doubt that one has left the key behind, that there is something wrong with one's clothes (fly of the trousers open !), that one has not put enough stamps on the letter. The physician has not written the prescription correctly. The dose of morphine was given in decigrams instead of centigrams. Such physicians often run into the druggist's in the greatest excitement and ask to be shown the prescription.[1] Lawyers think of an error in the form of the indictment, of a paragraph falsely quoted or applied. In short, every anxiety neurotic carries his fear into his occupation.[2] The disproportion between the object of the fear and the discomfort leads us to the diagnosis. There can be no doubt about the diagnosis if the other signs of anxiety neurosis are also present, viz., abnormal sensitiveness, palpitation, asthma, dizziness, paræsthetic congestions, numbness of a finger or of the arm, sick-headache, diarrhœa, vomiting, sleeplessness.

A knowledge of the psychic conflict will give us an indication for the diagnosis. I give only one example. A patient complains of a definite feeling of fear. He has bought a new *business* and is not satisfied with it. He fears it will ruin him—a fear with a logical basis and related to an object.[3] But we soon find out that the fear has no logical basis. The man is well-to-do, the business is comparatively good, there is no question of ruin threatening. It is only a secret anxiety which has been transferred to a definite object. It is a "false connection." He suffers under a compulsion : " *I must sell my old business and start a new business.*" What lies behind this one thought which pursues him, allows him no sleep, fills him with fears of all kinds ? Naturally a repressed wish. This riddle also is to be solved only with the help of Freud's key, sexual symbolism. *Business* is a popular expression for vagina. Now we can see the psychological solution. He is dissatisfied with his wife and would like to get another.[4]

[1] In one such case I was able plainly to show ideas of poisoning.

[2] Cf. my essay, " Berufsmahl und Kriminalität." (Gross' Archives, Vol. 41.)

[3] Griesinger speaks of " objectless fear." We see the nature of fear precisely in its relation to a certain object. Objectless fear is a contradiction in terms just like an " unmarried husband."

[4] " If we do not wish to admit a great sin, we bemoan a little sin with great emphasis." (Jung.)

The disproportion between the magnitude of the emotion and the fear-object led us in this case to the psychic conflict.

Many of the phobic conditions here discussed belong really to "compulsion neurosis." This is due to the fact that the two diseases, "anxiety-hysteria" and "compulsion neurosis" very frequently occur in combination. One very often finds compulsion neurosis with phobic phenomena and phobias with obsessions. In practice the distinction is not so important since both diseases, "compulsion neurosis" and "phobia" show almost the same psychic mechanism. The affect of the obsession is, according to Freud, a displaced or transposed one which is capable of reconversion into a sexual one. We have seen—in this point I find myself in contradiction with Freud—that all phobias also admit of the same reconversion. Freud originally found the essence of compulsory neurosis to consist in the following factors (1) An idea (overvalued) dominates the patient; (2) An affect attaches itself to this idea; (Anxiety, doubt, remorse, anger); (3) This affect is justified (the analysis shows this) and not to be got rid of by reasoning[1]; (4) The obsession is not the exciting idea, it takes the place of the repressed idea. It is of course not a case of one idea only; in a real compulsion neurosis there is a perfect maze of compulsory ideas which again may lead to the strangest compulsory acts.

In a later work Freud seeks to characterise compulsion neurosis in a simple formula : *Compulsive ideas are always transformed reproaches emerging after repression, and these always refer to a sexual action of childhood which has been attended by pleasure.*[2] The compulsion neurosis has three typical periods : (1) The period of childish immorality ; (2) The first repression at the beginning of the (often precocious) sexual maturity. As defensive systems, conscientiousness, disgust, shame, self-distrust, then appear ; (3) The return of the repressed memories in disguised form as compromise between impulse and repression. Freud recognises a number of anxiety conditions as belonging to the compulsion neurosis ; the social anxiety, the religious anxiety, the delusion of observation, the fear of temptation, the doubting mania, fear of treachery.

We see how two great circles, phobia and compulsion neurosis here intersect. Indeed, Freud says himself : " In all my cases of compulsion neurosis I have found a *sub-structure of hysterical symptoms.*

For the prognosis, the decision compulsion neurosis or anxiety hysteria is very important. The compulsion neurosis is the more obstinate trouble and requires much longer treatment. According to a fertile idea of Rudolf Reitler the *compulsion neurosis* is a heightened phobia (anxiety-hysteria, according to Freud), while this again is a development of an anxiety *neurosis*. There is a great deal to be said for this. It would confirm my view that between the various neuroses there are differences in degree but not in principle.

The case of the singer (Chapter XXV.) gives a characteristic picture of an anxiety-hysteria case combined with slight compulsion neurosis (washing compulsion, religiosity, etc.).

It may have struck many persons that there is nothing about neurasthenia in this book. I can only say once more : I know no neurasthenia. I can but confirm what Alfred Strasser[3] has found that neurasthenia is a very rare disease. Strasser, who is engaged in a large hydropathic institute, says that he sees only a few cases of genuine neurasthenia in a year. That will not surprise us because we have learned that there are only anxiety neuroses, phobias and

[1] " Zur Neurosenlehre." No. VI. "L'Etat emotif, comme tel, est toujours justifié."

[2] " Zur Neurosenlehre," No. VIII.

[3] " Die Behandlung der Neurasthenie im Hause." Blätler f. klin. Hydrotherapy, 1907.

compulsion neuroses. Therefore there is also no "neurasthenic anxiety" of which we read so much in the old text-books. The fear attacks in conversion hysteria may be of great intensity and be accompanied by hallucinations. In phobias attacks as such are rare. For the anxiety hysteric fears the attacks and the phobia is a protective measure against the anxiety attack. The agoraphobia, e.g., protects against the fear attacks to be expected during the crossing of the open space.

For the rest, the hysterical anxiety-attacks are extremely dramatic and frequently show, as has been mentioned, a characteristic disproportion between the anxiety-idea and the expression of the anxiety in actions.[1] Thus at sight of a mouse a hysteric may have an anxiety attack ; on the other hand she may relate with comparatively slight emotion the story of an attempt to murder or to violate her. This disproportion between anxiety-expression and the anxiety-idea is specially striking in paranoia, as Alfred Adler has pointed out. Paranoiacs show comparatively little anxiety. Because, no doubt, behind their hallucinations are hidden desires which originate partly in the erotic, partly in the megalomaniacal complex (ego-complex).

The highest degrees of anxiety attacks are seen in melancholia. It is very important in every severe anxiety-attack to ask oneself the question : Is it the beginning of a psychosis or the expression of a neurosis ? Many a suicide committed by a melancholic might have been avoided if the anxiety attack had been recognised in time as the beginning of a melancholia. The anxiety attacks in melancholia occur mostly in the morning after an anxiety dream ; they may reach the greatest intensity and rise to a fit of madness. In the lighter cases the patients localise the anxiety in the neighbourhood of the heart as heart anxiety, but feelings of lung anxiety are also not rare. Ziehen[2] describes also other forms of melancholic anxiety which are very similar to the forms of fear described by Freud in anxiety neurosis and probably arise from a combination of melancholia with anxiety neurosis ; a combination which is not at all rare, as the cases of melancholia analysed by me show.

Others feel the anxiety specially in the head or in the throat. In the former case I have heard it stated that the anxiety is accompanied by a feeling of giddiness or dizziness. Accompanying the throat-anxiety there is a cramp-like feeling of constriction in the neck. Very often one hears also that the anxiety from the breast rises in a hot stream to the head. The localisation of the anxiety in the abdomen is also not at all rare. In one case in which anxiety about a harmless and almost cured bladder trouble (cystitis) had caused the melancholia, the patient always localised the anxiety most definitely in the neighbourhood of the bladder. Rarer is localisation of the anxiety in the extremities. Thus, e.g., the above-mentioned patient suffering from retroflexio uteri felt the anxiety in the lower extremities. In one case, too, I have observed the

[1] "Pose, mimi and words either harmonise or are in closest contradiction." (Raemann).

[2] "Die Erkennung und Behandlung der Melancholie in der Praxis." Karl Marhold, Halle A. S., 1907.

localisation of the anxiety—without any demonstrable cause—in the arm. The duration of an attack of anxiety varies within very wide limits; it lasts sometimes a few minutes, sometimes hours.

In exceptional cases the anxiety is accompanied by neuralgic pains and then mostly by intercostal neuralgia on the left side. This happens also in cases which are not complicated with hysteria or neurasthenia." (Notice the striking similarity with the anxiety equivalents and anxiety localisations of anxiety neurosis !)

The differential diagnosis of " melancholic " anxiety is not always easy. Now and then anxiety neuroses occur which are accompanied by severe *tædium vitæ* or even by the delusion of guilt. The anxiety is never so intense as in melancholia. Yet in every case where self-accusations, micromania, or depression occur, great caution is necessary for frequently the anxiety neurosis may be a preliminary stage of real melancholia.

Now and then the chronic anxiety conditions in *dementia præcox* (schizophrenia) are taken to be " neurasthenic." All psychiatrists report that a great number of their *dementia præcox* cases had been treated under the diagnosis " neurasthenic " as " nervous." Evidences for "dementia præcox" are snappish, rude behaviour, motiveless affectivity, asocial deportment, brutal egoism, incorrigible " autistic thinking " (Beuler), impulsive running on and on, a general blunting of all ethical and æsthetic ideas, a striking indifference to the demands of life.

The most important differential diagnostic factor I consider to be the fact that in dementia præcox the conflicts are more evident than in hysteria. The repressions are overcome by delusion.

No. 136.—I am called to a twenty-four year old girl in order to cure her hysteria by psychanalysis. For some weeks the girl was under the observation of a noted psychiatrist in an institution. The diagnosis was hysteria. At the first conversation it struck me that she coarsely emphasised the thoughts of incest. She was afraid of her father. At the outbreak of the illness she had remained behind alone with her father, when the mother went to the watering place. Then she had first looked on the father with desire. Now she was afraid to be left alone with the father.

I declined the psychanalysis. My diagnosis was: Hebephrenia. The next day I saw the patient again. She talked with me for an hour without betraying a delusion. When she was going, I asked : " What about your fear of poisoning ? " She promptly replied : " I eat no soup. Mother wants to poison me ! "

Some days later a violent anxiety attack breaks out. She comes to the psychiatric clinic and there is introduced as a case of " hysterical delirium." Her condition grew worse from day to day ; she is transferred to the incurable section of a lunatic asylum with the diagnosis : Hebephrenia.

In another case I was able, in spite of the mad talk of the patient, from the way in which the real conflict was concealed from me to diagnose hysteria. Open psychic conflicts with the sexual incidents emphasised are not of the nature of hysteria and warn us to be cautious in diagnosing.

The anxiety attacks of schizophrenia manifest themselves in running on and on without plan or aim, which form one of the most important symptoms for recognising the illness. Anxiety conditions drive people to active vagabondage. Suddenly one night the patients get a fright and then run restlessly from place to place. The patient has no insight into his disease. He does not notice alterations in his psyche. Ordinary anxiety attacks also are by no means rare, likewise impulsive attempts at suicide, bizarre ideas of persecution, hallucinations.

Almost all who are early demented make endless complaints of various troubles, over-tiredness, mental exhaustion, which usually causes the physician to diagnose " neurasthenia."

Just the familiar characteristics of " neurasthenia," pressure in the head, sleeplessness, ill-humour, nervous muscular weakness, back-ache, and finally dyspepsia from gastro-intestinal atonia, may be found in the initial stages of *dementia præcox*. The differential diagnosis is nevertheless very easy, since the intelligence of the neurotic has not suffered and " as regards ethics " is rather over-sensitive.

The slight cases of melancholia (hypomelancholia) show a certain similarity with the severe anxiety neurosis we have described. But the anxiety neurotic is predominently irritable and has also merry moments. The melancholic is permanently sad. (Ziehen.)

I have already shown that Wernecke's anxiety psychosis cannot be accounted a specific form of disease. Also in maniacal depressive insanity there is in the melancholy stage a violent development of anxiety. Thus Specht[1] says : " Quite generally it seems to me that the anxiety in maniacal depressive insanity plays a much greater part than is admitted even by those authors who do not share Kræpelin's standpoint. The anxiety is accompanied by a flow of ideas and increased craving for motion so that the picture completely resembles the old ' melancholia agitata.' " The so-called anxiety psychosis is, according to Specht, only a form of the maniacal depressive insanity.

As is well-known many modern authors (Dreyfuss, Wilmann Kræpelin[2]) will not allow that melancholia is a disease *sui generis* and class it with maniacal depressive insanity.

In my practice I have observed a few cases which seem not to confirm this view. The clinical picture of cyclothymia is in severe cases very distinct. The slight cases may cause false diagnoses. The cyclic course of the depressions, the succeeding often only very briefly indicated high-spirited moods facilitate the diagnosis. The anxiety-development may be very great and lead to suicide.

It is noteworthy that the slighter cases can be influenced psychotherapeutically, but are apt to recur. The success occurs very quickly and is disconcerting, i.e., the depressed stage is succeeded

---

[1] " Ueber den Angstaffekt in manisch-depressionen Irresein. A contribution to the problem of melancholia." (Centralblatt für Nerv. and Psychol. 15th Juli, 1907.)

[2] Allgemeine Zeitschrift für Psychiatrie, 1907, Vol. 64, *p.* 680.

by slight mania. Frequently in the first weeks of the treatment there is depression. All these cases show enormously strong transference. It seems that here, too, the failure to overcome the homosexual component, or the consciousness of guilt in respect to wishing people dead, leads to psychosis.

As to *paranoia* I have already mentioned that its anxiety affects are in disproportion to the anxiety-idea. If, e.g., a lady appears in the consulting room and with cheerful, indifferent or mysterious mien, relates that she is surrounded by enemies who dishonour her by telepathic means and wish to put her out of the world, the diagnosis paranoia is very probable. The paranoic is always innocent, the melancholic a hardened sinner.

The anxiety conditions in *dementia paralytica* betray themselves by their absurd construction, by their boundless extravagance. Also the familiar objective symptoms (difference in the pupils, staring pupils, stumbling over syllables, alterations of hand-writing, anæsthesia of the lower legs, failure or heightening of reflexes) facilitate the diagnosis.

Of great importance also is an exact knowledge of the anxiety delirium of epileptics which may bring on anxiety dreams. Slight depressions also may precede the attack.

The hallucinations under which the patients suffer are very characteristic and have been clearly described by Kræpelin (l.c.) :—

" Often the introduction *is a quite definite regularly repeated deception of the senses;* especially noteworthy are the " black man " and the appearance of red objects, blood, flames, man in the red cloak. The patient completely loses his sense of direction ; his surroundings alter ; deceptions of the senses and anxiety-delusions occur. He has a very vague idea of what is going on around him, listens to the voices which scold and threaten him. He must be punished for masturbation, hears God speaking, and the death-car driving by ; must die, has done something wicked, feels something lay hold of him, sees himself surrounded by devils, spectres, wild animals, great masses of people who come out of the wall and often press forward from all sides. Before the fire stands a man who wants to shoot him ; already he has bullets in his body ; the physician has designs on him ; milk and bread taste of sulphur. Battles are being fought, a frightful blood-bath is being prepared, he is wading in blood and stepping over corpses ; mother and sister have been killed on the railway ; the home is blown up. He is led into an underground passage in which men and animals are torn to pieces on frightful instruments of torture. Everything is falling. Air and light are cut off from him ; the last judgment is upon us ; he is entering hell. At the same time he is overcome by the most intense fear of death so that he tremblingly awaits his end, he stammers one prayer after another or in solemn words commits his soul to God's keeping. Fabulous tales fill up the intervals ; the patient arrived in the post-chaise yesterday, joined the army, conversed with the Grand Duke. Sometimes God and Christ appear, give him his freedom, promise him pardon, crown him as prince of peace, take him to paradise in a splendid carriage. There his sacred mother appears. But these periods of joyful exaltation are always only interludes which rapidly pass.

While the melancholic in the fit of madness under the impression of tormenting self-reproaches, under the burden of his sins and of the hopelessness of his precarious position, commits suicide, the epileptic in the anxiety attack is inclined to terrible crime. Whole

families may be slaughtered. He may also attack strangers which is specially dangerous if he has a weapon.[1]
From what has been said the recognition of this anxiety delirium is not difficult. In epileptic delirium, as in the status epilepticus, fever has been observed. The recognition of all psychoses is just as important for the practitioner as the recognition of the neuroses. It is especially in the psychoses that the anxiety attack plays a very significant part. To be sure, the presence of a psychosis will not easily escape the attentive observer. In psychotherapy there is special need for a sympathetic pre-occupation with the psyche of the patient, and then alterations in the mental personality may be readily recognised. This can be acquired only by exact observation and a certain training of the perception. In one's practice one must remember not to be too pessimistic. In most cases behind the acute fear attack there is the familiar picture of the anxiety neurosis. All other anxiety attacks are comparatively rare. Only if melancholia is suspected is a certain pessimism advantageous. The supervision of patients suspected of melancholia is an important precaution which may prevent many a suicide.

[1] According to my analyses, true epilepsy is extremely rare ; most cases are parapathia and result from repression of an overpowering criminality. Cf. Chap. XXX, " The psychic treatment of epilepsy."

P

CHAPTER XXXVI

THE TECHNIQUE OF PSYCHOTHERAPY

BY psychotherapy is understood the use of mental powers for healing. Its technique presented at one time little difficulty. It was confined to exhortation, to promises acting suggestively, and to hypnosis. As Löwenfeld justly remarks, all therapy is really psychotherapy. No less than 2,000 years ago there were " soul doctors." Thus Plutarch was a renowned soul doctor who was sought out from far and near by people who wished to pour out their hearts and to beg for his advice. Our psychotherapy, however, represents a great advance on all the methods previously practised. Whereas formerly the psychic causes of the illness were not investigated,[1] or only superficially investigated, and one only sought to confirm in the patient the certainty that his trouble would soon be at an end, our therapy seeks out the roots of the disease. With our scalpel we go as it were down into the depths till we find the seat of the disease ; this we remove and thus effect a radical cure. The method formerly called the cathartic was re-christened by Freud the psychanalytic method,[2] and requires some practice before it can be employed with success. It does not do to use the psychanalytic method without having thoroughly studied it and having learned its mode of application. Unskilful soul doctors often do more harm than good. Therefore everyone must master the technique before he proceeds to treat severe cases.

Originally Freud employed hypnosis in order to penetrate the unconscious mental life of his patients, and it is an interesting fact that there are followers of Freud who even at the present day prefer this quick and convenient way to the laborious method of psychanalysis. Thus Dr. Arthur Muthmann, e.g., will not give up hypnosis, apparently because he saves himself the trouble of overcoming the resistances of his patients. Freud says : " It is the disadvantage of hypnosis that it conceals the resistance and prevents the physician from gaining an insight into the play of psychic forces. But it does not do away with the resistance, it merely evades it and secures only a temporary understanding and transitory results." Nevertheless, there are adherents of the Freudian theory, such as Muthmann, Frank Bezzola, and others, who give hypnosis

---

[1] In " Wilhelm Meister," Goethe describes an excellent soul doctor. There, too, we find represented incest as the cause of a psychosis (the old harper), a psychic trauma (the Count) and a case of secret guilt (the Countess).

[2] Freud says " psycho-analytic."

the preference. Brodmann, indeed, turns the tables, and prefers hypnosis because in his opinion the cathartic procedure in the waking state mostly has no enduring results.

I have shown by the records of numerous patients that we may achieve complete cures without hypnosis. More! I am of the same opinion as Freud, and use hypnosis only in very rare cases when for two reasons I am prevented from penetrating to the interior of the diseased mind : First, if for lack of time I want to help the patient quickly over a temporary condition ; and secondly, if the patient's lack of intelligence makes the psychanalytic method impossible. Moreover, we must take into consideration that hypnosis is very seldom successful, especially with the phobias. I have repeatedly witnessed Krafft-Ebing's vain attempts to bring about a deep hypnosis in obsessions, in phobias, and in psychic impotence ; even with the help of ether he could not succeed.[1] Only the pure conversion hysterics can be easily hypnotised,[2] those who are free from phobias and obsessions and who have in their nature a certain masochistic component which facilitates their subjection to the hypnotiser. But what do we gain by it ? We may for a moment alter a symptom or put an end to a conversion. But that is surely not our object. We want to liberate *all* repressions and to undertake an education of the patient in the direction of health. We, too, practise with the help of psychanalysis the *Ré-éducation* about which the French psychotherapists are now talking so much. To be sure, as I have already stated, the intelligence of the patient must be on our side. For the fundamental condition for the success of a cure is that the patient accepts the solution, that he brings it to us, that to a certain extent he acquires with us the technique of psychotherapy. He is then in a position to set free little repressions which may set in, even to analyse his unconscious tendencies, to become master of his unhealthy feelings and to overcome his internal resistances. In this education of the patient lies the chief value of the psychanalytic method. Now it is not every intelligence that is capable of going into the fundamental conditions of the method, and understand the connection between repression and illness. But neurotics present in general highly intelligent material, while persons of less intelligence—on the average—suffer much more frequently from dementia præcox. But as in the case of the mechanic, one can now and then achieve a brilliant if not a permanent result by some hypnotic sittings in combination with psychanalytic investigation.

We will now try to sketch the technique of the psychanalytic method. Here Freud employs a certain artifice. He lets his patients lie down during the consultation and sits behind them, so that he cannot be seen by them. This has some advantages.

---

[1] Janet and Raymond also found that the " psychæsthenics " are not hypnotisable (Les phobies et le psychasth. J.S. 124).

[2] Cf. Ferenczi, " Introjektion and Uebertragung." (Jahrbuch, Vol. I.).

Freed from all muscular activity the patient can devote the necessary attention to quietly following up his trains of thought ; also he speaks as it were into the air, because he does not see the analyst. Many women are shy of speaking about sexual matters while looking the doctor in the face.   So that in the way described the resistances of the patients are much more easily overcome.

After the patient has laid his complaints before us we make him a short statement, somewhat as follows : " All that I ask of you during the treatment is attention and sincerity.   You must not hesitate to speak out all that occurs to you.   Some of these ideas it will always seem to you have nothing to do with your illness, they are beside the point.   I beg you to abandon such a censorship of your ideas, and simply bring them before me as they arise. The decision as to whether the ideas are of importance for the understanding of your illness you will leave to me.   It is just such unimportant ideas that may contribute most of all.   Further, I ask you to bring me those ideas also which you may feel shy about repeating, and to do this in spite of all internal resistance.   I repeat that everything may be of importance, that no ideas are beside the point, that on the contrary precisely that on which you lay no weight may for me be most weighty."   One then leaves the patient perfect freedom of speech.

We have already seen in a number of cases what the patient usually begins to talk about.   Mostly it is about their relation to the analyst ; often they begin the story of their illness ; in certain cases again they sit quietly there, speak a few words, and again cease.   This means resistances to the revelation of their unconscious secrets, and these resistances become so strong that the patients fall into a state of momentary imbecility, and when the physician asks what occurs to them, they give the stereotyped answer :   " Nothing occurs to me.   I have nothing to say."   Only after some sittings does one succeed in moving the patient to speech. I prefer, however, to help the patients quickly over these painful first hours.   For there is a golden rule of psychanalysis and that is : Use the first sittings to win the confidence and friendship of the patient.   These once gained you can advance more energetically.   If one does not keep to this rule, but tries too energetically to clear up the resistances then it will often happen that on some pretext or other the patients absent themselves.

It is altogether wrong and incorrect to attack the patient with painful questions and to torment him.   We must not cross-examine the patient. The greater becomes my experience the more careful I become with my questions.   One must quietly leave the patient to make the advances. With patience, everything comes out spontaneously.   The idea that many psychiatrists have that the psychanalyst is a sort of Grand Inquisitor is as ridiculous as it is false.

If, then, one of my patients cannot freely repeat his idea, I set him in the first sittings certain tasks (a method somewhat different

from Freud's), e.g., " In order to cure you I must be thoroughly
acquainted with your life-history. Please tell it me at length.
Begin with your earliest recollection and try to give an epic breadth
to your narration." Then the patients will usually relate their
life-history, though in quite false and perverted fashion. Very few
patients try to be truthful in the first sittings. Most of them do
not like to make exact statements about sex matters that are
painful to them, and women especially have a way of denying in
the first weeks that passion has anything to do with their sexual
life. Thus one constantly hears that the patients have never masturbated, never suffered from sexual phantasies, never had to
contend with sexual temptations, and so on. Women usually add
that their nature is *cold*, " not like the others," that they are
truthful and sincere, that they never told a lie, etc. If the physician
asks about disturbances of the sexual life, he always hears a " No."
This persistent " No " must not disturb him. He must wait
patiently ; the truth will soon come to light. If he were satisfied
with these statements he would surely be duped. In this fashion
we get the false statistics which many physicians publish ; they
have investigated so and so many cases of hysteria and anxiety
neurosis and could detect a sexual origin only in a certain number.
But let him beware of violently trying to overcome this " No."
Let him be cautious in his questions and proceed very slowly.
Especially at first when as yet the patient does not know how
openly he may speak to the analyst.

When the patients have finished their life-history which
indicates what is essential only in a disguised, symbolic form
and tries to hide the truth, then begins the difficult work of the
analyst.   .

The first narrative has given the soul doctor superficial indications.
Freud aptly compares it with a non-navigable stream, its bed now
strewn with rocks, now divided and made shallow by sand banks.
The connections are broken, and the material must now be sifted and
arranged. A clear idea of the difficulty of this work may be gained
by studying the " Bruchstück einer Hysterieanalyse," by Freud
(Monatschr. f. Psychiatrie u. Neurologie, Vol. XVIII., Section 4).
For anyone who wishes to engage in psychotherapy this analysis
is a rich mine of information. But every new analysis presents
a new problem and every patient requires individual treatment.
Of most importance is probably a knowledge of *transference*.

A knowledge of the different forms of transference is for the
analyst the fundamental condition of successful work. Without
exact knowledge of transference the analysis sticks at a dead point
and advances no further. Especially for the beginner it is of the
greatest importance to know the different variations of transference
in order to be able to meet it effectually. I know that I am here
telling most of my colleagues what they have long known. But it
is the duty of those physicians who have long been engaged in

psychanalysis to lay their experience in the details of technique before a public forum and to invite discussion.

"Transference" is one of the most important of Freud's discoveries. It denotes the remarkable fact (whose psychological origins have not yet been investigated) that a patient treated psychanalytically projects all his emotions upon the physician. Chiefly it is the emotion of love, so that many psycho-therapists erroneously believe that transference simply amounts to the patient " falling in love " with his analyst. But in the course of an analysis we find that the patient also hates his physician, that he envies him and regards him as a rival, that he despises and abuses him just as he over-rates him and flatters him.

The question whether the transference is caused by the analysis must be answered with a decided negative. According to a striking phrase of Freud's : Psychanalysis does not create the transference, it only reveals it. We must assume that phenomena similar to transference of the emotions and fixing them on other people occur in every day life ; only so does life become comprehensible to us—an idea for which I have supplied evidence in my book, " The Language of the Dream."

We all have a number of freely floating affects which are always in search of an object to which they can attach themselves. In the neurotic many of these emotions are fixed, which may make him appear incapable of a certain affectivity. He cannot love, cannot hate, etc. Now in psychanalysis these old bonds are loosened and the patient finds himself with a number of affects to dispose of. To whom shall he transfer them when he is treated ? He must project them on to that object which is in the foreground of consciousness. During the treatment this object is, of course, the analyst. Care for his own health is always a person's weightiest interest. In the physician the patient loves and hates himself because he always either identifies himself with the physician or differentiates himself from him.

After these introductory remarks let us now see how in the practice of psychanalysis the transference expresses itself. Let us assume that we have begun to treat a lady with a phobia, who has expressed great doubt as to the success of the " cure," and has only submitted herself to treatment " for her husband's sake and because she will not leave any stone unturned " (lest she should reproach herself later). She comes to the treatment with evident resistances. She appears a quarter of an hour too late—always a bad sign for the future ; she makes merry over the various questions of the physician. She is asked to say what comes into her mind. Nothing occurs to her. Finally, she bestows on us a few scraps of the history of her disease, saying that is all she has to report. So it goes on for a few days, and one almost despairs of the possibility of an analysis. Then one day she comes a quarter of an hour earlier and declares that she finds herself already wonderfully relieved by the few interviews. All at once she has a number of ideas and various things to relate so that the sitting proves too short. This continues for some days and suddenly this lady, without any reason or for some absurd reason, stays away. Now what has happened? The patient has fallen in love with her analyst and unconsciously striving to save her virtue from all danger, the weightiest motive of most neurotics, she takes refuge in flight. The physician should have pointed out to her in good time that a displacement of affect had taken place. The first time she came to him "altered," he should have shown her that she was doing this out of love to him. That she is about to fall in love with him. That this love is a regular phenomenon in psychanalysis and really is a counterfeit love. The physician has taken over the rôle of a beloved person by the way of identification. On the day in question she must, for some reason or other, have identified him with her father or some other person. We all really loved but once and every later love was a substituted love. The physician must in the analysis substitute the objects loved in her youth, and thus make success possible. For one really did everything only from love or hate (defiance).

By the explanation the patient is tranquillised. She feels "that it is all just a game," and that she need not be alarmed for her virtue, since the physician steadily (more or less energetically) rejects her silent love advances and leaves only so much of the transference latent, as he needs to attain success. Once the patient is sure of herself she readily lets fall one protecting veil after another from her innermost soul life. She needs only to know two things : that the physician does not despise her, and that he does not love her.

The other case is much more frequent. A lady comes joyfully to the treatment. She has so much to tell that the time does not suffice. This continues for some days. One day she is silent. She has nothing more to say. She has told "everything." She has finished. The experienced analyst must then notice at once that transference is hindering the further course of the cure. He must beat the transference. Usually a dream will bring him the necessary material. Often the patients conceal these dreams because they are ashamed of them when they are about openly erotic relations between physician and patient.

With men it is the same thing. The never-failing homosexual component renders possible the same erotic projections and identifications as with women.

Without a knowledge of transference and the breaking of it and leading it back to the first love object any further treatment is impossible. I have given only the most important suggestions as to the kinds of ordinary transference because I wish to deal also with forms which are rarer and less known to my colleagues.

The most important form of transference, besides that already discussed—transference to the physician—is transference to the analyst's family. This usually takes a negative form. In dreams and phantasies the physician's wife is the object of much abuse and humiliation. She does not understand the physician, she is mean, ugly, quarrelsome, he ought to have quite a different sort of wife. The dreams show the wife in compromising situations. The whole family becomes the object of abuse. This is also the patient's mode of revenge. He finds the incursions into his family secrets painful, and acts on the principle of *tu quoque*. (If you slaughter my Jews, I will slaughter yours.) The daughter and the son are blamed and made the centre of humiliating phantasies. But the opposite also may happen. The whole family becomes the object of great reverence. We know this form of transference in practical life. A woman is married for the sake of the mother, the father or of the family.

A further variation of this transference is transference to another member of the household. The parlour maid, the cook, the nurse, the butler of the analyst become objects of the transference. This form shows plainly that tendency to revenge for rejected love about which we shall have to speak later. Thus ill-favoured, insignificant servants suddenly become the object of fervent, fanatical devotion. Indeed, it once happened that a patient of mine eloped with a Dulcinea of mature years because I had never thought of the possibility of such a fancy.

Transferences to other members of the household, e.g., to my dog, are not at all rare and admit of a great expenditure of caresses which are really meant for the analyst.

The most remarkable form of transference is transference to the dwelling. Once when I had to move into another house, it struck me how unhappy all the patients were about it. Indeed, one lady wanted to cease coming to me because it would not be so nice as in my " dear old red " room. The affects of the neurotic attach themselves to all the physician's surroundings ; but in his boundless need for love he is still careful to choose objects that are *safe* (dog, dwelling, pictures, Nature, etc.).

And during the treatment the patient's need of love is enormously increased. The old affects rise to the surface of consciousness and look about eagerly for objects. For married people the honeymoon shines again. Women come to the physician to give him thanks. For years their husband has never been so loving. But the business has also its unpleasant sides. In the patient's house, too, transferences to other members of the household take place, if this process is facilitated by an infantile prototype. Several times I discovered in patients as the source of the resistance a positively passionate love for a servant girl, in one case just in time to prevent a great piece of folly. Especially in the case of compulsion neurotics this form of transference seems to be specially favoured. The knowledge of this kind of transference to members of their own household is of extraordinary importance to the analyst. Many an inexplicable stand-still in the cure, many a sudden breaking off of the treatment comes from such a transference within the home-circle. The patient feels as a burdensome bond his unreturned fondness for and his dependence on the physician, and tries to get rid of it. In this effort he hits upon the strangest expedients. From rejected love he falls in love with some other object that happens to present itself. Thus the patient suddenly falls in love with any girl whom he had previously not noticed, and the beginning of many an analysis has, far more than the patient imagines, brought about a marriage. Repeatedly patients became engaged during the treatment, urged immediate marriage, and prematurely broke off the treatment, after having gained, by the result already attained, the degree of freedom which they felt absolutely necessary for life.

These are only a few small examples. I am convinced that there are many more forms of transference which we do not yet know and which, therefore, we cannot deal with in time. It is just experiences of this sort that we must collect and make available for the technique of psychanalysis. For countless are the obstacles which one has to avoid during a cure. And most failures prove nothing against the method ; at the most they reveal the inexperience of the disciples, and the fact that the technique is very difficult. It is important to warn the patients in good time and repeatedly about the transference, if it is not to bring the cure to nought. I remember having treated a lady many years ago who had shown me in her first dreams signs of transference. I thought this was all over because no further symptom indicated it. But I was surprised at her resistance, which was absolutely insuperable. She had no ideas, she had nothing to remember, in short we simply made no progress. Finally I urged her to tell me the cause of her silence, and she promised to write to me ; whereupon I received a glowing love-letter. Of course, it was all over with the cure. Since then, being on my guard, I warn the patients in good time, and explain this phenomenon to them, so that just enough of their affection remains as is indispensable for the cure. This fact was already well known to Feuchtersleben : " The soul doctor awakens love for himself when he gives it, gives it from a warm, true heart. It becomes a longing for him if he husbands it, which his duty demands, for he can hardly live for one patient alone. In this form it is one of the main departments of his treatment. Family life would form (through love) one of the worthy means if it were not, alas ! all too often the source of disease."

Enough of transference ! Let us turn to the interpretation of the " ideas." For this there are a few " rules." Thus the manner in which the ideas are uttered renders possible a sure conclusion

¹Paracelsus, too, is of the same opinion : " We physicians can give our patients nothing but our *love*."

as to the internal resistances. If the ideas come after long pauses, are brought forth with effort, with uncertain pauses one may be sure that they are produced under great resistances and *vice versa*. Often the ideas come in wild confusion and concern subjects apparently quite disconnected. But one must bear in mind that what is brought forth together must be intimately related and then one will never be deceived. Also one must pay no heed to the dubious utterance of reminiscences. As to this Freud says : " When the presentation is dubious one must entirely disregard this change of mind on the part of the narrator. When the presentation oscillates between two forms, it is rather the first expressed that one must consider as correct, the second for a product of repression."

When one gives an interpretation of the ideas one must not be misled by the first " No " of the patient, but listen to what he may say further. The material next produced often confirms the suggestion against the patient's will. The next dream also may bring the definite decision. The repeated " No " of the patient is often only a measure of the magnitude of the repression.

In general the patient exerts his greatest (unconscious) ingenuity in order not to let his secret be extracted from him. It is a continual secret fight between the analyst and the repressed *ego*. During this fight the patient accepts a number of facts which he had violently disputed, and this he does not or will not notice. The patient has a number of " dodges " for deceiving the analyst. Thus long trains of irreproachable thoughts rise up to conceal others which seek to withdraw from criticism and from consciousness (Freud). " A number of reproaches directed against others means a number of self-reproaches of the like content. This automatism proceeds after the pattern of the *tu quoque*."

The ideas have to be arranged, criticised, and employed according to these points of view, and this requires great attention on the part of the physician. The patient will and must feel that the physician is giving him kind attention and that he is noticing everything. In this way he sees what lies ahead and steers straight for his goal.

He must strive to find out the psychic conflicts through which the neurosis originated. During the first weeks and often during the whole cure there is a constant fight between the neurotic and the physician. Every inch of new knowledge must be wrested from the conflict of opinions. This happens most easily when the patient narrates a dream. As yet the patients have no notion that the psychotherapist is master of the art of interpreting dreams. Therefore the first dream is clear and reveals in fairly unequivocal fashion the secret of the neurosis. The exact technique of dream-interpretation is the key to the psychanalytical method. Without the exact knowledge of dream interpretation psychanalysis is simply impossible. The dream also enables us to understand the symbolism of the neurosis, which plays a much greater part than is generally supposed. The dream pictures are ambiguous (over-determined) and are a symbolic representation of unconscious repressed thoughts. To learn dream interpretation the stimulating book of Havelock Ellis, " The World of Dreams," should first be studied. Then my book, " The Language of the Dream," and finally the " Dream Interpretation " of Freud.

To master the technique one must above all investigate the wonderful symbolism of the dream.

He who does not understand the symbolic language of the dream will never be able to interpret a dream, or to perform a completely successful psychanalysis. Many people require a special training for this sort of thinking. At first many a connection seems un-natural, arbitrary and artificial and only the long series of ex-periences that one collects convinces the sceptic that this wit and artificiality is not made by the analysis but is caused by mis-representations of the dream.[1] The technique of dream analysis as well as the knowledge of certain fundamental psychic symptoms can best be learnt from one's own observations. A study of the works above-mentioned is absolutely indispensable. But every-thing cannot be learned from books and even the most experienced dream-interpreter comes across new symbols and new facts. The surest guide is the dreamer himself. At first one confines oneself to asking the dreamer to mention the ideas which occur to him in connection with the dream and to noting these down in the order in which they arise. Then it appears that after the manifest dream-content, the so-called " facade," we learn the latent dream-content only through these communications. For the dream is like a closely woven carpet of whose fine weft we have at the first glance no idea. If one undoes the different knots one sees how many delicate fibrils make up the whole. This phenomenon we call, with Freud, condensation, i.e., in the dream a person or a symbol may be welded together, " condensed " from several images. The whole dream is subject to this condensation and admits therefore of several interpretations. It is determined in several ways. Secondly, in the dream " displacement " plays a great part. The dream is misrepresented by shifting certain affects, qualities, wishes, etc., from one person to another. Thirdly, one must always bear in mind that the dream may deal in contrasts and that things are turned into their opposites. Indeed, the last fact has been a matter of popular knowledge for thousands of years, and even old women used to prophecy if one had dreamt something bad, e.g., of dying, that it meant happiness and *vice versa*. Many dreams

[1] Whereas my book on " Conditions of nervous anxiety " was very well received, my dream interpretations called forth the derision of my colleagues, and in many critiques I was ridiculed. If, however, anyone will give himself the trouble to test my works he will soon, from a Saul, become a Paul. The mastery of the technique of dream-interpretation is the fundamental condition of a rational psycho-therapy.

can be interpreted only if one reads them inverted, *i.e.*, from the end to the beginning. This is one of the strangest forms of dream exposition. Further, anyone who has read the histories of patients in my book will be able to exercise his own skill in various interpretations.[1]

But it is not only the dream from which we get knowledge of the unconscious tendencies. There are other stirrings of the unconscious as to which I must here speak in detail. These are symptomatic acts.; they may often in a lightning-flash, reveal more than a tedious analysis.

Little slips give the psycho-therapist valuable hints. If a patient comes late and misses the time appointed for him, one may be sure that he has resistances against the cure. The patients always excuse themselves by saying they had forgotten. Now forgetting and remembering are worth a special word.

I have shown by some examples that our recollections are biassed and must often be analysed as so-called masking recollections. For the psychotherapist there are no trifles. Even the smallest forgetting of a name may have a psychic motive. As a specimen of how far the repression of unconscious thoughts can go in forgetting I mention the following analysis :—

I once thought of my two Italian patients, whose names I could not recall. Their names have already been mentioned. They are called Askoli and Delorme, which I found it absolutely impossible to recollect. I strain my memory to the utmost ; the names will not come to me ; instead, two substituted names occur to me : Albori and Cantani. As to Albori, it occurs to me that that is the name of a great artist ; but presently I correct myself and say, " No, her name is Alboni." But the daughters of my Mr. A. who will not come to mind, are artists. Hence the connection. I recollect that Albori is the name of a field-marshal which leads me to his Excellence Dl., whom also I have treated, and, be it noted, with little success. I soon realise that I have forgotten the name A, because it is painful to me that he, like Dl., has not remained a faithful patient of mine. Along this track I get no further and I turn to Cantani. What do I know of Cantani ? As to him I have in my mind only a strict diet which may often do harm. He is a professor ; but on D., whose name fails me I, too, have imposed a strict diet and it failed, and even, as the patient falsely believes, did him harm. One of A's sons is also a professor. In the course of analysis Kant's (Cantani) " Macht des Gemütes " occurs to me. Right ! I wanted to act on D. through the Machte des Gemütes, and spoke to his sister about it. What is her name ? Marion—yes—Marie-on ; how beautiful that sounds, and yet only a Marie and an on. The name is really French and " mari " means, of course, husband. Now occurs to me the son-in-law of Mr. A., whose wife is also an artist. His name is Reissmann. I have sent Mr. D. a big account, there I, too, was the Reissman[2] seeing that I had not helped him. *This thought I wanted to forget, sought to repress.* Well now the whole secret is revealed, the names come back to me. They are Askoli and Delorme.

[1] Dream interpretation has received an unexpected impetus. We have penetrated deep into the nature of the dream and have gained abundance of new experiences some of which far surpass those discovered by the genius of Freud. When the " Störungen des Trieb-und Affektlebens " is completed I propose to follow up the " Language of the dream " with a second volume " Progress of Dream-interpretation."

[2] *Reissen* = to eviscerate. [Tr.]

Note the associations :—

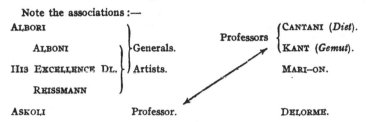

ALBORI
ALBONI } Generals.
HIS EXCELLENCE DL. } Artists.
REISSMANN

Professors { CANTANI (*Diet*).
{ KANT (*Gemut*).

MARI–ON.

ASKOLI   Professor.   DELORME.

I know by heart a glorious poem by Hieronymus Lorm (de Lorme) :—

" *Wass soll mir Freudelosen*
Der Zauber im Gemut "

Between Delorme and mind, then, double threads have spun themselves : Kant and Lorm. The bridge from Delorme to Cantani leads over the recollection of Lorm's poem. This explains how such an utterly different name as Cantani could occur to we.

Consider now the interesting diagram :—

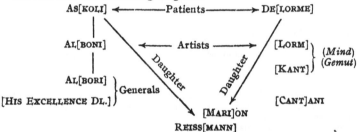

AS[KOLI] ←————Patients————→ DE[LORME]

AL[BONI] ←———— Artists ————→ [LORM] } (*Mind*)
                                [KANT] } (*Gemut*)

AL[BORI] } Generals
[HIS EXCELLENCE DL.] }   Daughter   Daughter

[MARI]ON
REISS[MANN]

[CANT]ANI

Other relations may be found. The three parts of words : koli—boni—bori are only apparently without significance. Koli = weights ; boni = the good. The whole business is with weighty (Koli), good (boni) patients whom I had lost.

The following is also noteworthy :—

ASK o L I.
ALB o R I.
ALB o N I.

The vowels, A, O, I, are in all three words the same. The consonants :—

S K L
L B R
L B N

give the words sekel, leber [liver], leben [to live] which seem to be not without relation to the whole psychic process. I will not dispute that it may be an accident ; but one comes uncommonly often upon such strange chances.

This sort of " running off the mental rails " may be of the greatest importance for psychanalysis. Thus, a patient comes under my care and tells of a lady who was *incomprehensibly* beautiful. He meant to say *indescribably*. I knew at once that for him the lady was *incomprehensible* in a double sense, and that was in fact the whole of his trouble. Then, too, the manner in which the patients come to the physician betrays a great deal of their secret purposes. If they come willingly to the cure then they are always a few minutes before their time ; if they are late or for any reason cry off, then one may be sure that this is caused by internal resistances, even when they have seemingly sound reasons. A strange symptomatic procedure was exhibited by a patient with compulsion neurosis, whose imagination was so filled with skatological things that I seemed to myself to be a cleanser of sewers in Neitzche's sense. This man always rushed into my room and begged me for a key[1]. That at once symbolised his train of thought. He also spoke of feeling as if there were dried fæces in his brain. He came to me to unload his dung. It is just through the elucidation of such little symptomatic acts that one may win the patient to oneself. The true psychotherapist passes unnoticed no phenomenon of the psychic life. Thus a lady tells me that she has occasionally had an hallucination.

No. 139.—" Oh, I very often have hallucinations. Only yesterday in a furniture shop I had a vision of a man."

" Can you give me any idea of what he looked like ? "

" I cannot describe him exactly. A light-brown pointed beard, velvet coat and grey trousers, like the officers wear in summer."

" As far as I know the trousers of our officers are always drab, not grey. Are you sure you mean the summer trousers ? "

" You are right, but my husband who was reserve-officer has had them dyed mouse-grey and the trousers of this phantom were of the same colour."

" Of whom did this phantom remind you ? "

" That is remarkable. Of a gentleman who is editor of a literary paper."

" What is his name ? "

" Kanner, the editor of a paper called ' The Hour ' "

" Had you previously spoken of an hour ? "

" Oh yes ! I said to the shopmen who served me : ' Make haste, my hour is up.' "

" Now, what about this Mr. Kanner ?[2]"

" When I was young he was supposed to be a great admirer of mine. I never spoke to him and do not know why he should have come into my head."

" That we will soon get at. He had a pointed beard, you say ? Now what did the shopmen look like ? "

" He was blonde and had a similar beard."

" Did he pay court to you ? "

" No—stop a moment, though, he said to me (when I bargained a long time about the price) : ' I did not know that such beautiful young ladies could be so naughty." —

" Three compliments then. Beautiful, young and naughty. For you know the Viennese ladies when they say to any one, ' Oh, you naughty one,' convey a secret, almost admiring recognition of ' naughtiness.' But we have not yet finished. Why should this hallucination choose a furniture shop for its appearance ? "

" I may be because since my childhood I have experienced an inexplicable fear in a furniture shop. I always think there must be someone in a corner, behind a chest or a sofa who might spring out. I was with my husband in such a shop, lately. He went on in front with the salesman, I remained behind alone. I suddenly experienced this inexplicable fear and hastened forwards."

" But the phantom that you saw, the editor who admired you, was surely not fear inspiring and frightful ? But how came this editor to have officer's trousers ? Is he a reserve officer ? "

" I think not, but now, strangely enough, something quite different occurs to me, namely a tall count, strikingly handsome, whose brother once courted me."

" Another silent admirer, like Mr. K., the shopman and others with light-brown pointed beards."

[1] Key—for opening lavatory door.
[2] Notice the question : Kann–er ? (Can he ?)

If we analyse this hallucination it appears that we have here the disguised fulfilment of a wish. The anxiety in the furniture shop has the same meaning as that fear which young girls experience when they are alone with the men they love, fear of the fulfilment of their longing, a contrast with the wishfulfilment called forth by the repression of various thoughts unpleasant to the waking consciousness. The phantom has been altered by condensation like a dream-picture. It has the features of three persons : of the admirer, of the husband in his most important character as trouser-wearer, and as officer. Her anxiety is well-founded, she is really attacked in the furniture shop and by a man, too, who combines in himself all the charms of manhood. A wish of the unconscious which has taken form and colour.

What then has happened in this hallucination ? The unconscious has projected its thought associations outwards as in a dream.

The four sets of thoughts—admirer—editor—husband—officer—are fused into one picture.

The further enquiry shows that the lady also suffers from anxiety conditions and anxiety dreams. She is afraid of burglars and robbers, looks every night under the beds, suffers from palpitation of the heart, and anxious expectation. In short she presents the typical picture of an anxiety neurosis. In consequence of the slight potency of her husband she is always unsatisfied.

With such artifices one may overcome the resistance of patients. There are, it is true, various round-about ways by which one may arrive at the truth. Such a method has been diligently studied by Bleuler and Jung—the association experiment. Jung has distinguished himself by the development of this method and has published several patients' histories which show that with the help of his association experiment he has arrived at the basis of the repressed complexes.

He takes a series of words which he calls " *stimulus-words,*" and then causes the person experimented on to say a second word which the stimulus-word suggests to him. This he calls the *reaction.* He notes the reaction period. Then he repeats the stimulus-word and here and there it occurs that the " reproduction " is incorrect. He knows now by the manner of the reaction whether with the stimulus-word he has come upon a complex or not. According to Kræpelin the probable average reaction in normal persons is 2.4 seconds. Jung thinks the figure too high and estimates the reaction period at 1.5 seconds. When the reaction occurs only after a long time there is evidently a great resistance which proceeds from the repressed complex. This resistance expresses itself also in the second reaction of the next stimulus-word which Jung calls " perseveration."

I consider this method as a laborious détour since the phenomenon of transference is concealed, and that therefore it is not to be recommended for psychanalytical practice. I have introduced a modification of this association experiment which seems to be indicated by Freud in the "Studien über Hysterie." Freud states there : " I had a patient who brought me her ideas in words. These words came out in jerks and only as a supplement she gave me their explanation."

As I have already shown, I manage this method thus : in the analysis of a dream, *e.g.*, when nothing occurs to the patient, I say to him the puzzling word in question, and ask him to name a number of words which then happen to occur to him. From these words the meaning of the stimulus-word can generally be found, and from it the whole series may be evolved. One may also use this expedient by asking the patient to say twenty, thirty or more words as they happen to occur to him. Usually he begins with objects which he sees in the room—to avoid this one may ask him to close his eyes—and then utters a series of words which mostly relate to the complex one wishes to discover. Often one of the words cannot be explained ; then one must quietly[1] wait. In the next few days the desired interpretation comes as by chance. With the help of this free association principle introduced into psycho-therapy by me one may circumvent many a patient's resistance and explain many a dark problem. But I am free to confess that now I very seldom have recourse to the method. I unearth the resistance more readily as transference, and can fully support Freud when he says that at the beginning of the cure the chief thing is combatting the resistance. Once the resistances are overcome the psychanalytic work proceeds in faultless fashion.

The cure is a ceaseless fight between the inertia of the neurosis and the progressive tendencies of the patient. The beginner in psychanalysis has no idea of the difficulties of the treatment which I have sketched in detail in the last two chapters of the fourth volume (appendix). Often the physician finds only when it is too late that the patient has got the best of him. He must constantly be on his guard and have an exact knowledge of all evasions and circumventions, all feints, parries and stratagems, all dodges and traps of the neurotic.[2]

Plain speech on sex subjects, especially with ladies, presents great difficulties to the beginner. Hence many a psychotherapeutic failure may be traced to the physician's neglect of that diplomatic procedure which alone can guarantee success. We must never forget that the whole of our modern system of society is built up on the principle of lying and suppression of the instincts. Especially in sex matters it is rarely that one person speaks the whole truth to another. That women at first never have the candour to discuss sex matters openly and freely is an established fact with which the physician must reckon. One would not think it possible with what decision and with what dramatic skill women ordinarily deny that of which they are ill and on which later they dilate in epic

---

[1] This method published in the first edition of the "Anxiety Conditions" (1908) has now been re-discovered and described by Neutra (Seelenmechanik und Hysterie. Leipzig, 1920. *p.* 200).

[2] An almost complete representation of the characterology of the neurotic is to be found in my collections of essays : " Nervous people " and " What there is at the bottom of the mind." " Disguises of Love." " The Beloved Ego." " The will to live."

style. The art of the psychotherapist consists in patiently failing to hear the " No," to investigate further without prejudice and to wait till the " No " changes to " Yes." The great essential is that the discussion of these things shall take place with high scientific earnestness. Once the patients understand that it is not a case of frivolities but of "material" which is necessary for understanding the history of this disease, they are very soon ready to respond to the open tone of the physician and to tell him the truth in all things without reserve. One must not try to force them, one must not make the psychanalytical interview into the inquisitorial rack. That is foreign to the nature of the analysis. He who has patience will find the ripe fruit drop into his lap. Women are happy when for once they can talk freely. Then one is amazed to find (and the analyses of disease-histories have proved this) with what force the hidden stream of sexuality pours through the minds of women. One must take care not to proceed too abruptly and thus expose oneself to the reproach of soiling the purity of an innocent being by forcing knowledge upon it. We never tell the patients anything new. We get the facts out of the patients. Often a week or two passes before the necessary contact is found and the patient has been educated up to the conviction that the physician does not despise him on account of his confessions. That is all most people care about. The stereotyped phrase after making a confession is : " I tell you this at the risk of your despising me," or " What ever will you think of me ? " The patients all seem to themselves wicked, abandoned, sinful. From this feeling of guilt, there grows in them an oppressive feeling of their own inferiority. The neurotic over-estimates the world around him and under-estimates himself. Often he exhibits the compensatory converse of this : contempt of the world and megalomania.

If with our patients we achieve only one thing : show them what in their individual fate is common to humanity—we have already rendered them a great service. I can, then, only advise every beginner once more to treat very carefully what through shyness has been carefully concealed. *The more gently one approaches the delicate tissue of neurotic fantasies, the more surely one avoids the danger of increasing the patient's resistance till it becomes stark self-defence, and of losing the patient. The tact of the man of the world, individual delicacy, imperturbable calm as well as great patience are absolutely necessary to attain the goal.*

The old Latin dictum, " *Primum non nocere* " holds for psychotherapy also. Freud has pointed out that a false psychotherapeutic procedure may do harm, and has called the methods of many colleagues who wish to conduct psychanalysis without the necessary schooling, " *Wild psychanalysis* " (Centr. f. P.-A. Vol. I.). I could cite quite a number of cases in which through misapprehension of its principles psychanalysis has done more harm than good. What shall one think of a colleague who says to a woman : " You are suffering from insufficient satisfaction. Your husband does not satisfy you ! " After the next coitus the woman raises a tremendous row with her husband. " Now I know what is wrong with me. You don't satisfy me ! " and she falls ill with a serious depression of spirits. That is psycho-therapy falsely conceived. For such things should be told at most to the husband, never to the wife. Mostly the relations are more complicated and the trouble has arisen through some psychic conflict which can be discovered only after some time. The man does not satisfy his wife because she loves another or because she is homosexual.

Equally incorrect is it to give patients advice which is beyond our competence. I can recommend a young man sexual intercourse and suggest all sorts of protective measures against infection. But I must not say to a young girl : " Get a lover, then you will be healthy ! " How easily through such false psycho-therapy one may drive an inexperienced girl into the gravest conflicts ! If she is frivolous she finds the remedy without our help. If she is hyper-moral like most neurotics, then by such advice we may make her illness worse. The fact is we must not say all we know. There are facts which one must keep to oneself.

I warn all my colleagues against taking psychanalysis so lightly and seeing a cure-all in sexual satisfaction when this is very difficult and to be attained through great moral sacrifices. The neuroses are complicated psychic fabrics. Clumsy hands must not touch them but rather keep to the old (though not approved) methods. Only a noble, a thinking person can be a good mental physician. Such a specialist must have a special aptitude and psycho-therapy can never be the work of the practising physician. He must know the connections and in slight cases give the proper advice. But never let one unacquainted with the perplexities of psychanalysis venture on a complicated psycho-neurosis before he has acquired the necessary knowledge. It would be best if every physician who wishes to learn psychanalysis would have himself analysed. For after all one always learns most quickly on one's own body and one's own mind.

We have already mentioned that a dose of philosophy certainly belongs to the gifts which the mental physician must possess. Often he can render a cure possible by widening the view of the individual shut within the narrow horizon of the neurosis. Finally the psychotherapist must take an interest in the patient's private affairs and, where permissible, interpose. The patients are work-shy and must with gentle force be got back into the habit of work ; work is everywhere recognised as a remedy. We make our task easier if we get the patient to deprive himself by regular work of the possibility of thinking about his illness. That we do not abandon all the other remedies of psycho-therapy goes without saying. We shall use the great power which we acquire over the patients to influence them favourably in every way, to strengthen their confidence, to restore

their joy in life. Often the neurotics are would-be suicides who are trying psycho-therapy as a last resort. Such patients must be helped over the most difficult days by the assurance that they can certainly be helped, they have only not to lose patience, and so on. The physician must not conduct a merely passive analysis as Freud and his school require. He must also take an active part, correct the patient's false notions, direct his gaze to an attainable goal. In my essay, "Die Ausgänge der psychoanalytischen Kuren" (Centralbl. für Psycho-Analyse, Vol. IV., *p.* 295, 1913) I say :
" To reconcile the patient with reality, that is the task of psychoanalysis. Thus the mental physician must act as educator and therefore the profession of analyst demands men above the average, to a certain extent creative artists, who in fact can form human beings. Analysis, according to the apt expression of Dr. Martin, must be followed by synthesis.[1]

We are frequently reproached for imputing to the patient things which he himself does not believe. Anyone who has gained some insight into the technique of psycho-therapy will admit that this is not possible. The patient brings us the material and this material itself contains the solution. If the solution is wrong, the patient does not accept it, and there is no result. The more passive the physician remains during the cure the greater the success. And all the time the physician must maintain his equanimity. The patient often identifies the physician with those persons of whom he cannot help thinking so often. To-day he feels love for him, to-morrow hate or distrust. But he must always feel that the physician understands his misery and is animated by only one wish —to help him. This feeling steadies him throughout the cure.

Yet a few words on the results of psychanalysis. Psychanalysis is a continual fight between the physician and the patient. It depends on his attitude of defiance or obedience (Alfred Adler) whether he ends the cure a healthy man or a sick one. For many patients do not let the physician have the triumph of having cured them, and leave him apparently not cured, and then get cured by some indifferent means—or indifferent physician. Again the patient must get used to doing without the physician, and also learn to get on without the "psychic morphia of psychanalysis." That is more difficult than one would believe. Hence most of the best results make their appearance only some time after the analysis. The patient, to defy the physician, retains some of the symptoms for a time until they have lost their meaning, that is their tendency to injure the physician. Considered from this standpoint, the successes of psychanalysis are far greater than has been here estimated. For after a psychanalytical cure many patients go to other doctors and complain of the wretched psychanalysis which

---

[1] The demand for a psycho-synthesis is now made with special energy by the Zürch school (Jung). Freud strongly opposes this demand and contents himself with the analysis.

has failed to help them.   This is their revenge because the physician has not fully met their exorbitant claims to love and attention. From these sources come the triumphs of the opponents of psychanalysis, who evermore repeat with scorn that patients have come to them whom psychanalysis had failed to help, and who were only cured by them.

These are only some of the most important principles of psychanalytical technique.   One should begin with the little easy cases[1] such as occur every day and proceed gradually to greater tasks. The difficulties once surmounted, one is richly rewarded by the possibility of assisting many people whom previously one could not help.   No expert comes ready-made into the world.

" The first of everything finds an abiding place in the child ; the first colour, the first music, the first flower, tinge the foreground of its life ; but here we can as yet lay down no law but this ; shield the child from all that is violent and severe even if these give sensations which at the time are pleasant."—*Jean Paul*.

---

[1] Jung (Die Freudsche Hysterienlehre, etc.) gives this advice : A perfectly harmless but extremely instructive exercise is, e.g., the analysis of the constellations of a complex association arrived at by experiment.   Dream— and hysteria—analyses are considerably more difficult and are therefore less suitable for the beginner.

CHAPTER XXXVII

PROSPECTS

I HAVE come to the end of my discussions of the origin and treatment of anxiety conditions. It remains to collate the numerous experiences we have collected and to answer the most important question of all : *What are the ways and means to prevent the occurrence of anxiety conditions ?*
Anyone who speaks of the regeneration of humanity, anyone who dreams of a better, more beautiful time, must first help to lighten the vast mass of foolish, senseless anxiety which burdens civilised mankind. We have only to look around us to see how tremendously widespread are these anxiety conditions which hinder as nothing else does the full development of one's powers.

If the affects could be measured, if mental tortures could be weighed, set before us in figures like a tangible material, a statistician might make it his life-task to reckon up the sum of all anxiety affects ; then we should have a gigantic total, a vast ocean of human suffering, ever filled anew by the tears of the wretched.

Humanity is over-burdened with anxiety. In whichever direction we look, everywhere we find anxiety. Anxiety for oneself and for others. All the joys of life are in danger of being drowned in this sea of anxiety.

The joy of life is a sensation felt only by the rarest of mankind, and by them only in certain moments. There is constantly interposed the dread spectre of anxiety, and this is fundamentally always fear of death or fear of annihilation. Mankind's consciousness of guilt is excessive. Anxiety is the manometer of this guilt consciousness.

I have striven so far as my weak powers permit to show that one may cure anxiety conditions by mental treatment. But more important than the therapy of anxiety conditions is their prophylaxis.

It is certain we are all suffering from repression. We are all suffering from moral hypocrisy. We are all suffering from the impressions of a lying age which hides the truth like a coward, and sets lies on the throne. The cause of all mental diseases including nervous anxiety conditions is repression. One sees in the cure with what relief the patients breathe again, how they seem to be freed from a great burden if they can speak out about everything *sine ira et studio.* Our society must be placed on an altogether different basis if we wish to carry out an active prophylaxis of the neuroses.

Is such a prophylaxis at all possible ? Is not the idea a utopian delusion ?

He who has carefully read the foregoing pages can himself give the answer. From them it is unmistakably plain that the cause of all anxiety is the repression and violation of the sex instinct as of the instinctive life in general. Thus if we wished to be consistent we should demand a freedom of sex relations which would make any repression or violation superfluous. Now that is certainly a demand whose fulfilment partly for ethical, partly for educational reasons is impossible. We have seen what a powerful part in the phantasies of the neurotic is played by incest thoughts and paraphilias as well as by criminal phantasies, how in the edifice of the neurosis they are as it were the foundation. We shall not be so rash as to plead for tearing down the barriers of incest and of ethics, and for setting free the criminal instincts. We can only show the way to hinder such incest thoughts from arising and to sublimate the asocial instincts, i.e., to transform them into social forces.

But we will deal later with pathological sexual emotions. First, what is the estimation of the normal feelings ?

Unfortunately, in our time sexuality is so intimately bound up with the idea of sin that even the normal feelings of the " modest " youth and the " pure " maiden are looked on as guilty and may lead to neurosis. *The consciousness of guilt is the chief cause of all neuroses and psychoses.* If we wish to prevent neuroses we must have a freer, more natural conception of sexual processes. For this one must get to know oneself, one must recognise, as Freud aptly says, on what hollow ground our virtues stand. Only the recognition of our own weaknesses enables us to understand the weaknesses of our fellow-beings, and that saying whose mild splendour has for thousands of years illumined our path, the saying : " He that is without sin among you, let him cast the first stone at her," ought to be the motto of every human being if he seeks to give judgment on sexual transgressions and the criminal aberrations of the miserable and the misguided. Even the criminal is, as Klages shows in his " Prinzipien der Charakterologie "[1] a product of his time.

A free natural world which does not anxiously hide these things but discusses them openly, will offer little or no occasion for repressions. Where there are no sins there are no neuroses. *This is not to say that we advocate a boundless sexual indulgence.* But it is just the secrecy with which the sex life is surrounded, the temptation of the forbidden which lends it its charm, the mystery of it all, all this serves to transform the sexual need from a natural act to a fall into sin. Frivolous and obscene talk are products of

[1] Published by Johann Ambrosius Barth, Leipzig, 1910.

a diseased age. Open transparent truth must prevail if the natural is to be viewed naturally.

But the most important thing is the revision of our moral code. A more healthy moral code would bring about a more healthy view of life. The present code has turned the natural sexual instinct into a source of vice. Are people then not aware of the importance of this instinct? Nietzche has somewhere stated it plainly: "*The degree and the nature of a person's sexuality reaches up into the topmost pinnacle of his spirit.*"

It is Freud's inestimable merit that in spite of the tremendous resistance of his fellow-experts he has spread abroad a knowledge of the importance of sexuality for our whole life.

This holds for humanity in general. But the prophylaxis of neurosis must begin in youth. We have seen what a damaging influence infantile traumas, and yet more the imperatives of the teacher, which act as traumas, and again especially the sharpening of his ambition and the spoiling by overtenderness have on the life of a human being. Indeed, one may confidently say : The sexual fate and with it the fate of the man are decided in childhood. Peter Altenberg, the bizarre philosopher, whose knowledge of mankind often shows flashes of positive genius, once uttered a wonderful saying, somewhat as follows : "When I see a mother who has brought her children in health through puberty to manhood, I should like to stand to attention before her, and take my hat off to her." Indeed, a teacher can have no greater merit than to have added to the ranks of the full-grown the child whom he has reared as a healthy human being. Now, hitherto we have made a sad mistake in believing that the sexual education begins only at puberty, that before this the child is a sexless being, with no idea of erotic things and no feeling for sexual things. That this assumption is ruinous, fundamentally false, I do not need here to argue over again. Twenty-four years ago, in my study on "*Coitus in childhood*," I pointed to infantile sexuality and its consequences to the individual. To-day, I can only repeat with the utmost emphasis that the sexual prophylaxis of an individual and therewith the prophylaxis of his anxiety ideas begins with the day of his birth. As early as that we notice in the child frequent sexual · excitations which demand increased attention. In the boys we notice erections ; we notice that the girl holds her hand to the vagina in order to produce pleasurable feelings by touching it. Generally it is peripheral stimuli which lead to these first sexual excitements. The experienced physician will seek out all those causes (eczema, worms, too tight clothing) which may bring about such conditions. But he will not omit to point out to the parents that unscrupulous nurses and wet-nurses frequently use stimulation of the genitals to quiet the infant.

Grown-up girls are carefully watched and it is a matter of serious consideration to whom they shall be entrusted. But in the choice of those who are to bring up little children many parents are unscrupulously easy-going, in fact, unconscientious. A strange servant girl just from the country, or from the slums of the great town, is given the care of the child ; the parents go their way and trouble themselves no more.

While the parents are blind to the traumas from the attendants, they fall upon the children with fury if they find they are masturbating. All the terrors of earth and hell are set in motion to keep the child from masturbating. Its hands are tied at night, a girdle of virginity is put on, bromide is ordered by the physician. The child is told that it will be imbecile and crippled if it continues this frightful " vice." *These are the most serious traumas for the children.* For the traumas through servants are not so dangerous. In certain circumstances they are borne quite well, and they prevent the child being too closely attached to the parents and the family. I confess openly that I have over-estimated the pathogenic power of the traumas caused by seduction. The traumas of the educators are much more serious.

Masturbation is harmless so long as human unreason does not make it a crime, and load it with the consciousness of religious and hygienic guilt. All children masturbate—some more, some less. Mankind would be a race of pitiable objects of utter imbeciles if masturbation were injurious. But the well-meant warnings of guardians and the false notions of physicians have turned many a masturbator into a neurotic. *I recommend all parents, physicians and educators not to trouble about masturbation in the children and at most to try by distractions and by tiring them out to get them to give up excessive masturbation.*

Yet more important is supervision of the children at a later age when they eagerly catch up every word and at once assimilate every new impression. For one thing must be kept in mind. *The later a child of the more cultured classes becomes familiar with the crude expressions of sexuality, the greater is its chance of becoming a mentally normal, happy human being.* Many parents are so anxious about this supervision that they never leave the child alone for a second ; they let it sleep in their bedroom until puberty and later. Now if coarse sexual trauma has its great dangers, it is not to be denied that the parents' excessive fondness has almost greater. Supervision of the children does not mean over-indulgence and blind partiality.

For one remarkable fact must be noted. In our time the tenderness of parents positively increases from year to year. Fanatics for tenderness among parents, now found everywhere, were formerly exceptions. To-day parents think of nothing else than the child : how they shall feed it, educate it, clothe it hygienically, harden it, how they shall impart facts about sex to it. A flood of books and periodicals scarcely meets the enormous demand. Can this be due simply to the fact that women's efforts for emancipation have

transferred the wife's interest from the husband to the child ?
That cannot possibly be the only cause.

The cause of hypertrophied love for children is to be found by
considering those cases where in former times parental fondness
was exaggerated to idolatry. Spoilt children were almost always
only children, called in popular language, "trembling joy."

Unhappily most modern families consist of such "trembling
joys." Neo-Malthusianism has permeated everywhere. In consequence of the countless, generally permitted means of anti-concep-
tion, the number of births continually decreases. The two-children
system is the rule, the more-children system, especially in well-to-do
families, the exception. Even the noted fertility of the Germans
which is constantly held up to the French as an example, will soon
belong to the past. In Berlin in former decades there were 220
births to 1,000 married women ; from 1873 to 1877 there was in
fact an increase to 231. Since then the number of births has
fallen from year to year, and in 1904 there were only 111 births
to 1,000 married women. In other great towns this proportion
is even worse than in Berlin. At the same time the number of
marriages does not decrease. In Prussia in the years 1901 to
1904 it was 8 per 1,000, while in 1850 it was a little less, viz., 7.8
per 1,000. Let us then note the fact that the two-children system
is the cause of excessive parental tenderness. Now what are its
evils ?

I will not here set forth the well-known evils at length. That
pampered children are seldom self-reliant, that they cannot adapt
themselves to circumstances, that they seem to be defenceless
against the blows of fate, all this is well-known. We need waste
no more words over it. More important is the fact that exaggerated
tenderness to the child, creates in the child a correspondingly great
need for tenderness. A need for tenderness that violently demands
satisfaction. As long as such children are little this need is completely met. The parents, and especially the mother, are so
overjoyed at the proofs of their children's love that they simply
lavish caresses upon them. And so the indulgences increase instead
of gradually diminishing. Now the child has to go to school.
For the first time in its life it is confronted with the will of a stranger
demanding neither tenderness nor love, only joyful work. How
easily then conflicts arise. The child thinks its teacher does not
love it ; at a rough word it shrinks, begins to cry. It begins to
hate the school ; it learns unwillingly. It wants another school,
other teachers. If its wish is granted, the same game soon begins
again.

When such children grow up the case is much worse. They have
an insatiable need of tenderness. From them come the women
who by their excessive love kill their husband's love. Daily, nay
hourly, they must receive sweet endearing terms, private pet-
names, kisses innumerable. If they are men they are very rarely

satisfied with their wives ; they make up outside the deficiency
of tenderness at home ; or they transfer this need to the children,
who thus inherit a sad burden. But that is not the worst.
*The greatest danger for the child is that it remains fixated to the
family and so becomes unfit for life.* The bipolarity of all phenomena
is maintained here. The servants really fulfil an important educative mission by directing the child to objects beyond the limits
of incest. We have in fact a false method in education. We try
to chain the children to the family by countless bonds of love,
when we should educate them for life. We educate the children
for ourselves, not for their own existence and their future. We
ought to make them into free human beings and to facilitate their
liberation from the family. Excessive severity and excessive love
are injurious. We should not give them occasion for overpowering
love and overpowering hate. Even at a very early age they must
be left a certain freedom of action and of choice, and above all
we must try to make them *self-reliant and free from any consciousness
of guilt.*
Let us be a little more careful with our indulgences and our
severity. Let us beware of over-strong imperatives. And let
us not burden the children with our claims on their love and
gratitude.

The greatest dangers of excessive tenderness consist in a premature excitement of the erotic sensations. We so easily forget
unpleasant experiences. Hence most adults have no recollection
of the erotic experiences of their youth. Parents especially excel
in this forgetfulness with regard to their children, a forgetfulness
that almost borders on hysterical amnesia. Hence most mothers
swear by the innocence of their daughters, the fathers by the purity
of their sons. They imagine that their children are an exception,
that they are unspoilt, that they still believe in the stork and other
similar nonsense.

*In sexual matters people's behaviour is incredibly naive. They
shut their eyes and will not see.* With what good reason does Frank
Wedekind scoff at a world which has secrets from itself. Thus
infantile sexuality is a secret which all the initiated know. If only
parents kept it in mind ! Then it would not happen that the
children until their tenth year and later must sleep in the parents'
bedroom so that the careful parents may observe the dear creatures'
lightest breath. That the children may get impressions there
which are extremely harmful for them, the parents do not choose
to think. I have given enough examples of this in the chapter
on the anxiety neurosis of children.

One might object that, among the lower classes, living together
is quite the usual thing and that nevertheless one seldom finds
neuroses among the workers. The explanation is simple. Poor
people have *many* children. Frustrated excitations are rare. All
these people are much more free from prejudice in their way of

looking at sexual life, so that repression plays a smaller part. With simple people quite other factors are decisive. When there is neurosis the repressions are caused by religious inhibitions. The idea of sin weighs heavily on the instincts of people who otherwise are not " sicklied o'er with the pale cast of thought." It is fear of the tortures of hell that drives them into the Inferno of neurosis. But in proportion to the educated upper stratum the great mass of the people contributes but a small contingent especially in the case of anxiety hysteria. Also the poor trouble far less about the children than do the rich. The child is left more to itself, has greater freedom to move about and can easily dissipate its exuberant energies in motor action. It is not tied to the family. It does not become a father's or mother's own boy. It does not attach itself to any sister or to a brother from whom it never more gets free. The oppressive narrowness of bourgeois family life, which tries to bring children to maturity in a pedagogically moral incubator is a factor by no means to be under-estimated in the etiology of the neuroses.

To those factors which may prematurely excite erotic feelings belongs also excessive tenderness. Between the tenderness of a lover and that of a mother there is really no difference. Both kiss, caress, press to the heart, pamper, embrace, squeeze, stroke. That stimulation of the peripheral nerves leads the excitations to the same central organs is clear. Thus the child gets its first erotic sensations from those who look after it. One may explain it as always, the wet-nurse, the nurse, the mother, the father, are the first love of the child, the first erotic love. This must not be taken to mean that I condemn affectionate intercourse with children. On the contrary ! A certain degree of tenderness is even necessary for normal development. *Only the tenderness must not be excessive.* Thereby the child is brought prematurely into a condition of erotic over-stimulation.

It cannot be too often repeated : we fuss over the children too much. There is too much theorising about bringing them up. We give them too much attention. Let us leave them their peaceful childhood, their merry play, the marvellous activity of their tireless phantasy. *Let us honestly admit that from our excessive tenderness we get great pleasure, the children great harm.* Let no mother be prevented from being tender with her children, from giving them loving attention, from making their youth as pleasant as possible. But parental tenderness should not find expression in mechanical actions. It should be an equable glow which warms but kindles no fire, and only on the great feast-days of life breaks into bright flame.

A further danger for the health of the child consists in the unhappiness of so many marriages. Unsatisfied women vent their need for tenderness on the children. Or they early drag the child into the quarrels of the adults. Freud observes : " The bad understanding between the parents excites the emotional life of the child, and causes it at the most tender age to feel intensely love, hate and jealousy. Strict bringing up, which permits no activity of the sexual life so early aroused, is a repressive force and this conflict at this age contains all that is necessary for a life-long nervousness."

That over-strictness presents the same dangers as over-tenderness, who will deny? The barbarous punishment of whipping in the parental home is responsible for many a neurosis.

Let the child be brought up with uniform energy, not too strictly and not too indulgently, for we have seen that strictness may be just as dangerous as mildness. Boys too strictly brought up, but indulged by the mother, look on the father as an oppressor and a torturer, which is a source of endless psychic conflicts for them. Also masochistic and sadistic tendencies arise in this way.

Little children should not be allowed to take part too often in the conversation of adults, and should be given the opportunity of mixing with children. Czerny justly remarks that the permanent company of adults constitutes for children a great burden on the brain. By every possible means one must try to avoid the premature stirring of erotic powers in the child. One will not always succeed. In many cases the impulses are so powerful that they break out without external stimulus. In infants one notices erections even in the first weeks, also various onanistic movements and manipulations. *Let us not take these phenomena too seriously.* Experience shows that, in the absence of external stimuli, this period of the first sexuality soon passes. It is part of the prophylaxis of anxiety feelings not to subject children to excessive fright, or to terrify them with gruesome stories and old wives' tales. They must early be trained to courage which can just as well be attained by a certain mental gymnastic as other mechanical and mental acquirements.

Education in fear is so thoroughly instilled by frightened mothers who tremble for the lives of their darlings, that the legion of anxiety-neurotics and hypochondriacs will never die out. Education through fear is itself a sad fault. This I say in opposition to Czerny who considers fear indispensable in the nursery. There is, however, only one education: through love and through one's own example.

It is injurious to spur on the child's ambition, to set great aims before it, to increase its self-love beyond bounds. The converse of this training, incessant blame, threats and grumbling produce an oppressive feeling of inferiority. It is of the greatest importance to inoculate the child early with social feelings and to educate it in sympathy, which alone can overcome the great enemy of mankind, brutal egoism, the egoism which in the world-war and afterwards broke out with such horrible force.

The task of the parents is to form free human beings, free from all superstition, free from all feeling of guilt, free from the fear of hell and the punishments of hell, of heavenly judges who weigh our every word. Let the child learn to do what is good—out of love to the good. Let it early learn to be truthful and courageous with itself; learn the courage to admit to itself its weaknesses and faults and to strive to convert them into strength and into advantages.

One important question cannot be avoided here, a question which is talked about everywhere, discussed in countless pamphlets, about which the greatest mental battles are fought: When and where shall we enlighten our children?

We have shown that one question is much more important and this is: How the children should not be enlightened? As to the positive question, I am a decided opponent of the enlightenment[1] system which is being advocated, and in which I see really a mental epidemic, a sort of psychic exhibitionism. This treatment of children is certainly a little perverse.

Enlightenment *en masse* in schools, as is proposed, is a monstrous idea, whose execution would certainly start countless sexual traumas. The method of natural science also seems to me impracticable. The question can only be solved individually, and best in this way: from the time the child reaches a certain age, the parents mingle sex subjects with their talk, taking them as matter of course, without solemn emphasis and mysterious ceremonies. The children should become acquainted gradually with the matter of course, and *everything* must not be too early explained to them. For let us not forget that the root of all desire to know is to be found in curiosity about sex and that a premature enlightenment of the children would certainly be injurious to the development of humanity.

And many impulsive powers would be lost to the individual which are absolutely necessary for the development of his personality. We should create certainly a race of healthy persons, but not persons of genius. The connections between genius and neurosis show this. The case is quite different when the children have passed the age of puberty and have come to be adults. Such children must be treated as adults, and the simplest way is to speak openly and freely with them about sex matters so that the stimulus of the hidden and forbidden shall disappear. It is of the greatest importance to avoid from youth up coupling the idea of sin with the instinctive life.

A timely enlightenment of every individual as to the importance

[1] " The stork story is at least harmless. No sensible child believes it. The story of propagation is a quarter-truth and therefore worse than a great lie. The natural science entrée to the sex-life appears to us objectionable. If an artificial enlightenment of early youth is really necessary the study of history is far more to be recommended. The most ennobling effect of history is that it shows on every side the fundamental power of love." (Fritz Wittels, Sexual enlightenment, Die Fackel [The Torch] No. 250.)

of the sexual instinct, and as to its different variations is a postulate of what is just and fair. For our analyses show that all human beings are at bottom alike, that the so-called perversions which fill cultured persons with such disgust, are indicated in rudimentary form in every human being. Iwan Bloch's researches have distinctly proved that these perversions are not the product of degeneration but that they exist among primitive peoples, and in fact far more frequently than among ostensibly refined decadent persons, who tired of normal enjoyments, crave new sensations. The whole lying show of our sexual life is *blatant in the fact that varieties of sex-instinct which are secretly practised by millions are punished in just that one who happens to fall into the hands of earthly justice.* Dr, Magnus Hirschfeld has rendered great service by drawing the attention of the civilised world to the enormously wide spread of homo-sexuality, for example. As my latest investigations show, these are cases of neurosis. Many a case of homosexualism improves remarkably after a psychanalytic treatment. Even if the homosexual does not cease to be a homosexual, yet the way to wife and marriage is often made clear for him. However, that may be, *no one should ever be punished for his individual taste in sexual life.* The sexual law which we have to decree must contain three points : Protection of youth up to a certain age ; protection from infection and protection of the individual will.

Whereas now an unscrupulous person who infects another with syphilis, making him miserable for life, remains a man of honour, under the new law he would be punished at least as much as anyone who intentionally inflicted on another a serious injury. Also the protection of the weak, the weak-minded, and of youth is necessary. What goes beyond this is a private matter with which we ought not to interfere. That would set society on a much sounder basis and liberate a great deal of repression. The double sexual life must be destroyed. Now every individual has sexually two faces, one for the outer world which corresponds to all the restrictions that are laid upon him, and another which he allows to be seen only on certain occasions. In this double life indeed lies the deepest cause of all neuroses. While then, on the one hand war must be waged on obscenity and frivolity, on the other hand, openness and honesty of sexual conviction must be recognised as matter of course. To the question raised by Freud,[1] whether our civilised sexual morality is worth the sacrifice which it exacts from us I would certainly answer with a mighty " No ! " Our experiences of peasants and workmen teach us the evils of our ridiculous make-believe in sexual things. What we need is to be freed from the oppressive burden of religious, ethical, and social inhibitions.

[1] Die "Kulturelle" Sexualmoral und die moderne Nervosität. Mutterschutz, Year 4, No. 3. Also in the " Beiträgen zur Neurosenlehre," II. Folge. Franz Deuticke.

It is sadly little that we have been able to say as to the prophylaxis of the anxiety conditions.   It is only incomplete indications,
only the start of a new science, which we can sketch in rough outline, the details being still a riddle to us.   This is connected with
the fact that our knowledge of peoples' sexual life is still very slight.
A later time will see more clearly the connections between sexuality,
criminality, and neurosis, and will thus be able to begin a prophylaxis conscious of its aim.
This will require infinite labour.   Thousand-year-old prejudices
must be overcome.   We must begin with the investigation of the
normal human being.
Our knowledge comes from observations of the diseased.   The
truth dawns upon us that the healthy are not different in their
nature.   We still fear to draw the conclusions from these facts and
to transfer the problem of anxiety from the individual to society.
What a mass of problems overwhelm us !   We leave their solution
in all confidence to the future.

For Product Safety Concerns and Information please contact our EU
presentative GPSR@taylorandfrancis.com Taylor & Francis Verlag GmbH,
ngerstraße 24, 80331 München, Germany

nd by CPI Group (UK) Ltd, Croydon, CR0 4YY
01/05/2025
01858533-0001